Cambridge Studies in Biotechnolo;

Editors: Sir James Baddiley, N. H. Carey, I. J. Higgins, W. G. Potter

8 Monoclonal antibodies in biology and biotechnology: theoretical and practical aspects

Other titles in this series

1 The biotechnology of malting and brewing
J. S. Hough

2 Biotechnology and wastewater treatment
C. F. Forster

3 Economic aspects of biotechnology
A. J. Hacking

4 Process development in antibiotic fermentations
C. T. Calam

5 Immobilized cells: principles and applications
J. Tampion and M. D. Tampion

6 Patents: a basic guide to patenting in biotechnology
R. S. Crespi

7 Food biotechnology
R. Angold, G. Beech and J. Taggart

Monoclonal antibodies in biology and biotechnology: theoretical and practical aspects

KENNETH C. McCULLOUGH
Institut für Viruskrankheiten und Immunprophylaxe
Basle, Switzerland

and

RAYMOND E. SPIER
Department of Microbiology, The University of Surrey

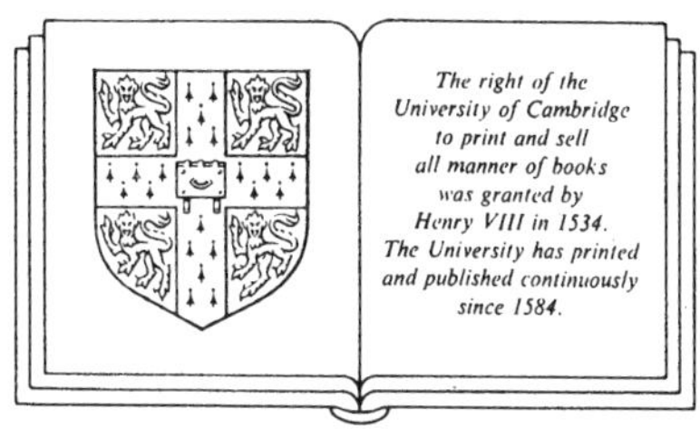
The right of the
University of Cambridge
to print and sell
all manner of books
was granted by
Henry VIII in 1534.
The University has printed
and published continuously
since 1584.

CAMBRIDGE UNIVERSITY PRESS
Cambridge
New York Port Chester
Melbourne Sydney

CAMBRIDGE UNIVERSITY PRESS
Cambridge, New York, Melbourne, Madrid, Cape Town, Singapore, São Paulo, Delhi

Cambridge University Press
The Edinburgh Building, Cambridge CB2 8RU, UK

Published in the United States of America by Cambridge University Press, New York

www.cambridge.org
Information on this title: www.cambridge.org/9780521103114

First published 1990
This digitally printed version 2009

A catalogue record for this publication is available from the British Library

Library of Congress Cataloguing in Publication data

McCullough, Kenneth C. (Kenneth Charles), 1951–
Monoclonal antibodies in biology and biotechnology : theoretical and practical aspects / Kenneth C. McCullough and R.E. Spier.
p. cm. — (Cambridge studies in biotechnology : 8)
Bibliography: p.
Includes index.
ISBN 0 521 25890 1
1. Antibodies, Monoclonal—Biotechnology. I. Spier, R. (Raymond)
II. Title. III. Series.
TP248.65.M65M33 1990
660′.63—dc19 89-914 CIP

ISBN 978-0-521-25890-6 hardback
ISBN 978-0-521-10311-4 paperback

To our parents and our wives, without whom we never would have had a hot meal.

Contents

Acknowledgements

We wish to express our gratitude and appreciation for their help to Patricia McCullough, Maureen Hodson and Beryl Hutchinson for the unenviable task of typing the manuscript; to Patricia McCullough for tirelessly preparing the original figures for Chapters 1–4; to all of our colleagues mentioned throughout this book for providing the experimental results essential for the text and figures; and to Jenny Federspiel for agreeing to be the guinea pig for testing the practical procedures in Chapter 2 and §§3.7, 3.8, 4.2 and 4.3. Thank you all.

1 Introduction: the immune response

1.1. Introduction

In order to develop a clear appreciation of the problems and processes associated with the preparation and use of monoclonal antibodies (MAb), it is essential that the structure and function of the immune system be understood. The initial evidence that the body possessed a defensive system against microbial attack first came to light in the nineteenth and early twentieth centuries. This knowledge has expanded during the past 20–30 years, to give a detailed biochemical and immunochemical insight into the structure and function of the antibody molecule, the bifurcation of the immune response against foreign material (antigen) into non-specific and specific mechanisms (which has been further subdivided into cellular and humoral responses), and the genetic control of antibody diversity.

An understanding of the structure and function of the immune system is necessary for a clear appreciation of the problems and processes associated with the preparation and use of monoclonal antibodies. The stimulation of antibody production *in vivo* (the humoral response) and the other components of the immune response will then be introduced, and the structure of the antibody molecule and its differentiation into classes and subclasses described and related, where appropriate, to immunological functions. This will assist with the understanding of the properties and functions of monoclonal antibodies, and of both how and why they can be produced. Although the immune system is a complex network of reactions and interactions, the antibody response will be described in the greatest detail, since it is the antibody response which is of direct relevance to the production of monoclonal antibodies.

Thus, the concept of the monoclonal antibody will be introduced in this chapter, and the specialised culture techniques required to produce them will be described and explained in the subsequent chapters.

1.2. A history of the early development of immunology

Table 1.1 summarises the early historical developments of immunology. Voltaire (1733)* remarked on the Chinese custom (a fifteenth-century

* Dates in this section refer to the dates of work, not those of publications; a numbered system of references is used from §1.3 onwards.

Table 1.1. *Chronology of early developments in immunology*

Date	Individual	Discovery
1733	Voltaire	Chinese inhalation of smallpox 'pocks' gave protection
1774	Jesty	'Pocks' from cattle to immunise his wife
1798	Jenner	Cowpox vaccine against smallpox
1885	Pasteur	Development of 'vaccination'
1886	Salmon & Smith	Cholera vaccine in chickens
1888	Roux & Yersin	Diphtheria toxin and antitoxin
1890	Van Behring, Kitasato	Tetanus toxin and antitoxin; term 'antibody' introduced
1893	Buchner, Calmette	Complement: heat-labile bactericidal and anti-venom component of serum
1894	Pfeiffer	Destruction of *Vibrio cholerae* by specific antibody and complement
1895	Bordet	Complement + specific antibody required for antimicrobial activity
1889 1896 1897	Charin & Roger Widal Kraus	Specific antibody agglutinated organisms or precipitated toxins
1890s	Metchnikoff, Wright & Denys	Blood phagocytic cells : complement + antibody enhances phagocytic cell function
1898	Pfeiffer & Marx	Antibody originates in spleen, bone marrow, lymph nodes and lungs
1900	Landsteiner	Differentiation of human blood groups using antibodies
1900	Nuttall, Wasserman & Schutze	Differentiation of human cow and goat milk using antibodies
1901	Uhlenhuth	Differentiation of egg whites of different species of bird
1902	Portier & Richet	Anaphylactic reactions
1903	Arthus	Manipulation of anaphylaxis
1900s 1930s	Ehrlich Heidelberg & Marrack	Physico-chemical characterisation of antibody: antibody–antigen reaction
1937	Tiselius & Kabat	Separation of albumins and globulins
1942	Chase	Immunity associated with lymphoid cells
1944–45	Medawar	Graft rejection
1946	Elek, Oudin, Ouchterlony	Antibody–antigen reactions and assays for precipitation reactions
1948	Fagraeus	Relationship between plasma cells and antibody
1949	Burnet & Lederberg, Burnet & Fenner	Clonal selection theory
1953	Graber & Williams	Electrophoretic separation of serum proteins
1955	Coons *et al.*	Antibody produced by plasma cells
1959	Porter	Antibody structure
1974	Jerne	Network theory

practice in fact) of prophylactic intranasal induction of smallpox infection. That is, they took dried powders of smallpox 'pocks', in a manner similar to taking snuff, in an attempt to 'immunise' (to use a modern term) against smallpox. This protocol was repeated in England, but with a 20% fatality. Benjamin Jesty (1774) used the pocks from cattle to successfully 'immunise' his wife.

The first scientific experiments were performed by Edward Jenner who, in 1798, published his first memoir, *An enquiry into the causes and effects of 'variolae vacciniae'*. Using the avirulent (causes mild or no illness) cowpox agent, he successfully induced long-lasting protection against the relatively lethal smallpox agent. Jenner termed this variolation, after the practice described by Voltaire (who also used the term variolation, from 'variola', the medical name for smallpox).

Pasteur demonstrated that virulent organisms (virulent describes an organism which will produce a severe or fatal illness) could be attenuated (made less virulent or avirulent). This was initially observed by accident; chicken cholera bacillus was left on a laboratory bench during a vacation, after which the organisms had lost their ability to produce disease in chickens (had become avirulent). However, inoculation of the avirulent organism protected the birds against the lethal disease induced by the virulent bacillus. This was similar to Jenner's observations on using vaccinia virus to protect against the virulent smallpox virus; Pasteur found that he could also induce protection using an avirulent strain of anthrax bacillus.

In honour of Jenner's work with vaccinia virus, Pasteur termed this treament 'vaccination'. Pasteur extended his work to produce 'vaccines' for sheep anthrax (by passage in rabbits); in July 1885, Pasteur vaccinated and protected a boy, Joseph Meister, who had recently sustained severe and multiple bites from a rabid dog.

The next advance was made by Salmon & Theobald Smith (1886), who successfully vaccinated chickens with heat-killed chicken cholera bacilli. In 1888, Roux & Yersin discoverd that a bacterium-free filtrate of the diphtheria bacillus contained the exotoxin ('poison') which would induce the production of an antitoxin in the blood of an inoculated animal. This antitoxin could be used to passively transfer immunity against the toxin. Van Behring and Kitasato both made similar observations with tetanus antitoxins in 1890 and introduced the term antibody. Ehrlich noted that 'antibodies' would neutralise the haemolytic and lethal action of the poison ricin.

Richard Pfeiffer (1894) observed that antibody specific for *Vibrio cholerae* would kill the organism, and Charrin & Roger (1889), Widal (1896) and Kraus (1897) discovered that specific antibody could agglutinate the organisms or precipitate the toxin from a bacterial filtrate (the so-called precipitin antibody).

Further to this, Buchner (1893) noted that serum lost the ability to kill certain bacteria after heating at 56°C. This heat-labile substance was called alexeine, now termed complement, and Pfeiffer showed in 1894 that such factors accomplished the dissolution of cholera vibrios. It was Bordet (1895) who demonstrated that both the thermolabile non-specific alexeine (complement) and the thermostable specific antibody were required for antimicrobial activity.

At this time, Eli Metchnikoff made his observations that phagocytic cells were present in the blood, and proposed that this was the mechanism by which microbial agents were destroyed. Almoth Wright & Denys then noted that both complement and antibody enhanced this phagocytosis, and Wright proposed that this antibody (and complement) reinforcement of phagocytosis should be called opsonic (Greek *opsono*, I prepare food for) and the substance (the antibody and complement) opsonin.

That antibody had a particular specificity was brought to light by Landsteiner (1900), who used antibody to differentiate human blood group (A, B, O) antigens; Nuttall, Wasserman & Schutze (1900), who distinguished human, cow and goat milk; and Uhlenhuth (1901), who differentiated egg-whites of different species of bird. However, not all antigen–antibody reactions are distinguishable; there exists related, or cross-reactive, antigen. Such cross-reactions between particular antibody and particular antigen were extensively studied by Nuttall. (The term antigen is used to describe anything which can be recognised as foreign to an animal and against which an immune response can be initiated.) Also, the binding of antibody with antigen (toxin, for example) was not the sole reason for the inactivation of the lethal effect of the antigen. Hans Buchner (1893) found that a tetanus toxin–antitoxin mixture was non-toxic to mice, but remained lethal to guinea pigs. Furthermore, Calmette showed that heating a non-toxic mixture of snake venom and antibody to 68°C restored the toxicity of the venom.

The research into immune responses diversified during the first few decades of the twentieth century. Studies on the hypersensitivity (anaphylactic) reactions (local inflammatory reactions to re-injection of substances which were harmless at their first administration) were initiated by the observations of Portier & Richet (1902), and the first description of the experimental manipulation of anaphylaxis was described by Arthus (1903). Medawar's observations (1944–45) have led to the acceptance that graft rejection phenomena are due to immunisation of the recipient by antigenic determinants on the donor's tissues.

The physico-chemical characteristics of antibodies and antibody–antigen reactions, pioneered by Ehrlich in the early 1900s, was further studied by Heidelberger & Marrack (1930s), and Elek, Oudin & Ouchterlony in 1946, from whom originate many of the tests for detecting antibody–antigen complexes.

Graber & Williams (1953) separated serum proteins by electrophoresis in gels, in advancement of the work of Tiselius & Kabat in 1937, who separated albumin, α, β and γ globulins in an electric field. The latter workers showed that antibody belonged to the γ globulin class, and R.R. Porter (1959) dissected these γ globulins further to reveal the structure of the antibody molecule.

On investigating the production of antibodies in response to antigenic stimuli, Pfeiffer & Marx (1898) deduced that antibody must originate mostly in the spleen, bone marrow, lymph nodes and lungs; Fagraeus (1948) showed a correlation between antibody formation and plasma cell development. The plasma cell is a morphologically distinct cell type found mainly in the spleen and lymph nodes. It is *c.* 1.5–2 times the size of the majority of lymphocytes and has a much greater cytoplasm to nucleus ratio. Coons and co-workers (1955) demonstrated that antibody was indeed associated with these plasma cells, and Chase (1942) was able to transfer a hypersensitive state to normal guinea pigs using spleen, lymph node or peritoneal exudate (washed from the peritoneal (abdominal cavity) cells of highly sensitised donors). Around this time, Burnet & Lederberg put forward their 'clonal selection theory', and Burnet & Fenner, in their monograph *The production of antibody* (1949), discussed the concept of immunological tolerance and the reasons why an animal did not respond immunologically to its own tissue antigens or those of a closely related animal.

Although much of today's knowledge of the immune response was stimulated by the theories propounded by Burnet & Lederberg, the hypothesis to which this knowledge is now most closely linked is the network theory of Jerne (1974). How this relates to the induction of antibody, and hence the production of monoclonal antibodies, will be dealt with in the following sections. But first, the work which revealed the structure of the antibody molecule will be described in more detail, and the relationship between this structure and the function of γ globulin will be given.

1.3. **The antibodies**

It was not until the 1960s that the basic structure of the antibody molecule was revealed by the work of Porter. Using an enzymic degradation of the γ globulin fraction isolated from serum, he determined the basic structure of the antibody, shown in Fig. 1.1. The figure also shows the cleavage sites of the enzymes used by Porter (this work is reviewed and presented by Hood *et al.* (1) and Humphrey & White (2)). Pepsin digestion resulted in the destruction of the F_c moiety. The various immunochemical processes associated with this portion of the antibody

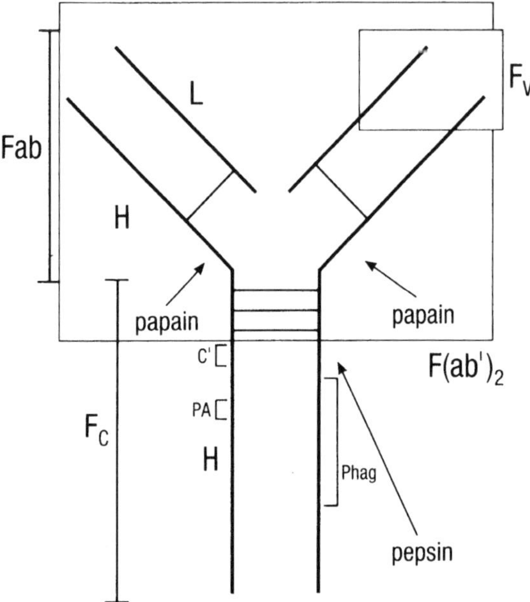

Fig. 1.1 Basic structure of the immunoglobulin molecule, showing the areas of interaction with antigen (F_v), complement (C′), protein A (PA) and phagocyte F_c receptor (Phag). Also shown are the site of cleavage with papain, yielding two Fab fragments and one F_c fragment, and the site of cleavage with pepsin, yielding the F(ab′)$_2$ fragment consisting of the two Fab and a small portion of the F_c. The disulphide bridges are shown as lines connecting the heavy (H) and light (L) chains near to the end of each Fab distant from the F_v end, and as lines connecting the two heavy (H) chains at the end of the F_c closest to the hinge region with the Fab.

molecule, such as complement fixation, binding to phagocytes and binding of staphylococcal protein A, were identified by comparing the reactions of whole antibody molecules with those after pepsin digestion. The pepsin-resistant fragment of the antibody molecule, F(ab′)$_2$, contained the antigen recognition site, or paratope. By using a second enzyme, papain, Porter showed that there were in fact two paratopes for every antibody molecule; papain cleaved the antibody at a site which generated two Fab fragments, in place of the single F(ab′)$_2$ obtained with pepsin digestion, and an intact F_c moiety. Each of the Fab fragments carried a paratope at the end furthest from the papain-cleavage site.

Subsequent to these early studies, knowledge of the structure of antibody progressed rapidly through the 1970s. The major immunoglobulin (Ig) classes – IgG, IgM, IgA and IgE – were shown to have unique structural arrangements of their chains and domains, as represented in Fig. 1.2 and Table 1.2 (1). A structure for IgD is omitted from Fig. 1.2 since its function as a serum protein is unclear; its major function is

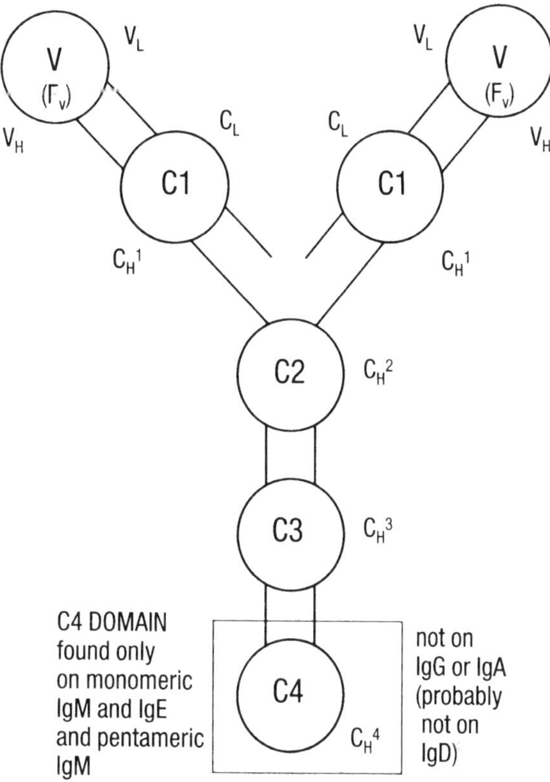

Fig. 1.2. Domain structure of the immunoglobulin molecule, showing the variable (V) and constant (C) domains. The V domain comprises the V domains on the heavy (H) and the light (L) chains: V_H and V_L respectively. The C1 domain comprises the first C domain of the heavy chain and the C domain of the light chain: C_H1 and C_L respectively. The C2, C3 and C4 (only on IgM and IgE) each comprise two heavy-chain C domains: C_H2, C_H3 and C_H4 respectively. (It is actually the C2 domain of IgM and IgE which are extra, and not the C4, probably corresponding to the hinge region of IgG, IgA and IgD.)

apparently as an antigen receptor on the B lymphocyte (see §§1.4.6 and 1.6.2). Physico-chemical properties of the Ig classes were also elucidated and these are shown in Table 1.3 (2). The relevance of these properties will be discussed below.

Reduction of the disulphide bridges with 2-mercaptoethanol (2-MCE) (in the presence of L-cysteine) or α-thioglycerol, demonstrated the presence of the heavy (H) and light (L) chains in the antibody molecule (3). Various enzymic treatments at different temperatures revealed further information about these 'chains'. Some of the fragments obtained contained amino acid sequences which were relatively conserved (constant) between different antibody molecules. Other fragments identified areas on antibody molecules which were variable (variation in amino

Table 1.2. *The chains and domains of the different antibody molecules in serum*

Antibody	Chains	Chain domains[1]	Molecule domains[2]
IgA	2 × heavy α	$2 \times V_L$	1 × V
	2 × light λ or k	$2 \times V_H$	
IgD	2 × heavy δ	$2 \times C_L$	1 × C1
	2× light λ or k	$2 \times C_H1$	
IgG	2 × heavy γ	$2 \times C_H2$	1 × C2
	2 × light λ or k	$2 \times C_H3$	1 × C3
IgM	10 × heavy μ	$10 \times V_L$	5 × V
	10 × light λ or k	$10 \times V_H$	
		$10 \times C_L$	5 × C1
		$10 \times C_H1$	
		$10 \times C_H2$	5 × C2
		$10 \times C_H3$	5 × C3
		$10 \times C_H4$	5 × C4
IgE	2 × heavy ϵ	$2 \times V_L$	1 × V
	2 × light λ or k	$2 \times V_H$	
		$2 \times C_L$	1 × C1
		$2 \times C_H1$	
		$2 \times C_H2$	1 × C2
		$2 \times C_H3$	1 × C3
		$2 \times C_H4$	1 × C4

Note:
[1] L refers to domains on the light chains; H refers to domains on the heavy chains.
[2] The antibody molecule domains are formed from the appropriate domains on the light and/or heavy chains.

acid sequence). Such areas are referred to as the constant (C) and variable (V) domains (1). IgG has one variable domain and three constant domains on each side of the antibody molecule (Fig. 1.2); IgA (7*S*) and IgE each have one variable domain and four constant domains, as does monomeric IgM. However, serum IgM is normally in a 19*S* pentameric form and IgA is found in secretions as a 9*S* dimer. Hence, the 19*S* IgM molecule also has a unique chemical structure – the J chain – while dimeric IgA contains a novel carbohydrate 'transfer piece'.

The variable domains form the F_v region of the antibody, and within this are found the hypervariable regions in which the major idiotopes (Greek, *idio*, self) of the antibody molecule reside. This is in comparison to the allotypic (Greek, *allo*, other) determinants, which are to be found mainly in the C domains (1). Of the idiotopes, that which is of most

Table 1.3. *The different immunoglobulin classes and subclasses found in the serum of different animals*

Animal	Immunoglobulin Class	Immunoglobulin Subclass
mouse	IgA	none
	IgD	none
	IgE	none
	IgG	IgG_1, IgG_{2a}, IgG_{2b}, IgG_3
	IgM	none
human	IgA	IgA_1, IgA_2
	IgD	none
	IgE	IgE_1, IgE_2
	IgG	IgG_1, IgG_2, IgG_3, IgG_4
	IgM	none
rat	IgA	none
	IgD	none
	IgE	none
	IgG	IgG_1, IgG_{2a}, IgG_{2b}
	IgM	none
rabbit	IgA	none
	IgD	none
	IgE	none
	IgG	IgG_1, IgG_2
	IgM	none
cow (and sheep)	IgA	none
	IgD	none
	IgE	none
	IgG	IgG_1, IgG_{2a}, IgG_{2b}
	IgM	none

importance in antibody–antigen reactions is the paratope: the part of the antibody responsible for interaction with the antigenic determinant for which the antibody is specific. Figs 1.1 and 1.2 show the F_v region and the V_L and V_H domains which carry the idiotopes. It is the uniqueness of the idiotopes (one of which is the paratope) which determines the uniqueness of each antibody molecule (which has been derived from a single clone). But how are these idiotopes arranged? Fig. 1.3 shows an example of the linear arrangement of the hypervariable regions (hv) in the light (L) and heavy (H) chains of the human IgG molecule (1). The light chain hv are termed Lhv_1, Lhv_2 and Lhv_3, and the heavy chain hv are termed Hhv_1, Hhv_2, Hhv_3, Hhv_4. The numbers signify the numerical position of the amino acids with respect to the carboxy-terminal amino acid. As can be seen, the hv are separated by sequences of amino acids

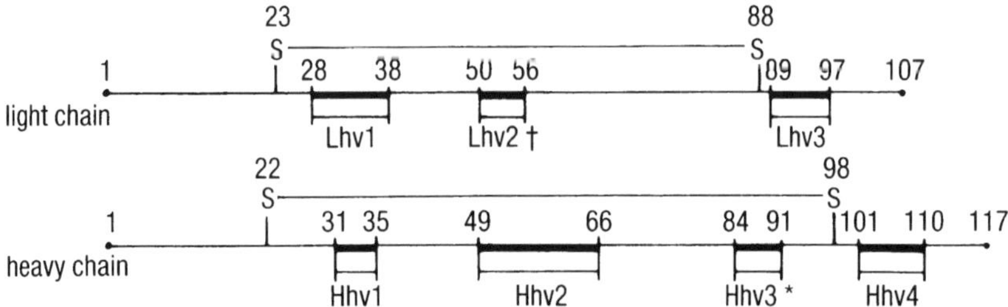

Fig. 1.3. A linear amino acid 'map' of the hypervariable areas in the variable regions of the light and heavy chains. Lhv, light chain hypervariable area; Hhv, heavy chain hypervariable area; numbers, positions of the amino acid residues; †, Lhv2 is *not always* part of the antigen–binding crevice; *, Hhv3 is *not* part of the antigen-binding crevice. (From Hood *et al.* (1).)

which are more highly conserved between different Ig molecules (Fig. 1.4). These relatively conserved regions are called the framework regions. It is the overall amino acid sequence (of both hv and framework regions) which determines the final structure of the Ig and hence the organisation of the idiotopes, including the paratope. This organisation brings most of the hv regions within a close proximity of one another, to form the paratope; Fig. 1.5 demonstrates this. The tertiary arrangement of the light and heavy chains juxtaposes Lhv_1, Lhv_2, Lhv_3, Hhv_1, Hhv_2, Hhv_4 within a cleft formed between the light and heavy chains at what is the extremity of the Fab portion of the antibody molecule. This cleft is the paratope: the antigen-binding cleft or crevice. The Hhv_3 region is always found outside the antigen-binding crevice, and the Lhv_2 region is occasionally found outside the cleft (1, 4). Each of these hv regions is a potential idiotope. Likewise, combinations of the hv regions (with or without framework regions) will also form potential idiotopes. The relevance of this will become apparent in §6.6. where iodiotope–anti-idiotope interactions will be considered with respect to the usefulness of the anti-idiotope monoclonal antibodies.

The idiotope differentiates each antibody molecule. An isotype differentiates the antibody class: IgM from IgA from IgE from IgG. The IgG molecules are further subclassified by isotype differences depending on the species of animal (Table 1.3). The isotypic markers are constant within a given species of animal, but are distinct between different species (xenogeneic: Greek, *xeno*, foreign). However, the closer the evolutionary relatedness of these xenogeneic species, the greater the antigenic relatedness of the isotypes. Rat IgM (or IgG, IgA etc.) will induce anti-isotypic antibodies in, for example, rabbit, which will cross-react with the respective mouse Ig, but will not react with bovine, rabbit or human Ig.

There are also allotypic determinants which identify certain Ig molecules of a particular animal species. Examples of these are shown in Table 1.4 (2). Allotypic determinants are found in the C_H1 and C_H2

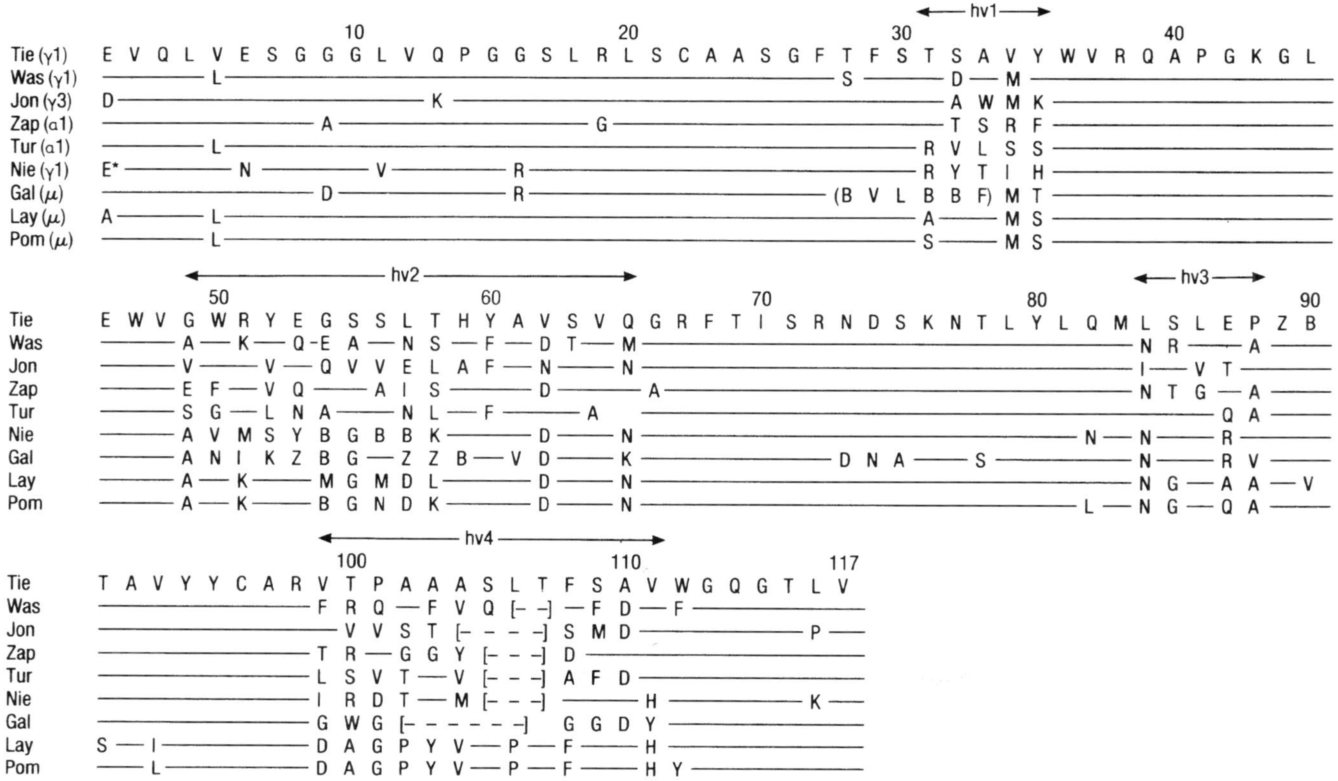

```
                                                                                  ←— hv1 —→
                              10                         20                        30                       40
Tie (γ1)   E V Q L V E S G G G L V Q P G G S L R L S C A A S G F T F S T S A V Y W V R Q A P G K G L
Was (γ1)   ———————— L ——————————————————————————————————————————— S ——— D — M ———————————————————
Jon (γ3)   D ——————————————————— K ————————————————————————————————— A W M K —————————————————
Zap (α1)   ————————————— A ——————————————— G ——————————————————————— T S R F —————————————————
Tur (α1)   ———————— L ——————————————————————————————————————————— R V L S S —————————————————
Nie (γ1)   E* —————— N ————— V ————— R ——————————————————————————— R Y T I H —————————————————
Gal (μ)    ————————————— D ——————— R ——————————————————— (B V L B B F) M T —————————————————
Lay (μ)    A ————— L ——————————————————————————————————————————— A ——— M S —————————————————
Pom (μ)    ———————— L ——————————————————————————————————————————— S ——— M S —————————————————

           ←——————— hv2 ———————→                                                          ←— hv3 —→
                50                   60                       70                    80                    90
Tie        E W V G W R Y E G S S L T H Y A V S V Q G R F T I S R N D S K N T L Y L Q M L S L E P Z B
Was        —————— A — K — Q-E A — N S — F — D T — M ——————————————————————————————— N R ——— A ———
Jon        —————— V ——— V — Q V V E L A F — N ——— N ——————————————————————————————— I — V T ————
Zap        —————— E F — V Q ——— A I S ——————— D ————— A ——————————————————————————— N T G — A ———
Tur        —————— S G — L N A ——— N L — F ————— A ———————————————————————————————————— Q A ———
Nie        —————— A V M S Y B G B B K ————— D ——— N ——————————————————————— N — N ——— R —————
Gal        —————— A N I K Z B G — Z Z B — V D ——— K ——————————— D N A ——— S ——————— N ——— R V ———
Lay        —————— A — K ——— M G M D L ————— D ——— N ——————————————————————————————— N G — A A — V
Pom        —————— A — K ——— B G N D K ————— D ——— N ———————————————————————— L — N G — Q A ———

                               ←——————— hv4 ———————→
                              100                  110            117
Tie        T A V Y Y C A R V T P A A A S L T F S A V W G Q G T L V
Was        ———————————————— F R Q — F V Q [– –] — F D — F ————————
Jon        —————————————————— V V S T [– – – –] S M D ——————— P ——
Zap        ———————————————— T R — G G Y [– – –] D ————————————————
Tur        ———————————————— L S V T — V [– – –] A F D ————————————
Nie        ———————————————— I R D T — M [– – –] ——— H ——————— K ——
Gal        ———————————————— G W G [– – – – – –] G G D Y ——————————
Lay        S — I ——————————— D A G P Y V — P — F ——— H ————————————
Pom        ——— L ——————————— D A G P Y V — P — F ——— H Y ——————————
```

Fig. 1.4. Amino acid sequence of the V_H regions of nine human heavy chains, showing the greater degree of variation in the hypervariable (hv) regions compared with the framework regions. (From Capra & Kehoe (66).)

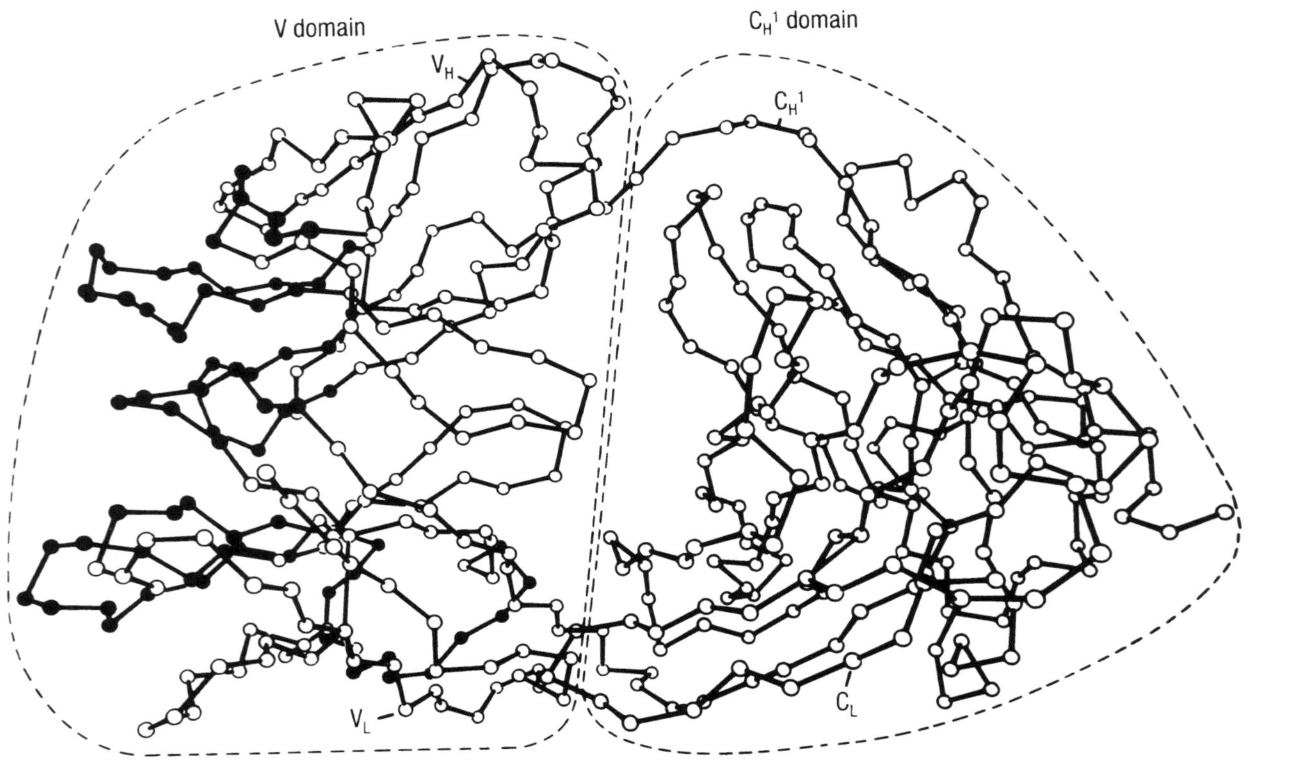

Fig. 1.5. The α-carbon backbone of the Fab fragment of the mouse myeloma protein McPC603, showing that all but one of the hypervariable regions (shaded circles) are brought together into the antigen-binding site. (From Davies *et al.* (67).)

Table 1.4. *Allotype markers found on human immunoglobulins*

Immunoglobulin isotype	Domain	Allotype marker found[1]
all with k light chain	$C_L(C_K)$	Km(1) or Km(1, 2) or Km(3) (previously Km = Inv)
IgG_1	C_H	G1m(1) or nG1m(1) G1m(3) or (17) G1m(2) or (18) or (20) nG3m(11) nG4m(a)
IgG_2	C_H	G2m(23) or nG2m(23) nG1m(1) nG3m(11) nG3m(21) nG4m(b) G3m(5) or nG3m(5)
IgG_3	C_H	G3m(11) or nG3m(11) G3m(21) or nG3m(21) G3m(6) or (10) or (14) or (15) or (16) or (24) or (25) nG1m(1) nG4m(a)
IgG_4	C_H	nG4m(a) or (b)
IgA_2	C_H	A2m(1) or (−1)

Note:
[1] Allotypic markers on immunoglobulin molecules characterise the light and heavy chains in terms of a particular form (allele) of the allotype gene. For example, a human IgG_1 molecule may have the Gm(1) or the Gm (non −1) allotype (G1m or nG1m) but not both. Nor will that IgG_1 molecule carry the Gm allotypes of IgG_2, IgG_3 or IgG_4. Mouse or rabbit immunoglobulins carry different allotypes from the human immunoglobulins. Therefore, allotypes are particular to an animal species, and vary between different populations of the same immunoglobulin subclass within that species. Outbred animals may have immunoglobulin populations with many of the different allotypes, whereas the immunoglobulin population of inbred animals will represent only a limited number of the allotypes.

domains (C_H1, constant region of the Fab portion of the antibody molecule closest to the hinge region with the F_c portion; C_H2, constant region of the F_c portion of the antibody molecule closest to the hinge region with the Fab portion). Thus, just as the variable regions of an antibody molecule are composed of areas of hypervariation within a framework of less variable (more conserved) regions, the constant regions have some areas of greater variation than others. These areas of variation within the constant region are still relatively conserved (compared with the hypervariable regions) but the low level of variation which they undergo gives rise to the isotypic and allotypic determinants.

Functions of the antibody molecule can also be related to the antibody structure (Fig. 1.6.). The antigen-binding site – the paratope – is situated within the combined V_L–V_H domain (1, 4). Binding of *Staphylococcus aureas* protein A occurs in an area of the C_H2 domain in the junction with the C_H3 domain (5). The initiation of the complement (C′) cascade is effected by binding of the first component (C1) for the classical pathway to an area of the C_H2 domain very close to the hinge region on IgG, or to areas on the C_H3 or C_H4 domains of IgM (4, 6). Normally, only altered Ig (after reaction with antigen for example) will bind C′. Presumably this may occur through alterations in the hinge region after interaction of the antibody with antigen or after heat-initiated aggregation.

The different antibody classes differ not only in their structure but also in how they effect protection against foreign material and infection.

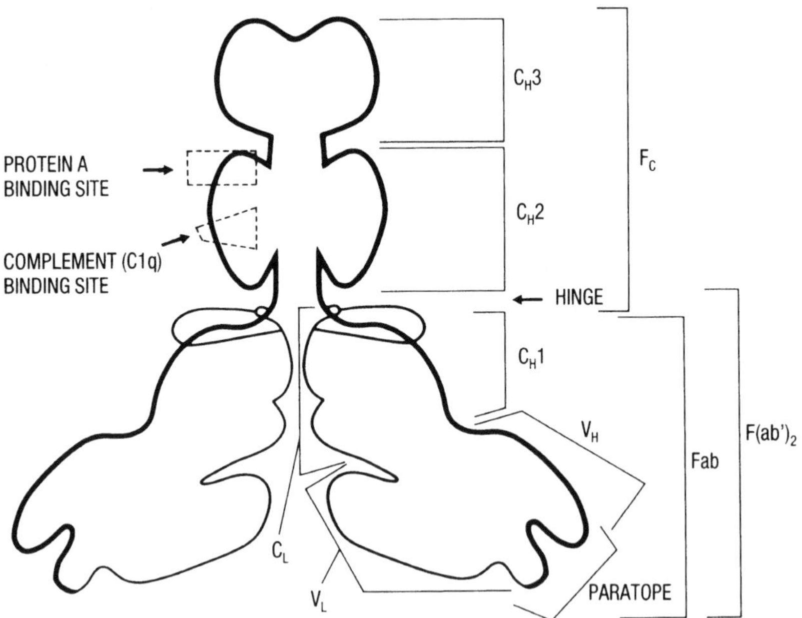

Fig. 1.6. A simplified drawing of the shape of the immunoglobulin molecule, based on data from X-ray diffraction studies. The heavy line is the heavy chain, and the light line is the light chain. The symbols are as Figs 1.1 and 1.2. The paratope is the antigen-binding crevice of the antibody molecule. (Drawn from the three-dimensional illustrations of mouse and human immunoglobulin molecules in Davies & Metzger (68).)

Diversity in this function is important because different pathogenic organisms are most efficiently destroyed by different immunological mechanisms. For example, many bacteria and parasites are destroyed by opsonisation or agglutination procedures followed by phagocytosis (Fig. 1.7) whereas intracellular infections (viruses and chlamydia) are often destroyed by the complement-mediated lytic processes, antibody-dependent cellular cytotoxicity (ADCC) reactions, natural killer (NK) cell activity, and cytotoxic T lymphocyte (CTL) activity (4, 7) (Fig. 1.7).

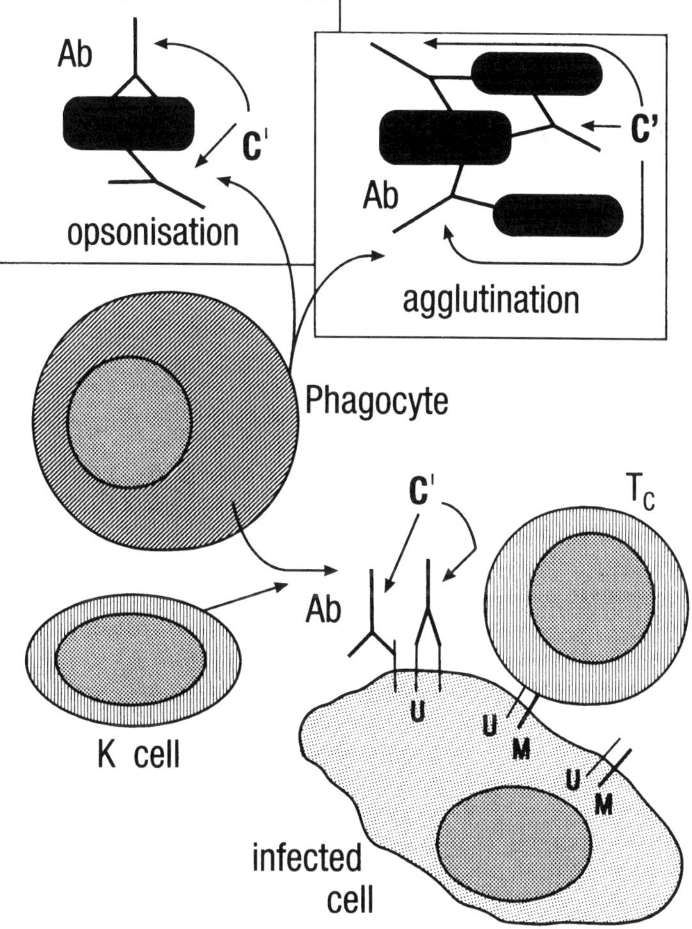

Fig. 1.7. Antibody (Ab) and complement (C′) based opsonisation and agglutination of bacteria resulting in enhanced phagocytosis by phagocytes; and the destruction of virus-infected cells, expressing on their surface viral antigens (U) and MHC class I molecules (M), by antibody (Ab) plus complement (C′), antibody-enhanced K cell (lymphocyte) or phagocyte (monocyte or polymorph–granulocyte) cytotoxicity, or cytotoxic T lymphocytes (T_c).

Table 1.5. *Physico-chemical properties and biological functions of different immunoglobulin isotypes*

Isotype	M_r	Sedimentation coefficient	Serum concentration (mg/100 ml)	Valency	Complement fixation	Enhances phagocytosis or ADCC
Human						
IgG_1	150 000 to 180 000	$7S$	800–1600	2	+	++
IgG_2					− (±)	+
IgG_3					+	++
IgG_4					+(±)	−
IgA (serum)	160 000	$7S$	150–400	2	−	−
IgA (secreted)	400 000	$11S$	0	2	−	−
IgM	900 000	$19S$	50–200	10	+	±
IgD	180 000	$7S$	0.3–40	2	−	−
IgE	200 000	$8S$	0.03	2	−	+
Mouse						
IgG_1	150 000 to 180 000	$7S$	800–1600	2	−	++
IgG_{2a}					+	+
IgG_{2b}					+	++
IgG_3					−	±
IgA	similar to human molecules				−	−
IgM					+	±
IgD					−	−
IgE					−	+
Bovine						
IgG_1	150 000 to 180 000	$7S$	800–1600	2	+	+
IgG_{2a}					+	+
IgG_{2b}					+	+
IgA	similar to human molecules				−	−
IgM					+	±
IgD					−	−
IgE					−	+

The relative differences in the function of the different Ig classes with respect to protection against illness are summarised in Table 1.5 and compared to their physico-chemical properties.

The structure of the antibody molecule is relevant to hybridoma technology and monoclonal antibody production since this structure is under genetic control. In any one antibody molecule, only one of the two types of light chain is found – either k or λ – coded for by the V_k and V_λ genes (1, 4). The allotypic determinants are constant within a species but the isotypic determinants vary, resulting in IgM, IgD, IgG, IgE or IgA. These determinants, which are found on C_H, are coded for by genes C_μ, C_δ, C_γ, C_ϵ or C_α (1, 4).

The genes responsible for these C-region sequences reside in specific locations on the chromosomes such that gene rearrangements will result in defined class switchings (1, 4). Fig. 1.8 shows the arrangement of these isotype gene loci and which class switches can occur. Only these switches occur, because they result from gene deletions and hence can never be reversed. Other genetic rearrangements associated with the loci responsible for the variable region sequences lead to the antibody diversity of the humoral immune system (Fig. 1.9). For further details the reader is recommended to consult Hood *et al.* and McConnell *et al.* (1, 4).

1.3.1. *Antibody production: response to antigen*

The cell with the genetic potential for the production of antibody specific for a particular antigenic determinant is the B lymphocyte or B cell. Receptors for the antigen, which are Ig in structure (monomeric IgM, IgD, or to a lesser extent IgG), are present on the surface of these cells (see §1.6.2). They have paratope-like regions which are specific for, and react with, the particular antigenic determinant. The antibody secreted by the progeny of the B cell has an identical paratope. In contrast, the isotype of the secreted antibody will not necessarily be the same as that of the receptor.

So where in the body are these antigen-specific B lymphocytes to be found, and how can antigenic determinants which can be as small as three amino acids (8) encounter such a cell? The antigen-responsive B lymphocytes are associated with the secondary lymphoid organs – spleen and lymph nodes – in what are described as the primary follicles of these organs. These follicles develop into the germinal centres after stimulation by antigen (Fig. 1.10). Although a minority of lymphocytes in the circulation are B cells (more so during an immune response) it is in the follicles that these lymphocytes are stimulated by antigen. This stimulation results from the interaction of antigen with the Ig receptor in the presence of the appropriate growth factors and accessory cells (see

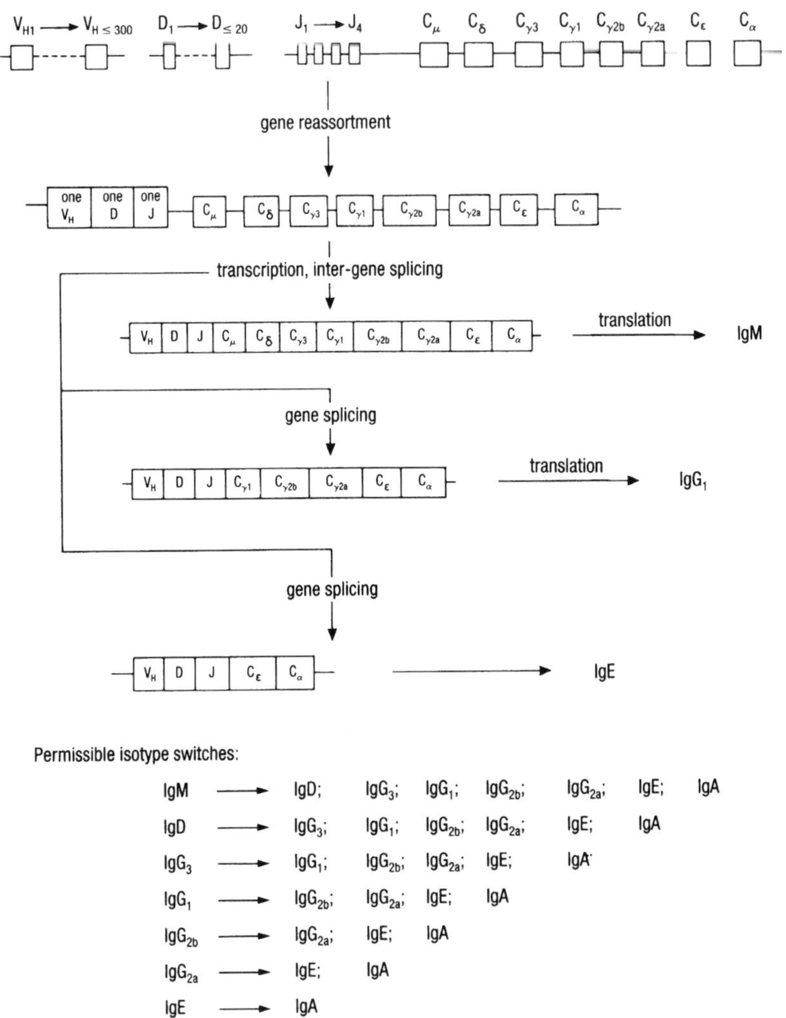

Fig. 1.8. Gene arrangements of the variable regions (V_H), joining regions (D and J) and constant regions (C) of the mouse immunoglobulin heavy chain. The figure shows how, through reassortment and splicing, the immunoglobulin isotype is selected, and which class switching is permissible (because of the order of the C region genes and the intergene splicing which will occur). (From Hood *et al.* (1).)

§§1.4.3–6 and 1.6.1–2). The B cell receptor will react with free antigen, but complete stimulation of the lymphocyte usually requires antigen to be presented on an accessory cell to helper (inducer) lymphocytes (T_h lymphocytes) (8). This aspect of the immune response will be dealt with in §§1.4.5 and 1.6.1. Not only antigen but also complexes of antigen with antibody, and antigen with antibody and C′ (to the C3 component) may

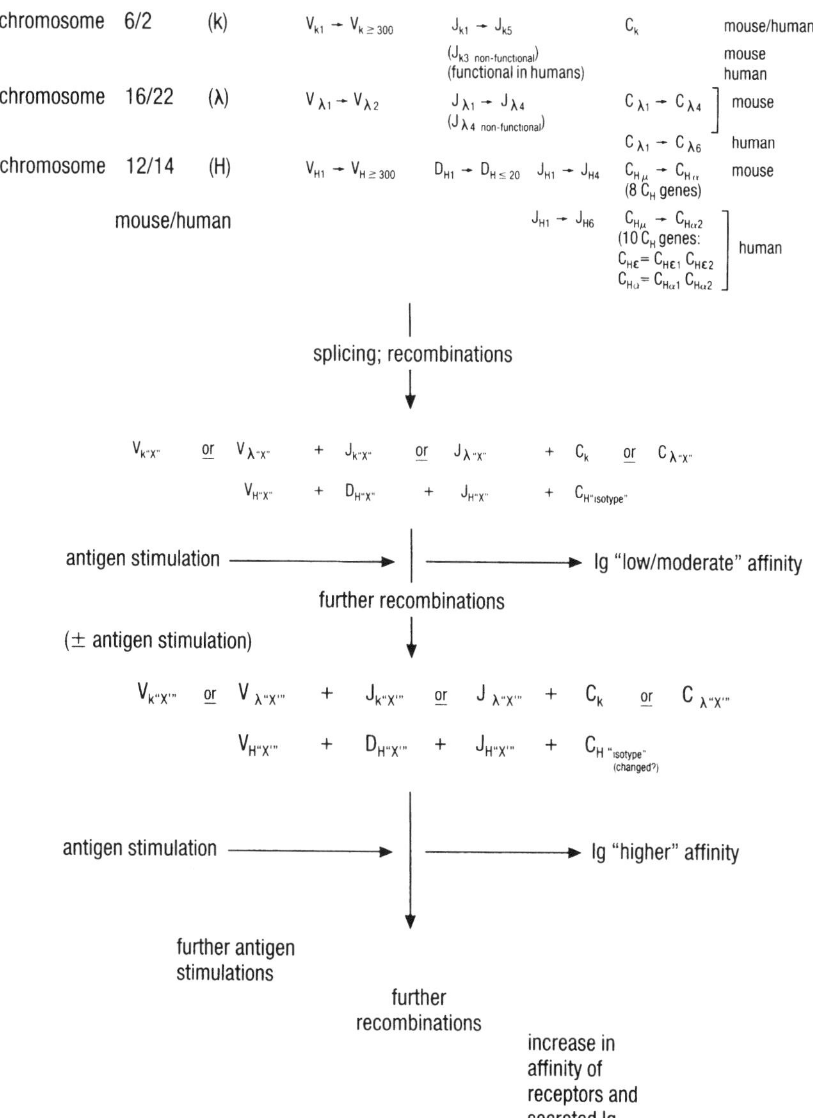

Fig. 1.9. The variable region (V), constant region (C) and joining region (J and D) genes of immunoglobulins; through splicing and recombinations at each antigenic stimulation of the B lymphocyte, the affinity of the encoded immunoglobulin molecule can be increased.

be presented (9). A very specialised cell found in the follicles and germinal centres of secondary lymphoid organs, the follicular dendritic cell (FDC), can trap and retain antigen–antibody or antigen–antibody–C′ complexes for long periods of time, resulting in a more efficient and prolonged

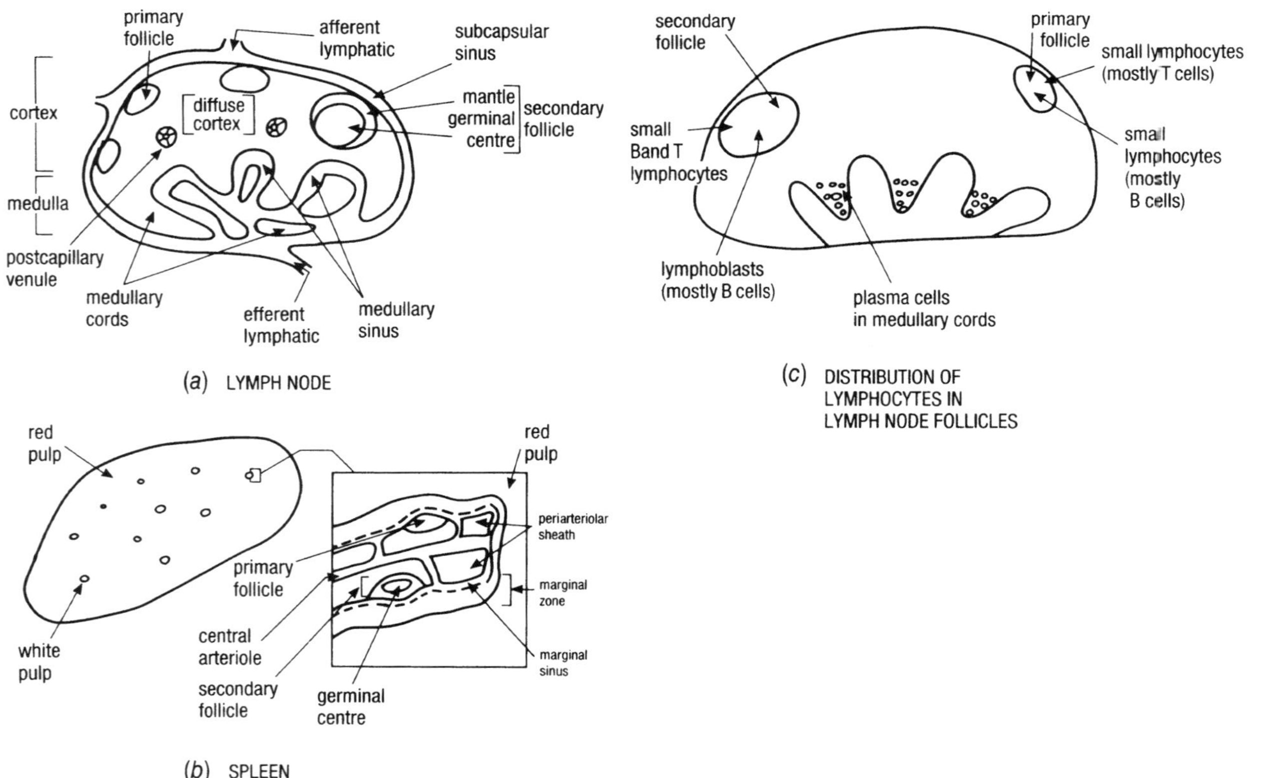

Fig. 1.10. Diagrammatic representation of the arrangement of primary and secondary follicles, and germinal centres in a lymph node (*a*) and the spleen (*b*), and the distribution of lymphocytes, lymphoblasts and plasma cells in the lymph node follicles and medullary cord (*c*).

stimulation of lymphocytes. These FDC are apparently of the monocyte lineage (related to macrophages) but are non-phagocytic. Stimulation of specific lymphocytes using antigen–antibody complexes preferentially results in the production of memory cells (responsible for the anamnestic response*) and not the antibody-secreting plasma cells (1, 2, 4).

1.3.2. *Other immunological processes*

Not all of the specific immune responses rely solely on antibody interacting with antigen and neutralising the effectiveness of that antigen (as in the case of diphtheria or tetanus toxin being neutralised with antitoxin antibody); this should be noted when using MAb to perform or study a particular immunological process. Reaction of antibody with antigen (opsonisation) alters the F_c portion of the antibody such that the complement cascade may be initiated (Fig. 1.11), phagocytosis (by macrophages and polymorphonuclear leukocytes) will be enhanced, and antibody-dependent cellular cytotoxicity mechanisms (effected mainly by a T-lymphocyte subset in humans, neutrophils in domestic animals or monocytes in rodents) will be initiated (Fig. 1.12). The involvement of particular cell types in these reactions results from the presence of 'F_c receptors' and 'C3b receptors' on their cell surface (that is, molecules on their cell surfaces which can bind to the altered F_c of antibody after reaction with antigen, or to the activated C3 (C3b) which has bound to that altered F_c).

There are also many important immunological processes which are independent of antibody: the cytotoxic T lymphocyte (T_c or CTL) and natural killer (NK) cell reactions. Such reactions are not of direct relevance to hybridoma technology, but as they are a compartment (see §1.4.8) of the immune system they must be considered in this context to appreciate the significance and relevance of any particular MAb in an immune response *in vivo*.

1.4. **The immune response**

The preceding section introduced the concept of compartments of the immune system. These compartments do, however, exhibit varying degrees of interdependence, and it is therefore necessary to understand how such compartments function and interact, to ascertain the relative role of any antibody species in that immune response, and to appreciate how antibody-producing cells, and hence hybridomas, can be produced.

* Anamnestic response: an antibody response (against a particular antigen) which is more powerful than expected, usually because the animal has already responded to a previous encounter with the antigen; the term is now generally applied to any secondary response, that is the antibody response that occurs after a second or subsequent encounter with an antigen.

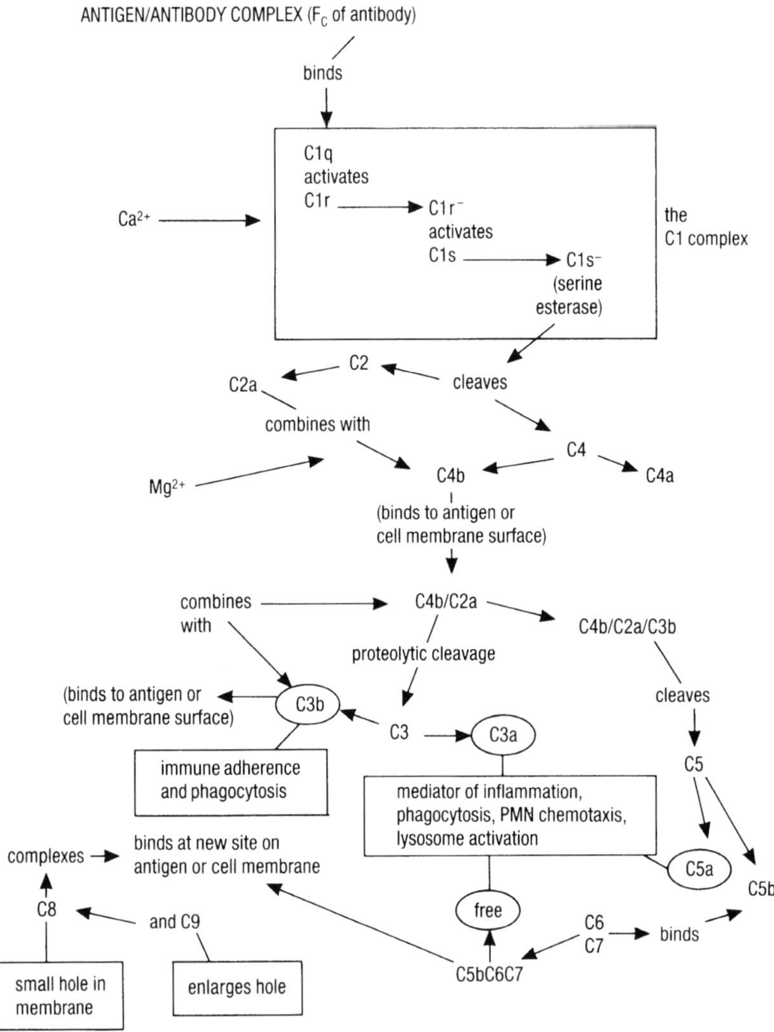

Fig. 1.11. The cascade of events which characterises the activation of complement by either the classical (*a*) or alternative (*b*) pathway. C1, C2, C3, etc., the different components of complement; C2a, C3a, C3b, C3bi, C4a, C4b, C5a, C5b, activation products of the different components of complement. The end-product of complete activation shows that activation of certain components can have a variety of other (sometimes more relevant or important) immunological functions. (See also Fig. 1.33.)

(*b*) Alternative pathway

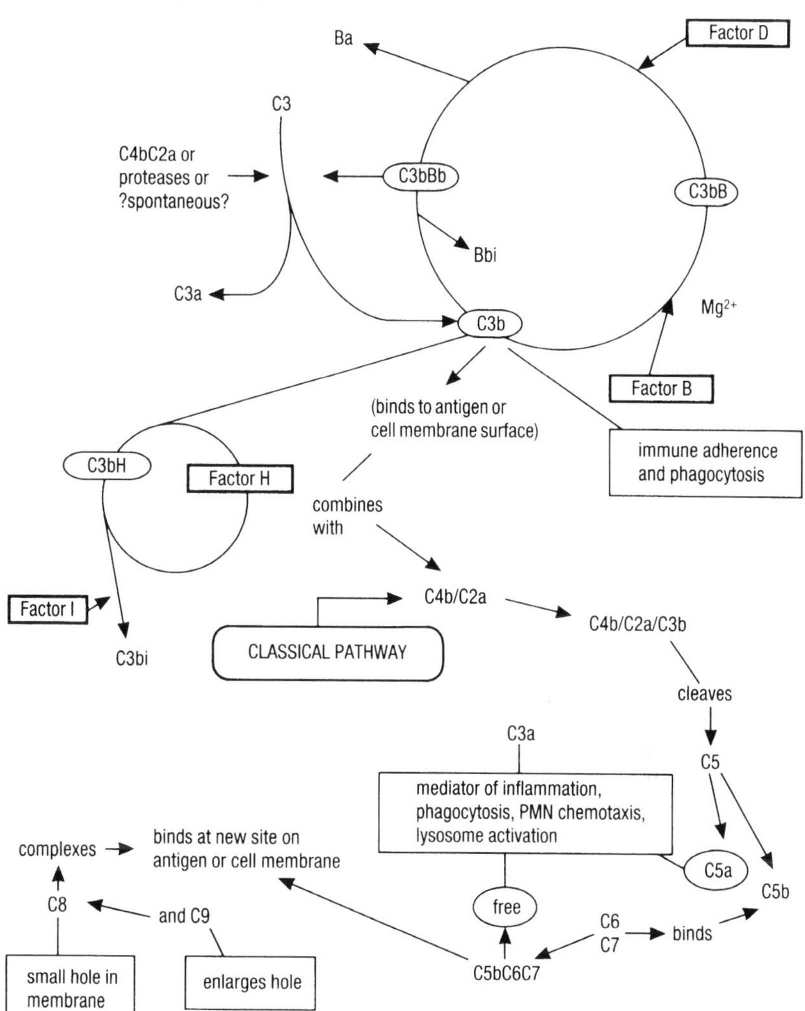

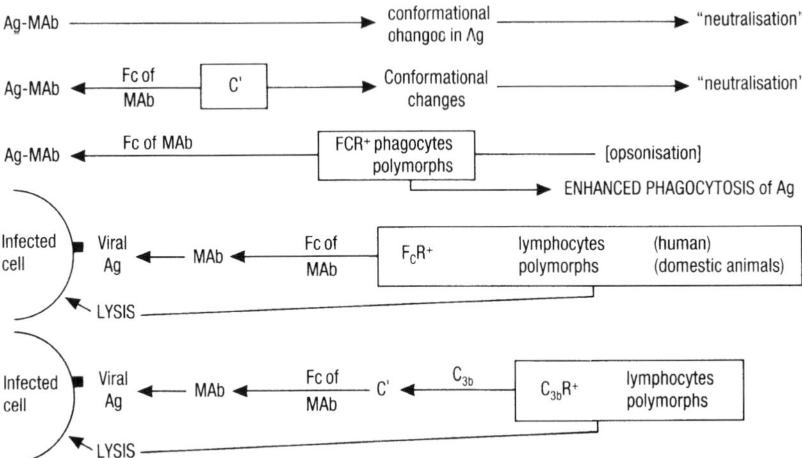

Fig. 1.12. The different antibody-based immune effector defence mechanisms against pathogen attack (from McCullough (39).).

The immune response can be broadly classified into non-specific and specific defence mechanisms. Through cells of the monocyte lineage (macrophages, Kupffer cells, astrocytes) and myeloid series (polymorphonuclear leukocytes – granulocytes or polymorphs – divided into neutrophils, eosinophils and basophils) in the 'non-specific compartment', antigens may be processed for presentation to the specific systems, or phagocytosed and thus neutralised as potential hazards to the host. The presentation is a relatively minor reaction in this compartment (effected by a small population of macrophages), which is primarily involved in preventing the antigen from reacting with and possibly damaging susceptible areas of the body. Antigen presentation is the major function of other cells of the monocyte lineage, termed dendritic cells and veiled cells, which are related to the macrophages but are non-phagocytic. In the 'specific' compartment are found the antibody response and the associated defence mechanisms, and the T_c cell reactions.

These two compartments of the immune response will be discussed separately to highlight their relative significance in the overall immune response and to emphasise their contribution to the eventual production and use of monoclonal antibodies. First, it is necessary to appreciate what is meant by the term 'specific' or 'specificity'.

1.4.1. *What is 'specificity'?*

The 'specific' immune response is directly related to the 'specificity' of the resultant antibody and can be defined as the extent to which the immune system recognises and attacks a particular antigen (the 'specific' antigen) compared with the extent to which a second unrelated, or closely related but not identical, antigen is recognised. An example of this can be provided from the work of Nisonoff *et al.* (10). Antibody was prepared against human cytochrome C and absorbed with rhesus monkey cytochrome C. These two molecules differed only at amino acid position 58, yet the absorption left antibodies which would bind only to cytochrome C of the human type with isoleucine at position 58 (the monkey protein had threonine 58). Smith-Gill *et al.* (11) showed that changing arginine to lysine at position 68 in chicken lysozyme C altered the reactivity of monoclonal antibodies. This phenomenon of specificity can be summarised as shown in Fig. 1.13, as can the related cross-reactivity of antibody.

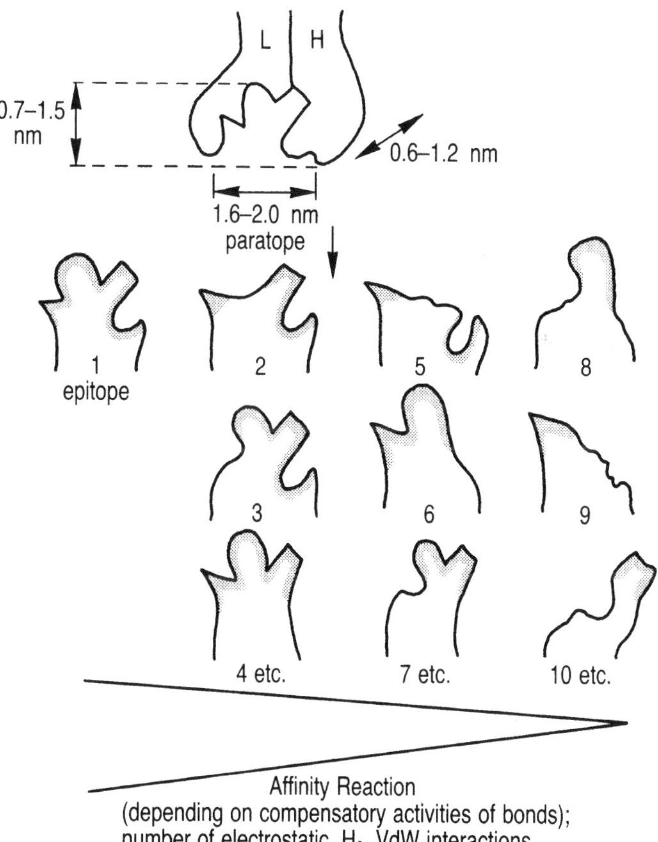

Fig. 1.13. Two-dimensional schematic representation of how affinity and specificity of antibody–antigen interaction can change with slight alterations of the antigenic determinant (epitope). (From McCullough (39).).

The cross-reactivity, and hence the specificity, of an antibody or monoclonal antibody (MAb) for a determinant on an antigen is due to the paratope of the antibody reacting with a particular antigenic determinant (epitope). The paratope is the antigen-combining site or antigen-combining crevice formed between the folded V_H and V_L domains (variable regions of the heavy and light chains) of the antibody. Fig. 1.13 shows a two-dimensional representation of the three-dimensional paratope–epitope interaction; to make explanations more simple, the antibody is to be regarded as homogeneous or monoclonal. The variations in the size of the paratope are also shown, and the shaded areas of the epitope represent the regions of binding with the paratope. This binding is effected by a combination of electrostatic, hydrogen-bonding and Van der Waals interactions, influenced by the spatial distribution of the amino acids and charges (on antibody and antigen) which are involved in the interactions. Each of the individual bonds is weak relative to the overall binding constant, which is due to the integrative interaction of the different bonds. The more bonds involved, the stronger the overall binding. However, in certain instances, some bonding can compensate for the absence of others, creating a higher affinity (stronger binding) than expected of an antibody for a related epitype*.

Considering in diagrammatic form the epitope patterns in Fig. 1.13, the type or paratope illustrated would have highest affinity (stronger binding) for epitope 1, and lowest for epitopes 8 to 10. However, the probability of finding complementary sequences or conformations between two epitopes is higher when using MAb raised against epitope 1 than when using MAb raised against, for example, epitope 8. Anti-epitope 1 MAb would cross-react with ten epitopes (1–10) (Fig. 1.13), whereas anti-epitope 8 MAb would only cross-react with six epitopes (1, 3, 4, 6, 7, 8) (Fig. 1.13). Conversely, an anti-epitope 1 MAb would have high affinity for only epitope 1, with decreasing order of affinity (strength of binding) as shown in Fig. 1.13. Anti-epitope 8 MAb, on the other hand, would have similar affinities for all the epitopes 1, 3, 4, 6, 7, and 8 (providing the conformation of the other epitopes did not sterically interfere with the binding of anti-epitope 8 MAb). Thus, in this example, anti-epitope 1 MAb would have a higher degree of cross-reactivity than anti-epitope 8 MAb. Conversely, when only affinities which are similar to those of the homologous reaction are considered, anti-epitope 8 MAb has higher cross-reactivity than anti-epitope 1 MAb. These considerations are most important when MAb are used in diagnostic and serological differentiation tests, since such tests can be designed to compensate against low affinity reactions. In an antiserum such reac-

* Epitope: an antigenic determinant of known structure, although now more generally applied to refer to any antigenic determinant. Epitype: a family of related epitopes.

tions, cross-reactions and 'specificities' would be expressed by a large number of Ab molecules. Likewise, they would be expressed by receptors on antigen-specific B and T lymphocytes. Although the structure of the receptors on these different cells may vary (only B lymphocytes carry receptors which can be recognised serologically as Ig molecules; the receptors of T lymphocytes are structurally related to the Ig molecule but are not immunoglobulin), the receptors will carry a 'specific paratope-like' region.

Specificity is therefore a relative measure of the capacity of an antibody molecule to recognise the antigenic determinant which induced it. Other determinants may also bind the antibody owing to amino acid sequences or conformational arrangements in common with the inducing epitope. The greater the number of these common regions, the greater the cross-reaction between the determinants. These cross-reactions are distinguishable from non-specific reactions which have no antigenic restriction (see §1.4.2). For example, an antibody may cross-react between two influenza type A viruses, but not between an influenza virus and mycoplasma. Non-specific phagocytosis would not differentiate these organisms, nor would it differentiate any antigen on the basis of the antigenic determinants.

As shown in Fig. 1.13, this closeness of stereochemical and electrochemical 'fit' between a paratope and epitope is concomitant with the strength of non-covalent bonds involved. This binding strength is measured as affinity: the property of the antibody which determines the rate of reaction with antigen and is measured by the free energy change of the reaction in kilojoules per mole. Just as specificity and cross-reactivity can vary between different MAb, so can the affinity (the term is avidity when used in the context of antisera, because this reflects the summation of the effectiveness of binding to a particular antigen by the constituent antibody molecules of different affinities). The relevance of affinity to the immune response will be dealt with in more detail in §§1.5.1 and 1.5.2.

1.4.2. *Non-specific defence mechanisms*

When dealing with invasive organisms such as viruses, bacteria and protozoa, the first line of 'immunological' defence is the non-specific secretions of, for example, the skin and mucous membranes. These are designed to make conditions for the survival of the invading organism as unfavourable as possible. The organism can, however, evade these conditions (either by encapsulating itself or penetrating the membranes) after which it will encounter the 'phagocytic' defence mechanisms. These are more readily recognised as 'immunological' in nature, and may be the first defence mechanisms encountered by certain antigens, such as

Table 1.6. *The mononuclear and polymorphonuclear phagocytes of the immune system – the reticuloendothelial system – and the non-phagocytic mononuclear (monocyte) cells*

Cell name	Site in the body	Monocyte (M) or polymorph (P)	Presentation of antigen
macrophage (blood monocyte)	blood, lymph	M	±
alveolar macrophages	lungs	M	–
peritoneal macrophages	peritoneal cavity	M	±
inflammatory (granuloma) macrophages	sites of injury or infection	M	–
activated macrophages	sites of injury or infection	M	–
cytotoxic macrophages	sites of infection	M	–
tumoricidal macrophages	sites of neoplastic growth; tumours	M	–
splenic macrophages	spleen	M	+
metalophil cells	lymph nodes, bone marrow and other lymphoid tissues	M	+
osteoclasts	phagocytic bone cells	M	–
Kupffer cells (histiocytes)	liver	M	–
cells of Langerhans (histiocytes)	skin, gastrointestinal tract, blood, lymph	M	++
connective tissue histiocytes	connective tissue	M	±
astrocytes	central nervous system	M	+
dendritic cells (non-phagocytic)	blood, lymph, lymphoid organs, skin, connective tissues	M	+++
veiled cells (non-phago-cytic)	blood, lymph, lymphoid organs, skin, connective tissues	M	+++
follicular dendritic cells (non-phagocytic)	lymphoid organs (in the lymphoid follicles and germinal centres – the interdigitating cells)	M	+ (if antigen complexed with antibody +++)

Table 1.6. *(cont.)*

Cell name	Site in the body	Monocyte (M) or polymorph (P)	Presentation of antigen
neutrophil, eosinophil, basophil (granulocyte[1])	blood, lymph, lungs peritoneal cavity, mammary glands, connective tissue	P	–

Note:
[1] A collective term for the three types of polymorph : neutrophil, eosinophil and basophil.

bacterial toxins and vaccine antigens, which are inoculated into the host. This compartment consists of the mononuclear and polymorphonuclear phagocytic cells of the body tissues and fluids (Table 1.6). As the name phagocytic would imply, these cells will engulf foreign antigens and also debris derived from death or destruction of the body's own cells and tissues. These observations promoted their initial description as 'immunological scavengers' by Metchnikoff (in the 1890s), who proposed the name macrophage. It is now apparent that the population of phagocytic cells is large and heterogeneous, although the 'immunologically' active phagocytes can be roughly divided into mononuclear phagocytes (of monocyte lineage) and polymorphonuclear leukocytes (granulocytes, of the myeloid series). These cells differ not only histologically but also in their phagocytic potential for different forms of antigen.

Table 1.6 also shows the important role played by the non-phagocyte cells of the monocyte lineage in processing and presentation of antigen to cells of the lymphoid series (see §1.4.4). A small subpopulation of macrophages (the 'Ia-positive macrophages', to use the term for the murine cells) can also present antigen, but unlike the macrophage population as a whole, presentation is the major function of the non-phagocytic dendritic cells, veiled cells and follicular dendritic cells. Because these presentation reactions are obligatory for the activation of many of the 'specific' immune responses, it is appropriate that they should be discussed in detail with these 'specific' reactions. Further discussion of the role of phagocytes in immunology will be made with reference to the 'specific' reactions, because these two compartments are considerably interdependent.

1.4.3. *Specific reactions*

What are 'specific' immune reactions? They are those in which the response is stimulated by and directed against a relatively narrow range of antigens. This is in contrast to the non-specific reactions, such as phagocytosis, which do not experience this degree of restriction. The term specific is, however, relative. There is no such event in immunology as the highly specific reaction of 'lock and key fit'. The reaction of antibody with antigen depends on the spatio-temporal relationships between the interacting molecules. These molecules are not fixed in space; there is a degree of fluidity. Considering this in terms of the lock and key, the gate of the lock is not rigid, but has a degree of free movement; and a number of keys, which are also non-rigid, can fit. In addition, the key does not have to be fully compatible for there to be an interaction with the lock. These different degrees of fit, and the spatial alterations occurring in the structure of the interacting portions of the antibody and antigen, result in the so called cross-reactivities of antibody and antigen, and the different affinities (strengths of binding) of antibody molecules. This has become most apparent through the use of monoclonal antibodies. The humoral properties of an antiserum are a reflection of a heterogeneous population of antibody, and may in fact be disproportionately influenced by a dominant minority of antibody functions (see §§1.4.1 and 1.5.1).

Thus the term specific is only a relative term, and several apparently unrelated antigens may show unexpected cross-reactivities (12). Despite these idiosyncrasies, the specific immune responses are considerably restricted in their spectrum of recognition. These responses also consist of a large diversity of mechanisms. These mechanisms or subcompartments, in approximate order of when the antigen will encounter them, are (i) the processing phenomena mentioned in §1.4.2; (ii) the regulatory networks (T_h, T_s cells and Id–anti-Id); (iii) the B lymphocyte and the antibody-producing cells; (iv) antibody-mediated cell-effector mechanisms; (v) antibody-independent cell-effector mechanisms (T_c, T_d); (vi) immunological memory. Appreciation of the function of these subcompartments and their interdependence will highlight the relevance of antibody, and hence of monoclonal antibodies, to the immune response. Owing to the individual complexity of each subcompartment, and the importance of each to hybridoma technology, they will be dealt with under individual headings.

1.4.4. *Antigen-processing cells, APC*

There have been three excellent reviews or collections of reviews on this subject (8, 13, 14). The non-phagocytic dendritic cells (DC) and veiled cells (VC) are probably the most important of the APC, because this is apparently their major function and they are extremely mobile cells *in vivo* (15) (but see also below). After stimulation, mononuclear phagocytes are also apparently relatively mobile, but the major role of

Table 1.7. *Comparisons between dendritic cells and macrophages*

Characteristic	Dendritic cells (and veiled cells)	Macrophages
phagocyte	–	+++
esterase	±	++
phosphatase	–	+
peroxidase	–	++
destruction (degradation) of antigen	–	++
destruction of infected or tumour cells	–	++
Ia antigen expression	++	± (only a small percentage of the population)
antigen processing (*not* degradation)	++	± (related to Ia expression)
antigen presentation to T_h lymphocytes	+++	± (related to Ia expression)

these phagocytes (in particular the stimulated or 'recruited' phagocytes) is the engulfment and intracytoplasmic degradation of antigen (Table 1.7). The APC will therefore trap, transport and present antigen to the appropriate ('specific') B and T lymphocytes in the follicles of secondary lymphoid organs more efficiently than if lymphocyte stimulation relied on resident (in the lymphoid organs only) APC. There is evidence that APC will transport antigen to the follicles (13) but whether this is due to a single cell travelling from the site of encounter with the antigen to the follicles or to transfer of the antigen along a series of APC is unclear (13, 14).

One well characterised property of APC, from an *in vitro* aspect at least, is the obligate requirement for a group of chemically defined glycoproteins (the Ia molecules of the class II major histocompatibility complex) to be in association with the presented antigen. Only through this association can T_h lymphocytes bearing the homologous Ia be stimulated and hence support the differentiation of antigen-specific B lymphocytes into antibody-producing cells (see §§1.4.5 and 1.4.6). This requirement of the Ia glycoprotein is probably of relevance *in vivo* and not merely an *in vitro* phenomenon (Table 1.8); firstly, short-term *in vitro* culture of Ia-bearing phagocytes results in the loss of both surface Ia glycoprotein and the ability to function effectively as an APC (16); secondly, antigen-pulsed monocytes can only be used to stimulate antigen-specific T_h cells *in vivo* if the monocytes carry an Ia glycoprotein

Table 1.8. *Evidence that Ia glycoproteins function* in vivo *and are not* in vitro *artifacts*

in vivo	*in vitro*
Resting monocytes always contain a percentage of cells with Ia.	Culture of resting macrophages results in the loss of Ia expression.
Transfer of Ia^+ monocytes to deficient animals results in restoration of antigen presentation.	Only when Ia^+ cells are present in a population will antigen presentation occur.
Ia^+ monocytes can be pulsed with antigen and transferred to an animal with the same haplotype of Ia, resulting in antigen stimulation. If the haplotypes are not matched, no antigen stimulation is seen.	Mixed populations of monocytes and T lymphocytes co-operate in antigen presentation, only when the Ia haplotypes are the same.
Only with animals in which there are populations or subpopulations of monocytes and lymphocytes carrying the same Ia haplotype will antigen presentation be seen.	

homologous with the T_h cell Ia molecule (8, 13, 14); thirdly, F_1 progeny* of parents differing in their Ia glycoproteins contain populations of cells carrying each but not both of the Ia serotypes, but only those APC and T_h lymphocytes with homologous Ia glycoproteins will co-operate in antigen presentation (8, 13, 14, 17).

Finally, a cell-free filtrate from antigen-presenting macrophages contained a substance with both Ia glycoprotein and presented antigen specificities (an Ia–antigen complex?) which replaced antigen present on APC as an immunostimulatory substance for T_h lymphocytes (18).

This stimulation of the antigen-specific immune reactions by antigen presented on APC involves several cellular interactions and the use of a range of biomolecular growth-regulatory substances. Fig. 1.14 shows how these pathways are related. The suppressor 'circuits' are also shown to a limited degree, as they are a very important regulatory system which can be considered as antigen-specific. These circuits will be dealt with in more detail below. The figure shows that the APC will produce monokines (lymphocyte and growth regulatory factors). These factors,

* F_1 progeny: the first-generation offspring, in this case the first generation of cells, derived from defined parents.

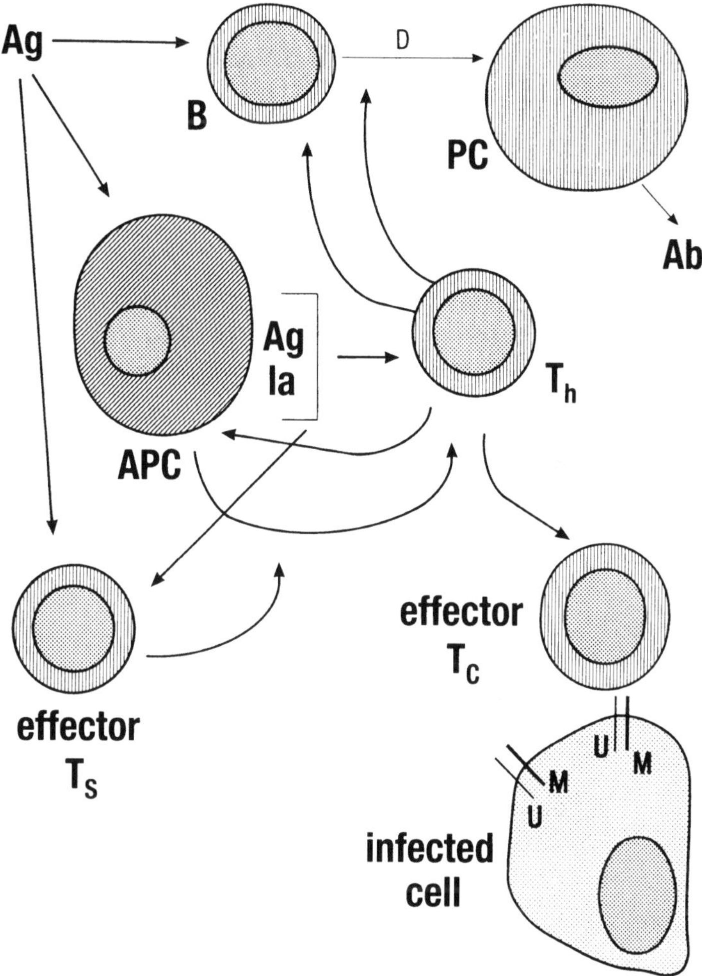

Fig. 1.14. Stimulation of B lymphocytes (B) by antigen (Ag); presentation by antigen-presenting cells (APC) of the antigen in association with MHC Class II molecules (Ia) to T helper lymphocytes (T_h), which assist the differentiation (D) of B lymphocytes to antibody-secreting (Ab) plasma cells (PC), and assist the differentiation of effector cytotoxic T lymphocytes (T_c) which have responded to viral antigens (U) in association with MHC class I molecules (M) on virus infected cells; and antigen stimulation of T suppresssor cells (T_s). Heavy straight arrows, stimulation reactions; light arrows, differentiation or synthesis pathways; heavy curved arrows, production of soluble mediators of immunological function.

coupled with the antigen presented by the APC, induce the T_h cells to produce lymphokines, which in turn will regulate monocyte, T lymphocyte and B lymphocyte growth and activity. These substances, or at least those which are characterised, are listed, along with their known functions, in Table 1.9. This interactive production of monokines and lym-

Table 1.9. *The major characterised regulatory factors produced by monocytes (monokines), lymphocytes (lymphokines) and other cells (cytokines)*

		Effects		
Factor	Producer cells	Stimulation/enhancement	Regulation	Harmful
Interferon (IFN_{α})	Leukocytes Fibroblasts	Polymorph/monocyte/NK cell cytotoxicity IL-1 production Anti-viral state in cells	The IFN_{α} induction of Ia antigens	Lymphocyte depression
IFN_{β}	Fibroblasts (leukocytes)	as IFN_{α}	$IFN_{\beta 2}$ (IL-6) responsible for anti-viral effects (at least) of TNFs	
IFN_{γ}	T lymphocytes (particularly T_h and NK)	T_h cell activity Polymorph/monocyte/NK cell cytotoxicity Phagocytosis Proliferating B cell differentiation Ia antigen expression IL-1, IL-2, TNF production	Antibody production (at high dose) T_s cell induction	Immune suppression

Interleukin-1 (IL-1) (= LAF)	Monocytes	Monocyte cytotoxicity	Prostaglandin induction	Severe pyrexia (inflammatory cell induction)
		T cell maturation	Prostaglandin-regulation of immune function	Induction of inflammatory cells in arthritis
		Effector T_h cell generation after antigen stimulation	ACTH induction: thus cortisol production and regulation of immune function	Bone/ cartilage resorption
		Amplification of IL-2 production (does *not* induce IL-2 production)	T_s cell generation	Islet cell damage
		Antibody production (via enhanced T_h cell activity)	Pituitary function	
		Astrocyte growth		
		TNF induction		
		GM-CSF production		
IL-2 (= TCGF)	T lymphocytes	Antigen-activated T cell proliferation	IFN_γ production	Immune suppression
		IL-2 and IL-2 receptor production in activated T_h cells	T_s cell generation	Toxic at moderate concentrations
		Phagocyte maturation		
		Late differentiation signal for B cells		
		NK cell proliferation (also requires IFN_γ)		
		Precursor T_c cell activation		
		IFN_γ induction		
		TNF_β induction		

Table 1.9. *(cont.)*

		Effects		
Factor	Producer cells	Stimulation/enhancement	Regulation	Harmful
IL-3 (Pleuripotent CSF)	Various, including T lymphocytes	Myeloid cell growth (+ other proteins results in differentiation of all leukocytes) IL-2 receptor increase		
IL-4 (see B cell growth factor I)	T_h lymphocytes	= B cell growth factor I (BCGF I) = B cell stimulating factor 1 (BSF1) = B cell differentiation factor (BCDF)		
IL-B4 (see B cell enhancing factor)	B lymphocytes	= B cell enhancing factor (of growth/differentiation)		
IL-5 (see B cell growth factor II)	T_h lymphocytes	= B cell growth factor II (BCGF II) = T cell replacing factor (TRF) = Eosinophil differentiation factor (EoDF)		

B cell growth factor I (BCGF I, BSF1, or IL-4)	T_h lymphocytes	Proliferation of antigen-induced B lymphoblasts Preparation of B cells for 'differentiation phase' (BCGF II/IL-2 dependent) Mast cell growth		
B cell growth factor II (BCGF II, TRF, or IL-5)	T_h lymphocytes	Induces further differentiation of B cells after 'BCGF I' phase Promotes eosinophil differentiation	Prostaglandin induction in eosinophils	Prostaglandin-induced tissue damage
B cell differentiation and maturation factors (BCDF;BCMF)	T_h lymphocytes	Probably synonymous with the BCGFs ($BCDF_\gamma$, BCGF I or BSF1 or IL-4)		
B cell enhancing factor	B lymphocytes	T_h cell function due to the effects on T_s cells	Reduces precursor T_s cell induction Inhibition F_c receptor expression	

Table 1.9. *(cont.)*

Factor	Producer cells	Effects: Stimulation/enhancement	Regulation	Harmful
T cell growth factor 1 (TCGF1)	T_h lymphocytes	= IL-2		
TCGF2	T_h lymphocytes	Probably = BCGFI (BSF 1)		
Mast cell growth factor 2 (MCGF2)	T_h lymphocytes	Probably = BCGFI (BSF 1)		
Tumour necrosis factors:				
TNF_α	Monocytes	Polymorph/monocyte/NK cell cytotoxicity	Prostaglandin induction	Pyrexia (inflammatory cell induction)
TNF_β .... (Lymphotoxin)	Lymphocytes	IFN_γ-induced cytotoxicity Fibroblast growth	Prostaglandin-regulation of immune function	Tissue damage in arthritis
		IL-1 production GM-CSF production Anti-viral state in cells Cytotoxic for tumour cells	Pituitary function	Hypoglycaemia, augmentation of Islet cell damage by IL-1

Macrophage activating factor (MAF)	T lymphocytes	Activates monocytes to macrophages Similar effects on macrophages to IFN (may be same factor as MIF and MCF with different effects being due to different concentrations)	'Suppressor macrophage' induction (induction of prostaglandins)	Tissue damage and inflammation if over-stimulation of macrophages
Macrophage inhibition factor (MIF)	T_h lymphocytes	Enhances F_CR expression	Controls macrophage movement	
Macrophage chemotactic factor (MCF)	T_h lymphocytes B lymphocytes	Monocyte and macrophage chemotaxis Monocyte complement stimulator (of the C2 component)		
Macrophage aggregation factor	T_h lymphocytes	Aggregates macrophages (enhances function?)		
Macrophage suppressor factor (MSF)	T lymphocytes	Suppresses macrophage function		

Table 1.9. *(cont.)*

		Effects		
Factor	Producer cells	Stimulation/enhancement	Regulation	Harmful
Macrophage cytotoxicity inducing factor (MCIF)	T lymphocytes	Macrophage cytotoxicity inducing factor		
Platelet activating factor	Large lymphocytes	Platelet activation F_c receptor cross-linking (leading to enhanced phagocyte activation) Polymorph functions (e.g. adherence)		Over-production of platelets Endothelial cell damage due to polymorph adherence
Colony stimulating factors (CSF)	Fibroblasts Endothelial cells T lymphocytes Monocytes	Myeloid cell growth Differentiation of mature monocytes/ macrophages (M-CSF or CSF1, and GM-CSF or CSF2) and granulocytes or polymorphs (GM-CSF)	Is another MIF	

CCDF	T_h lymphocytes	T_c cell differentiation factor
Proteoglycan	T_h lymphocytes	B cell proliferation
Prolactin	Pituitary gland	Maintains T cell immunocompetence
Keratinocyte-derived T cell growth factor (KTGF)	Epidermal epithelial cells (keratinocytes)	T cell growth
Thymosin fraction 5	Thymus (from thymosin$_{\alpha 1}$)	Lymphoproliferation IL-2 production by antigen-stimulated T cells
Polymorph chemotractant	Monocytes	Polymorph chemotaxis

Table 1.9. *(cont.)*

		Effects		
Factor	Producer cells	Stimulation/enhancement	Regulation	Harmful
Prostaglandins	Monocytes	IL-1 production (if already induced)	Inactivate polymorph/ monocyte/NK function	Anaphylactic (prostacyclin)
	Polymorphs	Enhance monocyte activation, particularly phagocytosis (prostaglandin E_2)	Inhibit lymphocyte proliferation	Inflammatory (pyrexia)
			Inhibit platelet aggregation	
Leukotrienes (LT)	Monocytes	Polymorph chemotaxis (LTB_4)	Stimulation of prostacyclin production	Anaphylaxis and inflammation ($LTC_4/D_4/E_4$: = slow-reacting substance of anaphylaxis)
	Polymorphs	Enhanced macrophage cytotoxicity (LTB_4)	Inhibition lymphocyte function	
	Mast cells	Endothelial cell production of platelet activating factor		
Glucocorticoids	Adrenal gland		Inhibits lymphocyte proliferation and function	Immunological non-responsiveness
ACTH	Pituitary gland		Induces glucocorticoids	

Table 1.10. *Localisation of accessory cells in the body*

Cell name	Site	Function
macrophage	blood, lymph, lymphoid organs, lungs, peritoneal cavity, skin, connective tissues, mammary glands	phagocytosis and degradation (destruction) of antigen; cytotoxic for infected and tumour cells; some antigen processing and precipitation.
cells of Langerhans	skin, blood, lymph	as for macrophage, but possibly with more antigen processing and presentation capacity.
astrocytes	central nervous system	as for cells of Langerhans
dendritic cells	blood, lymph, lymphoid organs, skin, connective tissues	antigen processing and presentation
veiled cells	as for dendritic cells	as for dendritic cells
follicular dendritic cells	germinal centres and follicles of secondary lymphoid organs	capture, retention and presentation of complexes of antigen with antibody (and also complement)

phokines is of extreme importance to all 'non-specific' and 'specific' immunological reactions. Whether it is the monocyte which presents antigen that also produces the required monokines, or whether two cell populations are required (a non-phagocytic presenting cell and a monokine-producing activated macrophage, perhaps) is as yet undetermined.

Accessory cells, whether functioning as APC or phagocytes, are to be found in most areas of the body, as shown in Table 1.10. The exception is the follicular dendritic cell. There is no evidence that this cell is transient within the follicles; in fact, it may be permanently resident. Furthermore, it is apparently involved in the presentation by simple trapping (i.e. no processing) of antigen–antibody–C′ complexes but not free antigen (9). It does, however, form a major part of the APC family. Whether T_h-cell-dependent antigen or the T_h-cell-independent mitogens for B or T cell polyclonal activation are used, APC are apparently required for the maturation of the immune response. The specific response is regulated, in the majority of antigens, by T cell–T cell, monocyte–T cell, monocyte–B cell and T cell–B cell interactions, often through the production of the soluble growth-promoting or regulating factors known as cytokines. These cellular interactions will be described in more detail in §1.4.5.

Table 1.11. *Characterisation of T-dependent and T-independent antigens*

Classification	Example[1]	Reason for classification[2]
T-independent (TI1)	TNP linked to either enterobacterial lipopolysaccharide, *Brucella abortus* or *Nocardia* water-soluble mitogen	Little or no requirement of T_h lymphocytes or APC for the stimulation of B lymphocytes[3]
T-independent(TI2)	TNP linked to either Ficoll, dextran, polyacrylamide or type III pneumococcal polysaccharide	Limited requirement of T_h lymphocytes[4] and an obligate requirement of APC for the stimulation of B lymphocytes
T-dependent (TD)	Most antigenic substances (protein, glycoprotein, lipoprotein, nucleoprotein, polypeptide in nature)	Obligate requirement of both T_h lymphocytes[4] and APC for the stimulation of B lymphocytes

Note:
1 The TNP is the hapten, and that to which it is linked is the carrier molecule.
2 The classification is determined with respect to the antibody response against the hapten (TNP) and the characteristics of the control of the response mediated by the carrier molecule (57–62).
3 The requirement for APC (57, 58) and limited T lymphocyte (59) involvement depends on the type of response. A mitogenic response will generally not require T lymphocytes or APC, although their presence may improve the response (59, 61).
4 The T_h lymphocyte help appears to be in the form of antigen non-specific soluble factors for TI antigens (61); for TD antigens, the help is in the form of both the antigen non-specific T cell factors and the antigen-specific T_h lymphocytes themselves. When using hapten-carrier conjugates (e.g. TNP–Ficoll), carrier priming (e.g. by Ficoll) can be used to generate T_h lymphocytes which will 'help' the subsequent B lymphocyte response against the hapten in the hapten–carrier (e.g. TNP in TNP–Ficoll) (60). T lymphocyte help can also be stimulated directly by already activated B lymphocytes; this was shown when B lymphocytes were activated (primed) with antigen, and then mixed with non-activated (resting) T cells, after free antigen had been removed (62).

1.4.5. *Regulatory networks*

Antigens can be classified into T-dependent and T-independent antigens (Table 1.11). As the T-cell-dependent antigens are in the majority and more relevant to the application of hybridoma technology, this section will deal primarily with T-dependent (TD) antigens. Firstly, however, it is necessary to describe some of the properties of T-independent antigens. These can be subdivided into TI-1 and TI-2 antigens (Table 1.12), based on their requirements for monocyte and T lymphocyte involvement. The table shows that endotoxin B cell mitogens, such as bacterial lipopolysaccharide, belong to the TI-1 class. These mitogens are substances which aspecifically stimulate all B cell clones (polyclonal B cell activation). This is in contrast to other T-independent and all T-dependent antigens,

Table 1.12. *Examples of TI-1 and TI-2 antigens*

(For reviews, see (63).)

Antigen type	Examples
TI-1	bacterial lipopolysaccharide
	Brucella abortus
	Nocardia water-soluble mitogen
	liposomes containing lipid A
TI-2	Ficoll
	Dextran
	polyacrylamide
	type III pneumococcal polysaccharide
	pokeweed mitogen
	liposomes without lipid A

which stimulate a small proportion of B cells (less than 1% of the unstimulated or 'resting virgin' B lymphocyte population) bearing receptors 'specific' for determinants (epitopes) on the antigen. The major differences between TD antigens and TI antigens is in the role of accessory cells and the subclass of antibody induced (Table 1.13). The APC (see previous section) are required for processing and presenting TD and TI-2 antigens but not TI-1 antigens. An IgM response is most common against TI-1 antigens, whereas the class switch from IgM to IgG, which becomes the dominating antibody class, is seen with TD and TI-2 antigens. This class switch is controlled by regulatory T_h lymphocytes, which are involved with the B cell response against TD antigens and, to a limited degree, with TI-2 antigens. It is therefore misleading to refer to TI-2 antigens as being T-independent since the response against them does require T lymphocyte help. The difference between TD and TI-2 responses lies in the degree of T cell help, with the TI-2 responses requiring lower levels of help than those of TD. It is likely that only a few mitogenic substances (substances that may react with receptors on lymphocyte surfaces which are distinct from the antigen receptors) are truly T-cell-independent; most, if not all, antigenic substances stimulate responses which are, to different degrees, dependent on T lymphocyte help.

The regulatory lymphocytes are the T helper subset (T_h) and T suppressor subset (T_s) of the T lymphocyte family. The T_s population is divided into precursor, stimulator and effector cells. It is beyond the scope of this book to adequately review the current state of knowledge regarding T_h and T_s cells and the regulatory factors they produce; the reader is therefore advised to consult the reviews on this subject (19–23). With respect to hybridoma technology, these T_h and T_s cells are of relevance in two areas. Firstly, they regulate the B cell response to the

Table 1.13. *Immunological differences found with the response against TI-1, TI-2 and TD antigens*

Antigen type	Concentration		Presentation by APC	Requirement for T_h lymphocytes	Requirement for T_h lymphocyte 'helper' factors	Immunoglobulin isotype[1] induced	Memory response generated
TI-1	low	(i)	none	none	none, but their presence will enhance	IgM (virgin B cells specific for the TI-1 antigen)[1]	usually not
		(ii)	none	not normally[2]	not obligatory, but their presence will enhance[2]	IgM (virgin B cells specific for the TI-1 antigen) + some IgG (low level of isotype switching)[1]	at a low level
	high		none	none	none	IgM (virgin B cells) + IgG (already existing memory B cells specific for any antigen)[3]	no[3]
TI-2	low		yes	can help, but not absolutely necessary[4]	yes, but a low level of B cell reponsiveness in their absence may be possible[4]	IgM + IgG (virgin B cells specific for the TI-2 antigen)[5]; in absence of T cell factors, IgM only[5]	yes (but less than with TD antigen)[5]
	high		probably not necessary	probably not necessary	probably not necessary	as for TI-1 at high concentrations	no

TD	low	yes	yes	yes	IgM + IgG + IgA (virgin B cells specific for the TD antigen, with considerable isotype switching); mainly IgG with memory cells, and probably some subclass switching of isotype	yes, very efficient
	high	not necessary	will depend on the type of tolerance induced	will depend on the type of tolerance induced	none; tolerance induced	only in the T_s lymphocytes, since tolerance is induced

Note:

[1] The TI-1 antigens can be divided into those which do not induce class switching from IgM to IgG or a memory B cell response (e.g. TNP–LPS) and those which induce a low level of both (e.g. TNP–*Brucella abortus*) (63, 64).

[2] T_h lymphocytes and the 'helper' factors which they produce are not normally required for B lymphocyte responses against TI-1 antigens, but the presence of either T_h cells (59, 60) or T cell factors (61) could enhance the response.

[3] TI-1 antigens do not efficiently stimulate memory cell production, but high concentrations of these antigens function as mitogens or polyclonal activators of many subsets of B cells which are specific for other antigens (particularly the TI-1 antigens which give the reaction shown under (i) (64).

[4] T lymphocytes can be primed by Ficoll to perform a 'carrier' function with respect to B cell responses against TNP–Ficoll (60). Extensive T cell depletion greatly reduces B cell responses to TI-2 antigens, whereas such depletion only occasionally diminishes the responses to TI-1 antigens, and then to a much lower degree compared with TI-2 antigens (59).

[5] Some IgM to IgG class switching, and memory cell development, can occur with TI-2 antigens under the correct conditions of stimulation (63–65).

majority of antigens. T_h cells provide the necessary factors to facilitate B cell differentiation (after B cell activation by antigen). T_s cells also respond to T_h cell activation when that activation reaches a minimum threshold level (T_s precursors are either stimulated by factors such as T_h cell IL-2 or the IL-1 which monocytes are induced to produce by antigen plus activated T_h cells, or stimulated by the idiotopy of the T_h cells). This results in a feedback inhibition of the function of T_h lymphocytes, and thus the differentiation of B cell clone(s) dependent on that T_h subset will also be suppressed (this prevents excessive generation of T_h cells, T_h factors and antibody). T_s cell-dependent regulation is dealt with in more detail below (see Fig. 1.15). The second area of relevance for T_h and T_s cells is in the production of hybridomas. Although the majority of work cited in this monograph will deal with B cell–myeloma cell* hybridomas, T cell–T lymphoblastoid cell hybridomas have also been produced (24–26). Many of these latter hybridomas have used T_s cells and produced T_s cell factor (T_sF). There are also some reports of hybridomas with T_h cells secreting 'helper' factors, such as IL-2 (TCGF), BCGF I and BCMFII (24–26). The topic of T cell hybridomas will be dealt with in detail in §§2.7 and 6.1.4.

Lymphocyte receptor-based regulatory networks (idiotypic networks)
B lymphocytes, T_h lymphocytes, T_s lymphocytes and the other lymphocyte-dependent antigen-specific mechanisms of the immune response (T_d, T_c; see below) can 'communicate' with one another, and hence are regulated, by a network of lymphocyte receptor–anti-receptor reactions. The receptors on the surface of lymphocytes, such as the immunoglobulin-like molecules (see §1.3) bear epitopes unique to that particular clone of lymphocyte. These epitopes are called the idiotopes (Id). Expansion of particular B cell or T_h cell clones, and the production of antibody following antigenic stimulation, increases the relative concentration of the Id carried by these cells, and antibody molecules secreted by the stimulated B lymphocyte carry the same Id as the receptor molecule of that B cell. When Id reach a particular concentration, termed their immunogenic level, anti-Id-bearing cells are stimulated (Jerne's network theory, (27)). These anti-Id-bearing cells carry receptor molecules which recognise the inducing Id as foreign, and are stimulated in similar fashion to the stimulation of lymphocytes by the antigenic determinants, for example, on a virus. Id–anti-Id reactions are primarily involved in the regulation of an immune response. During such a response, T_h cells will be stimulated by antigen to provide the necessary help to the development of the protective immune response (antibody production; cellular

* Myeloma cell: a transformed plasma cell which consistently secretes a structurally and electrophoretically homogeneous or monoclonal Ig molecule.

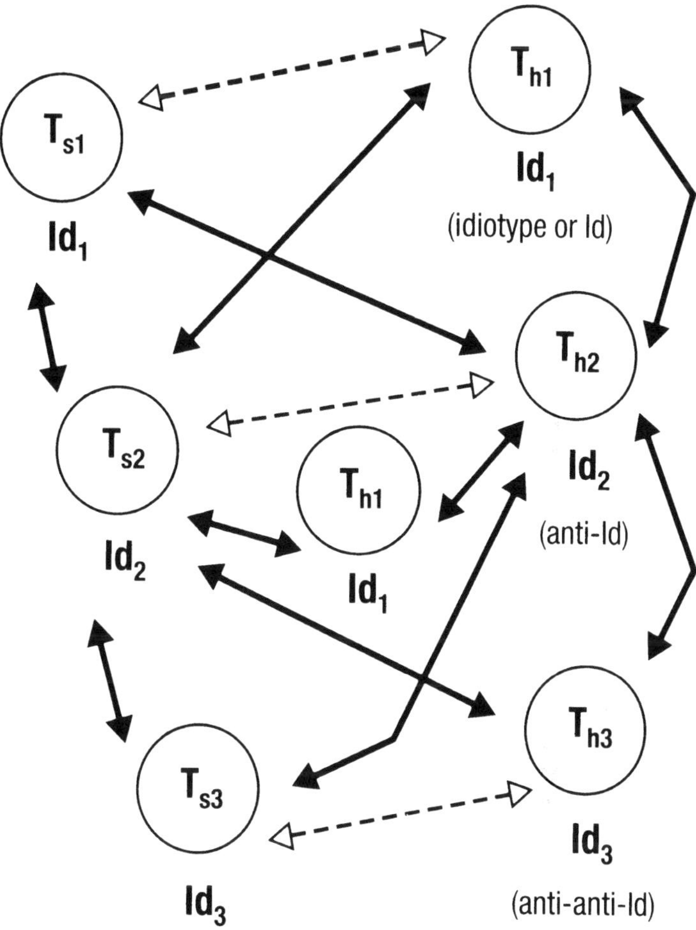

Fig. 1.15. Idiotype (Id)–anti-idiotype interactions between helper (T_h) and suppressor (T_s) lymphocytes, either directly (solid lines) or through factor production (broken lines).

cytotoxicity). When the threat posed by the antigen has been overcome (the antigen has been 'neutralised') this response must be down-regulated. This is achieved through the Id of the receptors on the T_h cell stimulating anti-Id receptors on T_s precursor cells. This results in the production of T_s cells, which suppress the function of T_h cells and thus inhibit the differentiation of the appropriate B cell clone (Fig. 1.15). The suppressor networks are complex multi-pathway systems with subsets of T_s cells (Id-bearing or T_{s1}) stimulating other T_s cell subsets (anti-Id or T_{s2}); see, for example, Greene *et al.* (28).

There are also anti-Id-bearing T_h and B cells. Stimulation of these cells by the appropriate Id may result in the production of anti-Id antibody or more Id-bearing antibody as shown in Fig. 1.16. This aspect of the Id–anti-Id networks will be dealt with in more detail in §6.6, where the relevance to hybridoma technology will be discussed.

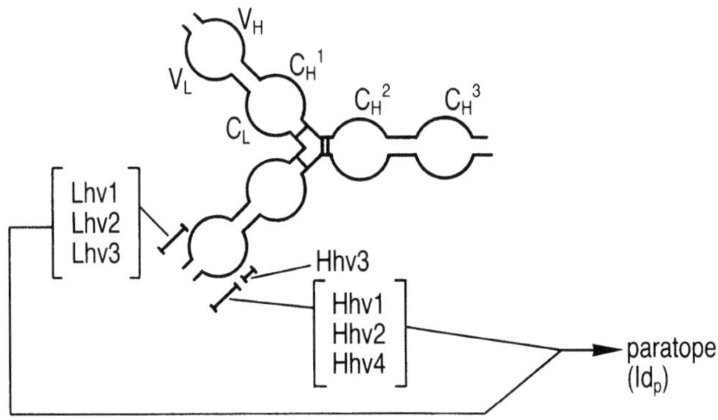

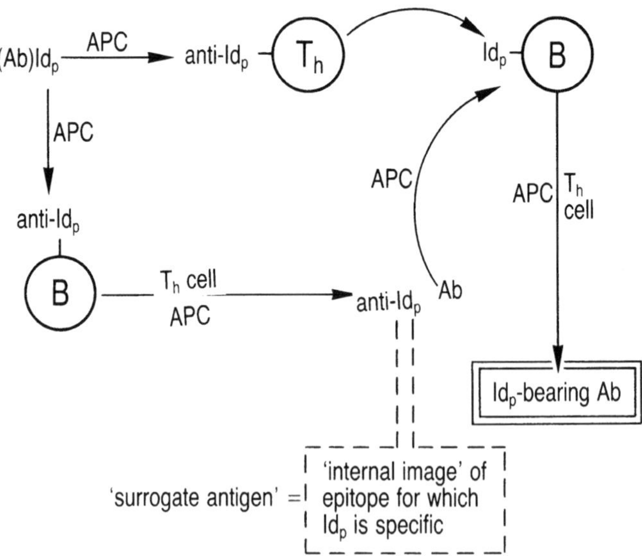

Fig. 1.16. Idiotype (Id)–anti-idiotype interactions between Id or antibody molecules (Ab), B lymphocytes (B) and T helper lymphocytes (T_h), resulting in the production of anti-Id bearing or Id-bearing antibody. Id_p, the idiotope(s) associated with the paratope; APC, antigen-presenting cell (required for its accessory factors and not so much for antigen presentation). (From K. C. McCullough and D. Langley (33).).

Id–anti-Id reactions can be complex. Hood *et al.* (1) have shown how a single Id-bearing B cell clone can stimulate at least three different anti-Id clones (Fig. 1.17). Each of these could, in turn, behave as the 'Id-bearing cell' and thus induce their own 'anti-Id'. This network of stimulations could continue expanding for as long as the Id-bearing molecules were at immunogenic levels. This topic is reviewed by Bona (29), Bona & Cazenave (30), Urbain *et al.* (31), Kelsoe *et al.* (32) and McCullough & Langley (33), who explain how and why Id–anti-Id stimulations are limited.

In order to alleviate the problem of talking about Id, anti-Id, anti-anti-Id, etc., these authors use the terms Id_1, Id_2, Id_3, etc., where Id (Id_1) stimulates Id_2 (anti-Id_1) which in turn stimulates Id_3 (anti-Id_2) and so forth (Fig. 1.18). Id_3 could in fact be identical to Id_1. This is because not only is Id_2 the anti-Id against Id_1, but Id_1 is also an anti-Id against Id_2 if both Id_1 and Id_2 are within the paratope of the appropriate antibody molecule. The reasons for the maximum of six Id specificities shown in Fig. 1.18, and fuller details of the complete network system, so far as is currently understood, are given in the reviews of Urbain *et al.* (31), Kelsoe *et al.* (32), Bona (29) and Bona & Cazenave (30). Concerning MAb, the interactions shown in Figs 1.16 and 1.17 are of most relevance, because it is due to these that monoclonal anti-Id antibody and anti-Id

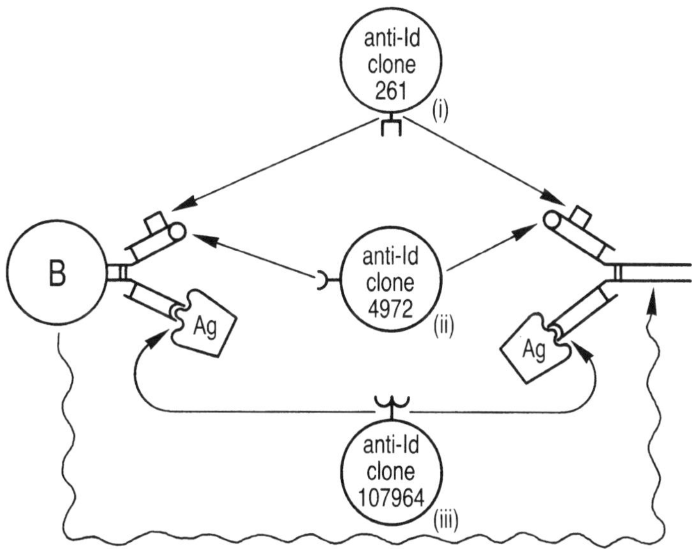

Fig. 1.17. The three major families of idiotypes (Id) which can be induced by an antibody molecule or the receptor of a B or T_h cell. Symbols represent: (i), anti-Id against Id outside the paratope; (ii), anti-Id against paratope-associated Id; (iii), anti-Id against Id formed by interaction between paratope and antigen. (Adapted from Hood *et al.* (1); see also McCullough & Langley (33).)

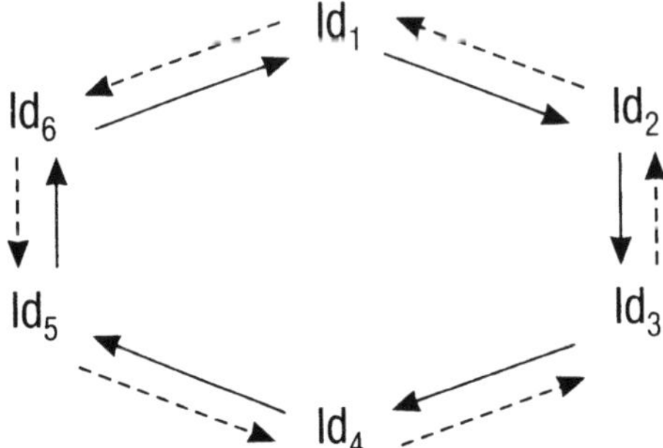

Fig. 1.18. The chain of idiotype interactions which can occur, in which idiotope, anti-idiotope, anti-anti-idiotope, etc. are represented by Id_1, Id_2, Id_3, etc. The cycle could be complete after Id_2, Id_4, or (as shown) Id_6.

antibody against MAb may be produced (33). The usefulness of these anti-Id antibodies will be dealt with in §6.6.

1.4.6. *The B lymphocyte and antibody production*

The subset of lymphocytes which bear surface Ig-like molecules – the B (bursa-derived of birds; bone-marrow-derived of mammals) lymphocytes – are a heterogeneous population of cells subdivided depending on their specificity for antigens or the epitopes (antigenic determinants) of the antigens. Determinants on the antigen bind with particular B lymphocytes through the Ig-like 'receptors' on these cells. The specificity of this reaction is governed by the regions on the receptors which are identical to the paratope (antigen-binding site) of antibody secreted by the B lymphocytes *after antigen-driven differentiation*. This differentiation is obligatory for successful antibody production. The stimulatory signals involved are shown in Fig. 1.19. Exceptions to this scheme are the TI antigens, which include the polyclonal B cell activators or mitogens. Such substances, e.g. lipopolysaccharide (LPS) from certain strains of enteric bacteria, and pokeweed mitogen, do not selectively stimulate a small population of B cells (clones), but stimulate all clones (hence the term polyclonal activator). These substances can prove useful tools in immunology, and even in hybridoma technology (polyclonal stimulation of *in vitro* enriched 'antigen-specific' B cells can be used to produce the B lymphoblasts required for the production of hybridomas; see §§2.5.7 and 2.7.1). However, mitogens do not use the same surface molecules on lymphocytes as do antigens; hence there is no relationship between the mitogen receptor and the antibody molecules secreted by stimulated B lymphocytes.

The majority of antigens used in both immunology and hybridoma technology stimulate a restricted number of B lymphocyte clones by the

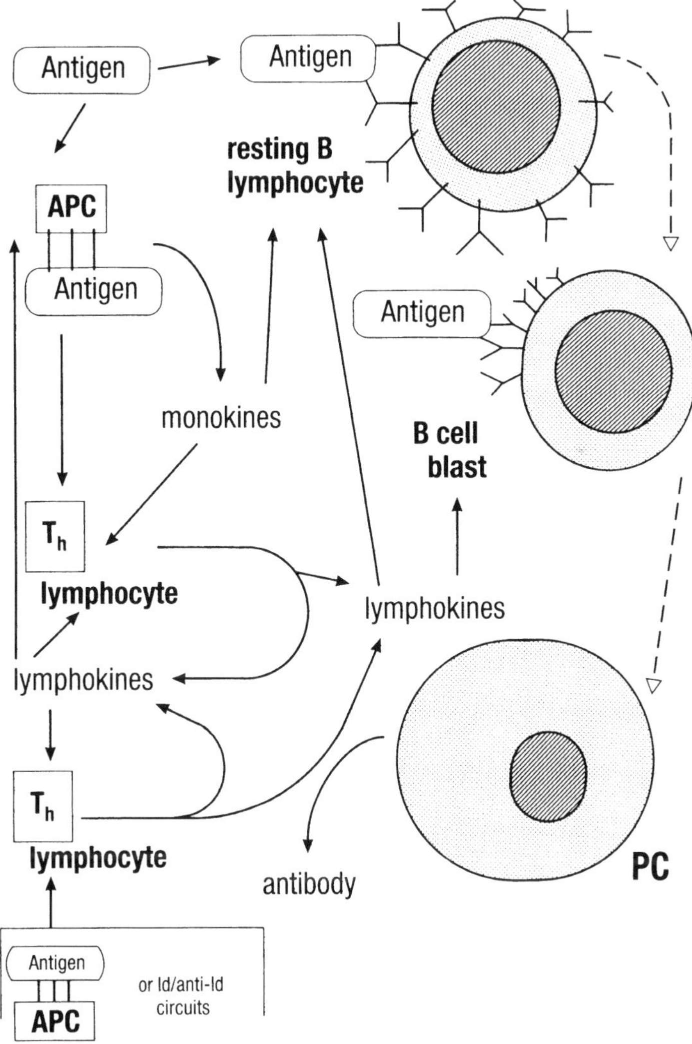

Fig. 1.19. The various signals and interactions required to stimulate B lymphocytes with antigen, and drive the differentiation to antibody secretion by plasma cells. APC, antigen-presenting cell; Id, idiotype.

scheme shown in Fig. 1.19. The antigen cross-links the Ig-like receptors, which results in 'capping': the receptors migrate to a small area or pole of the cell surface. These receptors are then internalised. It is the capping, however, which is responsible for inducing the B cell to enter into the physiological state in preparation for further differentiation (should the correct T_h cell growth factors be present). Reaction of the B cell receptors with antigen *without* cross-linking results in internalisation but not capping. The B lymphocytes cannot undergo differentiation into the antibody-secreting cell, but just regenerate receptor molecules.

Following antigen-induced capping of B cells, further cell division and differentiation will *only* proceed if the appropriate T_h cell-derived and monocyte-derived factors are present. The TD antigen (termed T-dependent or TD antigen owing to the dependence of the reaction on the appropriate T_h cells) is presented by the APC to 'antigen-specific' T_h lymphocytes. The B cells are stimulated by antigen alone or in association with APC, resulting in capping. Stimulated T_h cells are stimulated to produce a variety of substances, including immune interferon (IFNγ), interleukin 2 (IL-2), B cell growth factors (BCGF I and II), B cell differentiation factors, B cell maturation factor and other lymphokines which act as stimulators and regulators of both macrophage and lymphocyte activity and movement (see Table 1.9). How many of these represent individual molecules with individual functions, and which are multifunctional factors or combinations of a number of molecules acting synergistically, is still unclear. Such T_h cell actions are termed 'antigen non-specific help'. The term 'antigen-specific help' comes from the contact between T_h cell, B cell and antigen, through the 'antigen bridge' found when using 'carrier–hapten' compounds; the T_h cell recognises determinants on the 'carrier' molecule, while the B cell recognises 'hapten' determinants. With complex antigens such as viruses, bacteria or protein molecules like toxins and toxoids, this 'carrier–hapten' type of recognition can also be seen; that is, the T_h cell and B cell recognise different determinants on the antigen. However, a T_h cell which recognises a particular determinant is not necessarily restricted to helping only one clone of B cells. The restricting factor is that the B cells and T_h cells must be a minimum distance apart for this antigen-specific type of help. It has been proposed that the two cells must actually come into contact, although the validity of this is still uncertain, and recent evidence is suggesting that the antigen-bridge is an artifact of artificial carrier–hapten systems not found with complex antigens. The 'help' can still be regarded as antigen-specific since, under most network conditions of stimulation, both the T_h cells and the B cells interact with and respond to antigen. Although the T_h-cell derived B lymphocyte growth factors are 'antigen non-specific', they can only 'help' the B cell growth and differentiation *after* that B cell has been stimulated by antigen. Similarly, monocytes only produce their cytokines (monokines) after stimulation either by antigen or by T_h cell lymphokines produced after response of the T cells to antigen; furthermore, the monokines most effectively promote growth and stimulation of the T_h lymphocyte when those cells have been stimulated by antigen. For example, monocyte-derived interleukin 1 (IL-1) can enhance the generation of IL-2 receptors on T_h lymphocytes, rendering them more responsive to T_h-cell-derived IL-2, but only if the T_h lymphocytes have been activated by antigen.

The antigen-stimulated (capped) B lymphocyte will, depending on the conditions of stimulation, follow one of two differentiation pathways. This results in the production of either memory cells (morphologically indistinguishable from the original B cell) (see §1.4.9) or the major antibody-secreting cells, the plasma cells. The morphology of this differentiation pathway to the plasma cell will be dealt with in §1.6.3. The plasma cell is a terminal cell (half-life 8–12 h) whose sole function is to produce antibody reactive against the antigenic determinant (epitope) which stimulated the original B lymphocyte. This is the reason why the *paratope of the secreted antibody is identical to that on the B lymphocyte Ig-like receptor.*

The above cellular interactions which can occur in B lymphocyte stimulation are summarised in Figs 1.14 and 1.19. In addition to these are the interactions in which T_h cells recognise cell membrane determinants on B cells (Fig. 1.20); T_s cells are stimulated by either antigen or T_h cells and effect indirect suppression of B lymphocytes (Fig. 1.21), Id–anti-Id networks are induced (Figs 1.15–1.17) and B cell differentiation is suppressed directly through the cross-linking of the F_c receptor (F_cR) and Ig-like antigen receptor on the B cell by antigen–antibody complexes (Fig. 1.22). One such series of effector pathways involving these compartments is demonstrated in Fig. 1.23.

These pathways are important for the efficient induction of the B lymphoblasts required for hybridoma production. They are also of relevance for the efficient induction of anti-Id antibody (§6.6) and the T_h and T_s lymphocytes which can be immortalised by T cell hybridoma

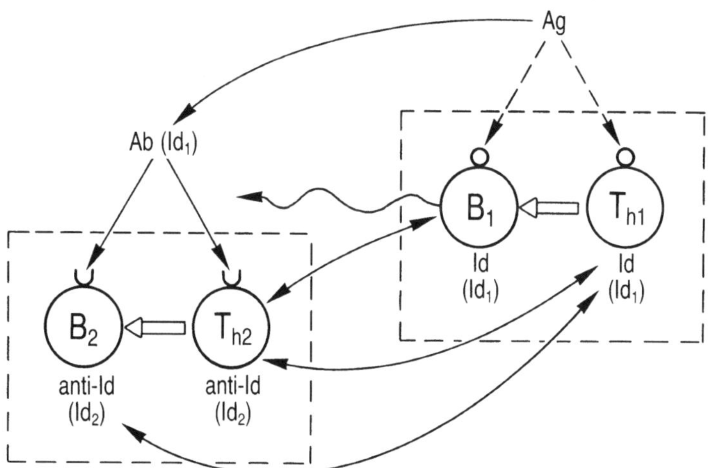

Fig. 1.20. Idiotype and non-idiotypic interactions between subsets of B and T_h lymphocytes. Broken arrows, antigen-specific stimulatory pathway; open arrows, non-idiotypic 'help'; double arrows, idiotypic 'communication' network. (From McCullough & Langley (33).)

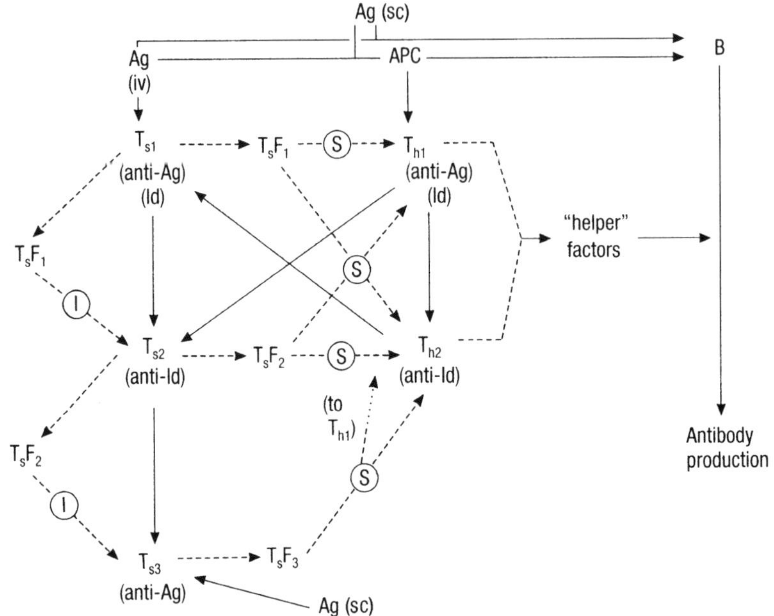

Fig. 1.21. Stimulation of T suppressor lymphocytes (T_{s1}, T_{s2}, T_{s3}) by antigen (Ag), other T_s subsets, T_s cell suppressor factors (T_sF_1, T_sF_2, T_sF_3) and T helper lymphocytes (T_h1, T_h2). I, induction by T_sF; S, suppression by T_sF; - - →, effector pathways by factors; →, cell–cell or cell–antigen interactions and lymphocyte differentiation pathways. The figure shows how the stimulation of T_s cells and T_sF can indirectly suppress the differentiation of B lymphocytes to produce antibody.

techniques (§§2.7.1 and 6.1.4); but the immune response does not end with the production of antibody. Other leukocytes have a role, which is either dependent on (the antibody-mediated or antibody-dependent cellular cytotoxicity reactions, ADCC), or independent of antibody (cellular cytotoxicity and hypersensitivity reactions).

1.4.7. *Antibody-dependent cellular cytotoxicity reactions (ADCC)*

Fig. 1.24 shows, in a simplified form, how ADCC and complement (C′)-enhanced ADCC reactions may function. These reactions are controlled by the specificity of the antibody; the cellular component (the effector cell) has no inherent specificity. Effector cells bind through a receptor on their surface to the altered F_c portion of antibody which has reacted with antigen. Thus, the receptor on the effector cell is termed the F_c receptor or F_cR. Similarly, in the C′-enhanced ADCC reaction, antibody reaction with antigen stimulates the complement pathway, and effector cells bind to the activated third component of complement, C3b, via the C3bR. Such reactions are directed against cellular organisms such as bacteria, protozoa and other parasites, and against cells infected

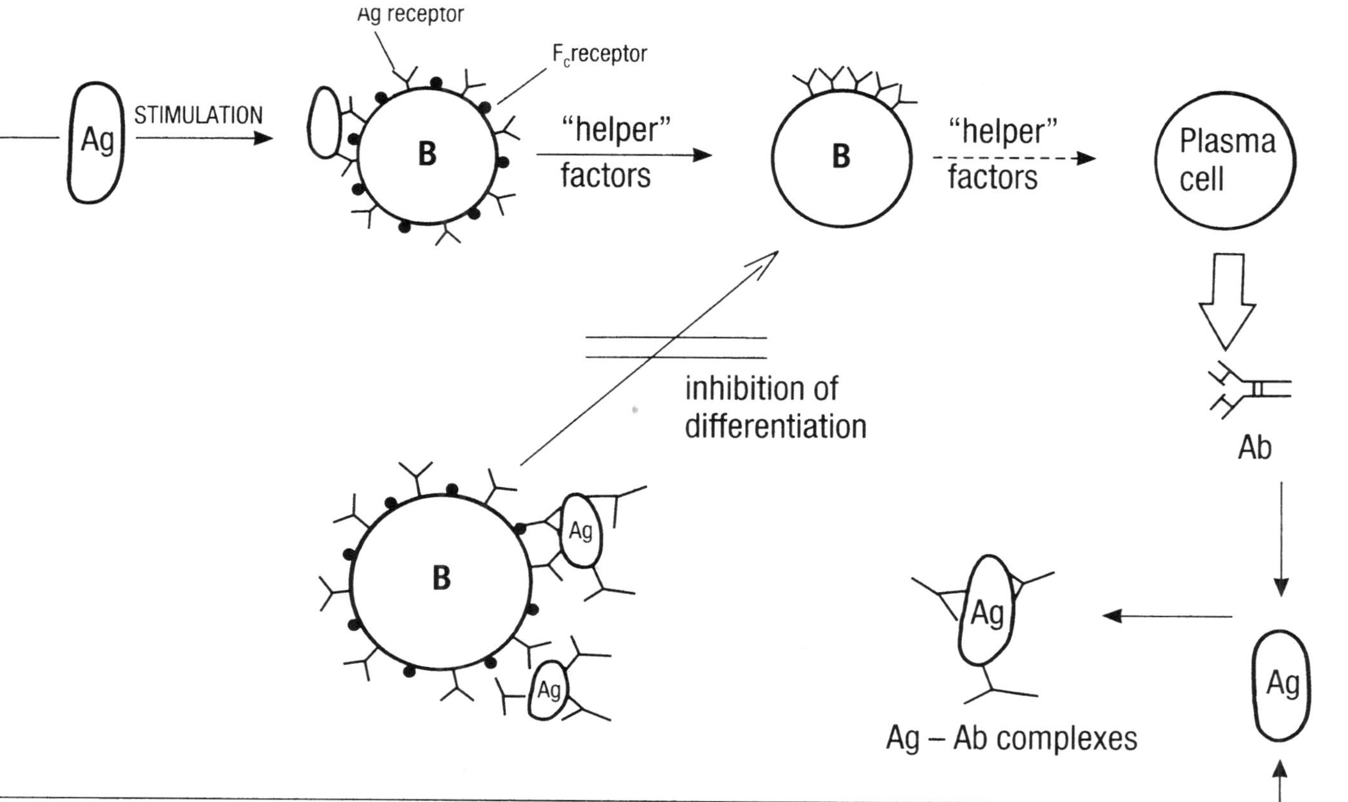

Fig. 1.22. Cross-linking of antigen receptors and F_c receptors on the surface of B lymphocytes by antigen–antibody (Ag–Ab) complexes inhibits the normal differentiation pathway of B cell lymphoblasts into antibody-secreting plasma cells.

(a)

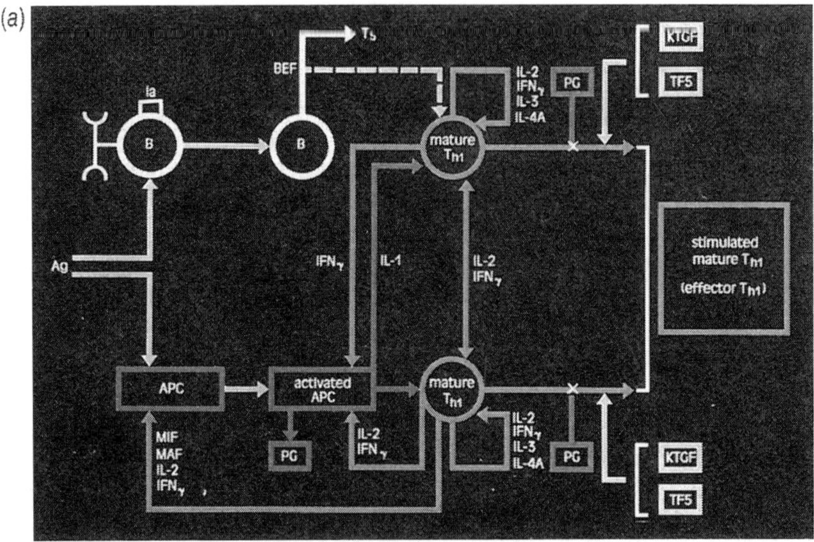

(b)

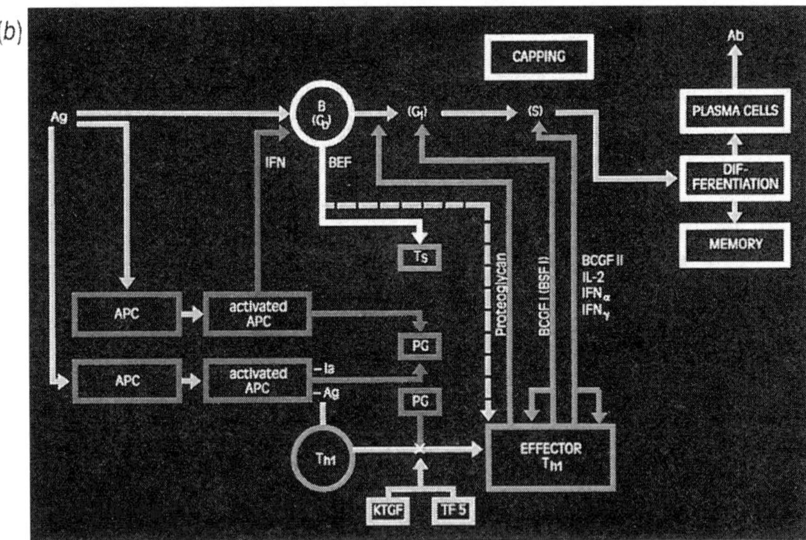

Fig. 1.23. The cellular interactions and the role of leukokines (monokines and lymphokines) in the different compartments of the immune response. (*a*) Antigen-driven, antigen-specific immune responses of B lymphocytes and T_h lymphocytes; (*b*) antigen-stimulation of B lymphocytes and the differentiation to antibody-producing cells or memory cells; (*c*) activation of macrophages and granulocytes (polymorphs); (*d*) activation of cytotoxic immune defence mechanisms; (*e*) induction of regulatory suppressor T cell circuits; (*f*) induction of regulatory (suppressive) B cell activities; (*g*) T cell–B cell idiotype–anti-idiotype responses. Ag, antigen; B, B lymphocyte; APC, antigen-presenting cell (monocyte); T_h, T helper lymphocyte (T_{h1}, anti-antigen; T_{h2}, anti-idiotype); T_s,

(c)

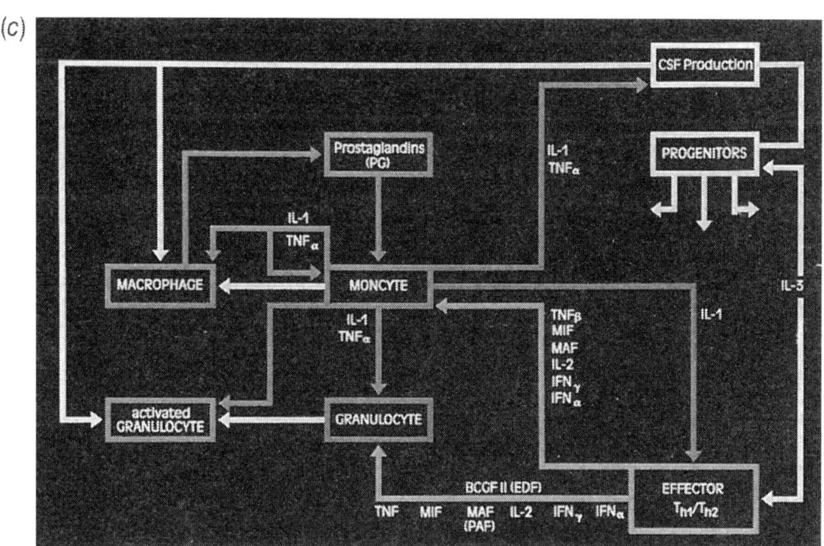

(d)

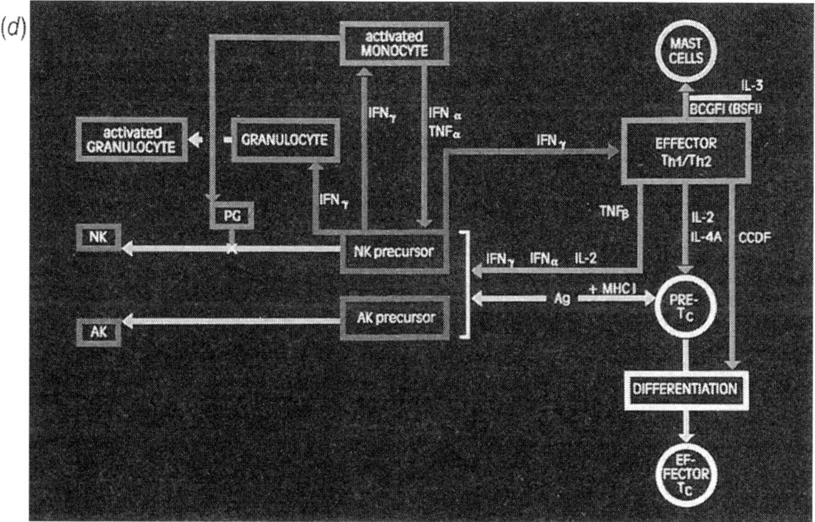

T suppressor lymphocyte (T_{s1}, anti-antigen; T_{s2} anti-idotype); G_0, G_1, S, phases in the growth cycle of cells; Ab, antibody; Ia, MHC class II molecules; NK, natural killer cell (large granular lymphocyte); AK, activated killer lymphocytes; T_c, cytotoxic T lymphocyte; pre-T_c, precursor T_c; MHCI; MHC class I molecules; pre-T_s, precursor T_{s1} or T_{s2}; T_sF and SRIS, suppressor T cell factors; Id, idiotype; TRF, T cell replacing factor (BCGFs, IFNs, IL-2, etc); EIR_B, IgE-induced regulant of B cells; SFA, suppressive factor of anaphylaxis; SBF, suppressive B cell factor; F_cR_γ, F_c receptor for IgG; F_cR_ϵ, F_c receptor for IgE. For an explanation of the monokines, lymphokines and other cytokines, see Table 1.9.

(e)

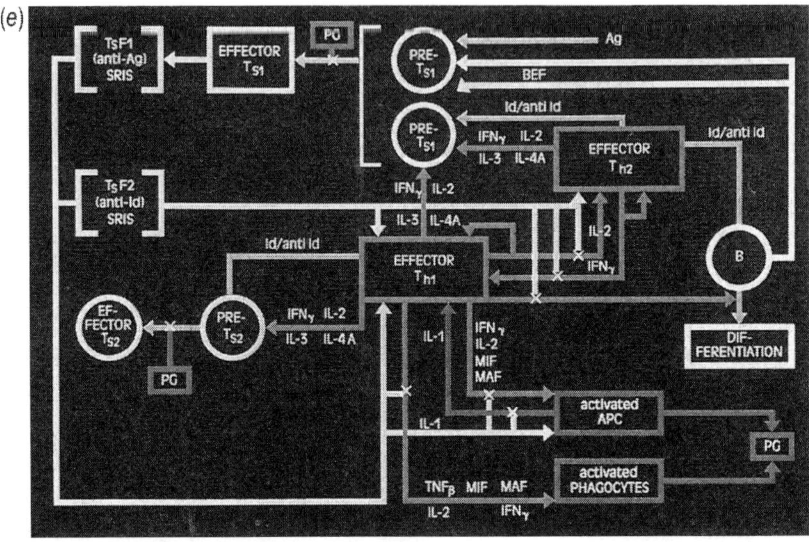

(f)

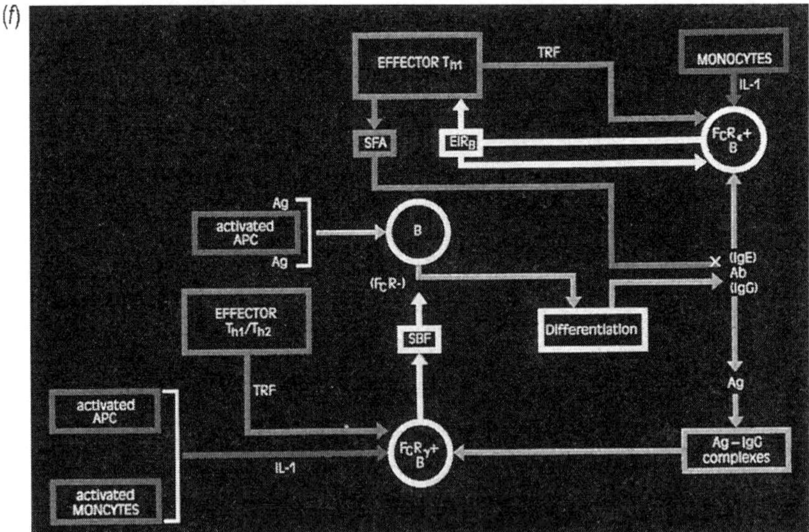

Fig. 1.23 (*cont.*)

with viruses or other intracellular parasites, which express 'foreign' proteins on their surface. The physiology of these effector cells varies between animal species. The major effector has been shown to be a T lymphocyte in humans, neutrophils in domestic animals and a monocyte in rodents. All of these cells contribute to ADCC reactions to some degree in most species, but the major effector varies. The distinguishing characteristic of these reactions is that they are antibody-mediated

(g)

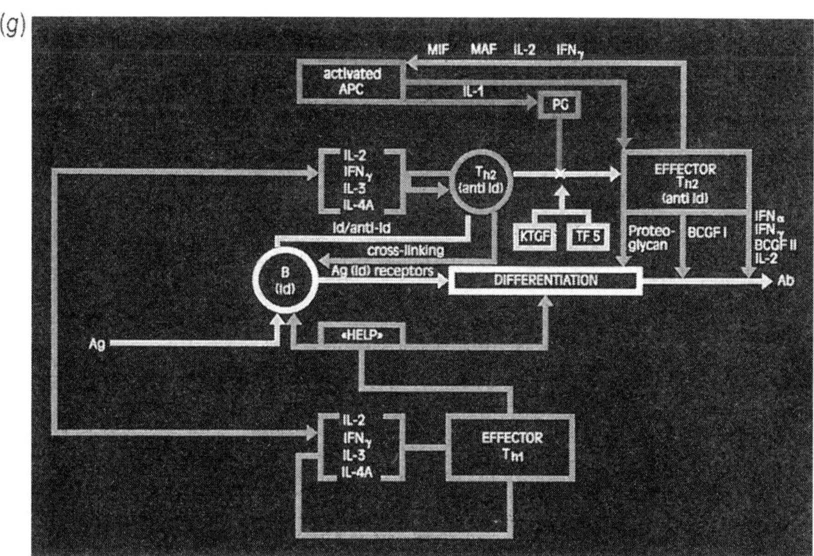

cytotoxicity reactions, and should not be confused with opsonisation resulting in antibody-enhanced phagocytosis and the antibody-independent cellular cytotoxicity reactions.

1.4.8. *Antibody-independent cell-effector mechanisms*

In contrast to ADCC, these are independent of antibody, and it is the cell effector which is specific for a particular antigen. Antigen is presented to the T_h cells in a manner similar to that of B cell stimulation. (T_s cell stimulation is similar.) A precursor cell is stimulated by antigen and the effector cell stage develops with the help of T_h cell factors. The antibody-independent cell-effector mechanisms fall into two categories; delayed-type hypersensitivity (DTH) and cytotoxic T lymphocyte activity (CTL). The effector cells are the T_d and T_c respectively. The function of the T_d circuit is to attract phagocytic cells to the site of antigen invasion (and hence stimulation) and to promote phagocytosis of that antigen. This results in classical hypersensitivity reactions (described in detail by Humphrey & White (2)). The T_c circuit under normal physiological conditions does not usually produce noticeable clinical symptoms. The function of these cells is to destroy host cells which have been altered to carry surface 'foreign' antigens, for example virus-infected cells and tumour cells.

These two circuits have little direct relevance to hybridoma production, but the T_d mechanisms are of importance when considering immunisation protocols, especially when using subcutaneous inoculations and cellular immunogens. It is not desirable to induce T_d circuits at the expense of B cell circuits. The T_c mechanisms can also influence

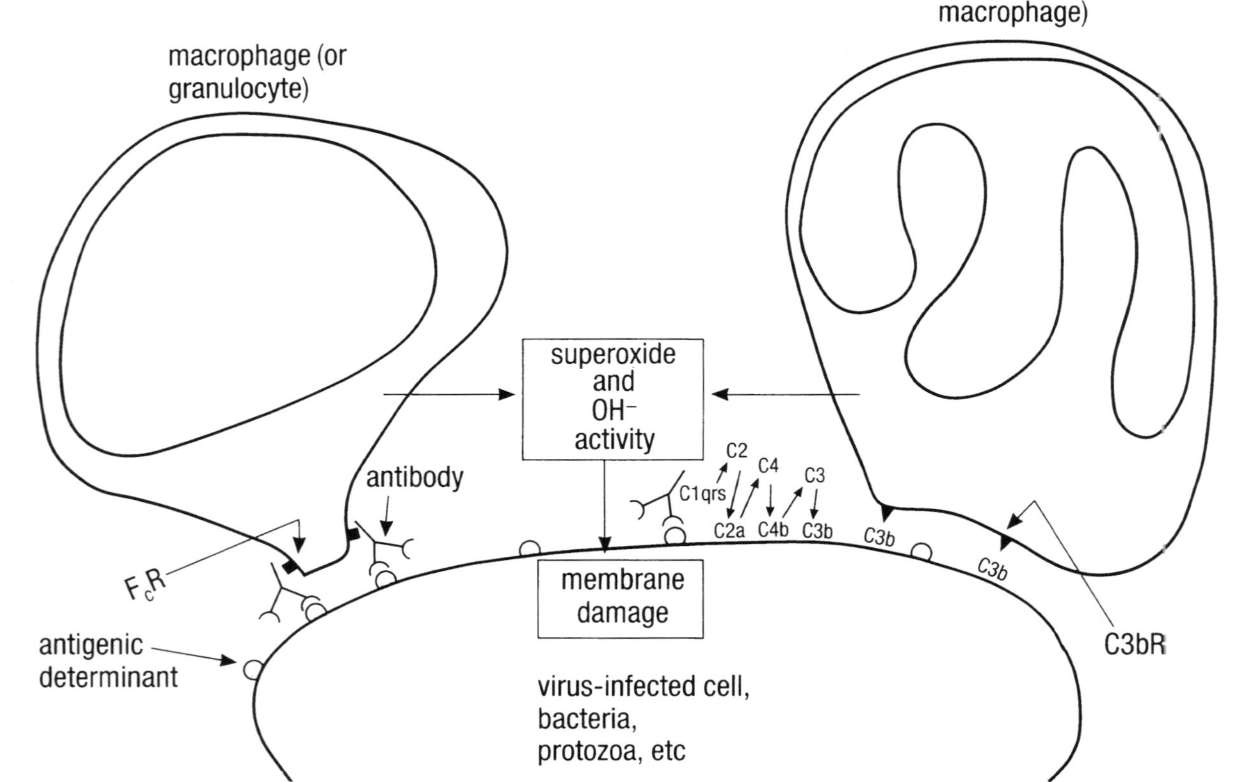

Fig. 1.24. Antibody-dependent cellular cytotoxicity (ADCC) and complement-enhanced ADCC reactions. F_cR, F_c receptor; C3bR, C3b receptor; C1qrs, C2, C4, C3, the first four components of complement.

the outcome of an immunisation using cellular immunogens, or pathogens which can infect and alter the surface of host cells, but they are of most direct relevance to hybridoma technology when attempting to induce ascites tumours with a hybridoma cell line. The hybridoma will be recognised as a tumour cell, and for this reason, a minimum number must be inoculated to overcome the T_c and T_d defences.

1.4.9. *Memory*

Memory is the name given to the process by which the host immune defence prepares for a subsequent attack by an immunostimulatory antigen. This memory development is apparently confined to the antigen-specific or Id-specific lymphocyte populations (B cell, T_h and T_s cell, T_d cell and T_c cell). Since the B lymphocyte and T_h–T_s lymphocyte activities are of the greatest direct relevance to hybridoma technology (hybridomas have been successfully produced using these cells), the memory response with such cells will be described.

As mentioned previously, the antigen-specific B lymphocyte has two alternative differentiation pathways along which it may progress after antigenic stimulation. One pathway leads to the terminal plasma cell and antibody production (§§1.4.6 and 1.6.3). The other pathway does not directly result in antibody production. Feedback mechanisms 'inform' the immune system that the invading antigen has been effectively dealt with and no more antibody is required. Klaus & Humphreys (34) have described what is apparently just such a mechanism. Within the germinal centres are cells of the monocyte lineage which have recently been characterised (35, 36). An important characteristic is the numerous processes interdigitating the B cells and the T_h cells. They are termed follicular dendritic cells (FDC). The FDC in germinal centres of secondary lymphoid organs have a preference for trapping antigen–antibody and antigen–antibody–complement complexes. When levels of circulating antigen are low, these complexes can be trapped and held by FDC for several days. In contrast, when free antigen levels are high (flushed through the germinal centres relatively rapidly), complexes are also rapidly turned over. With the latter situation, plasma cell production is preferentially stimulated. In the former situation (antigen–antibody complexes retained by FDC) memory is preferentially initiated. Miller & Nussenzweig (37) and Klaus (9) showed that antigen–antibody–complement complexes most efficiently stimulated memory, followed by antigen–antibody complexes. Antigen alone tended to stimulate antibody production in preference to invoking the memory response. These experiments were performed with a very potent immunogen, keyhole limpet haemocyanin. Whether or not all TD antigens are similarly effective has yet to be resolved.

The induction of immunological memory results in an expression (growth) of the stimulated B cell clone without differentiation into antibody-secreting cells such as plasma cells. There are concomitant changes in some of the B cell surface receptors. Some or all of the antigen-receptors acquire an IgD-like as opposed to IgM-like isotypic determinant, but the paratope or antigen-specificity of the receptor does not change, although it can increase its affinity for the inducing epitope. Overall, these memory cells are similar morphologically and physiologically to the original B cell.

The T cells never differentiate into terminal cells. Stimulation of these by antigen results in expansion of particular clones concomitant with the generation of the T cell function (T_h cells provide 'help' to B cell differentiation; T_c and T_d cells are responsible for antigen-specific cytotoxicity and DTH respectively). Thus, the effect of memory induction is to greatly expand the clones of antigen-specific B cells and T cells (in particular T_h, T_c and T_d cells) in order that the immune response against subsequent encounters with the antigen may be more rapid and more intense. In the case of pathogens, this is aimed at providing a more efficient and effective protection. This enhanced response is termed the anamnestic response (see §1.3.1), and this is of prime importance to the operation of antigen-specific lymphoblasts relative to the production of hybridomas. The relationship between the memory response and the efficiency of hybridoma production will be dealt with in §§2.5.2 and 2.5.4.

1.4.10. *Concluding remarks*

The immune response is a complex interaction of stimulatory, regulatory, assistant or helper, and suppressor functions. These must be considered with respect to the induction of the appropriate cells for hybridoma production. Furthermore, when the MAb has been produced, the function and relevance of this must be interpreted in the light of the various immune defence mechanisms which may operate. It is the interactions between the different immunological pathways during the response to antigen which determine the properties of any subsequently produced MAb. The most relevant of these properties is how well the antibody reacts with the antigen; that is, the affinity of that reaction.

1.5. **Affinity of antibodies and the immune response**

The affinity of different antibody or MAb for a particular epitope has implications for hybridoma technology in two respects. Firstly, there is the relationship between the avidity of the antiserum and the constituent affinities of the individual antibody; related to this is the degree to which affinity, and other properties (specificity, cross-reactivity and the various immunochemical reactions; see §4.1 and Chapter 6), of the MAb reflect the summated properties of the autologous antiserum. These properties are directly influenced by the immunisation protocol used to generate the immune splenocytes, and this leads to the second implication. What influence does affinity play in the efficacy of the immune response? Lymphocytes bearing low affinity receptors are stimulated at a different rate from 'high affinity' lymphocytes. However, the immune system will progress towards a more avid memory with re-stimulations by a particular antigen; but this avidity does not reflect the relative roles played by high affinity and low affinity receptors and antibody molecules in the immune response. The high affinity reactions can dominate and hence confer a disproportionately high avidity to the memory or the antiserum.

1.5.1. *Affinity of MAb and its relevance to the avidity of antiserum*

MAb selected from a particular fusion may show lower affinities and/or more cross-reactivity than would have been expected from studies on the autologous antiserum (the antiserum from the mice whose spleens were used for the fusion). This is because the MAb derived from a fusion are not representative of the antibody population of the autologous antiserum. Neither are the hybridomas produced representative of the spleen cell population, or even the B lymphocyte population of that spleen (see Table 2.13, and the review by Milstein (38)). What these hybridomas express is representative of the genetic potential of the B lymphocyte–lymphoblast population.

After one or two immunisations, the plasma cells present in the secondary lymphoid organs may represent the antibody population found in an antiserum. With multi-boost immunisations, the relative proportion (in the antiserum) of antibody molecules which have resulted from previous inoculations will not necessarily be reflected in the population of B lymphoblasts of the spleen or lymph nodes. Hence, antisera will reflect the proportion of antibody-secreting cells, in particular the plasma cells, in all secondary lymphoid organs which were present both at the time of bleeding and during at least the previous 21 days (the half-life for IgG is 21 days). In contrast, the MAb derived from a fusion reflect the number of immature (excluding plasma cells; see §§1.6.3, 2.3.1 and 2.5.6) lymphoblastoid B cells in the particular lymphoid organ used for fusion. MAb derived from a particular fusion are therefore representative of an antibody population which is likely to have arisen during a short period of time from a single lymphoid organ. Antisera, by contrast, represent the antibody production over a number of days in all lymphoid organs.

Similarly, the affinity of a group of MAb molecules may not reflect the avidity of the autologous antiserum. If that antiserum is of high avidity, this reflects the dominant reaction rate and binding constant among the different antibody molecules present in the antiserum. Individual antibody molecules may not exhibit such an affinity. (It is for this reason that 'affinity' will be used to describe the binding capacity of individual and monoclonal antibodies. 'Avidity' will be used to describe the cumulative affinities of antibody molecules as seen with antiserum.)

A higher avidity may be observed with the antiserum than with the constituent antibody molecules for several reasons, not all of which are mutually exclusive. Synergistic reactions of lower affinity molecules could enhance the binding and hence affinity of each antibody (39). An antiserum will also contain antibody molecules of varying affinity, and the affinity of some of these antibodies may be similar to the avidity of the serum. Such high affinity antibody molecules may, however, be in the minority (perhaps less than 5%), but could exert a greater influence on the avidity of the antiserum than the low affinity molecules. Biphasic reaction curves (as described, for example, in the review by Mandel (40)) may exemplify such mixtures. As the high affinity molecules are diluted, the avidity of the antiserum is reduced to reflect the remaining reactivity of the majority population of lower affinity molecules.

The constituent affinities of antisera vary considerably with time after immunisation (41) as would the proportion of MAb with particular affinities derived from each fusion. Furthermore, if fusions are performed using X63 or NS1 mouse myeloma cells or Y3 rat myeloma cells, some of the hybridomas will secrete monovalent antibody (see § 2.4); monovalency can greatly alter the reaction rate and binding constant of a particular antibody for a particular epitope (see Icenogle *et al.* (42)). Mandel has reviewed this topic (40) in which he reports on the work of Hornick & Karush (43) who showed a 10^4-fold enhancement of the multivalent reaction over the monovalent reaction.

A simplified diagram of how high affinity and low affinity antibody might interact in an antiserum is shown in Fig. 1.25. For ease of explanation, all reactive antibody will be of either a single low affinity or a single high affinity. Some low affinity antibody would react with the antigen but be displaced by the higher affinity (higher binding constant and stronger binding) antibody. Free antigen and free antibody would continue this displacement phenomenon with high affinity antibody being bound preferentially to the antigen. This high affinity antigen–antibody interaction could, however, influence the binding of the lower affinity antibody, rendering its binding stronger than if that low affinity antibody were used alone. Under the appropriate conditions, complexes of antigen with high affinity antibody and low affinity antibody would be found at equilibrium. The normal situation is of course more complicated, but the figure demonstrates how a minor population of high affinity antibody could influence the reaction by displacing low affinity antibody and

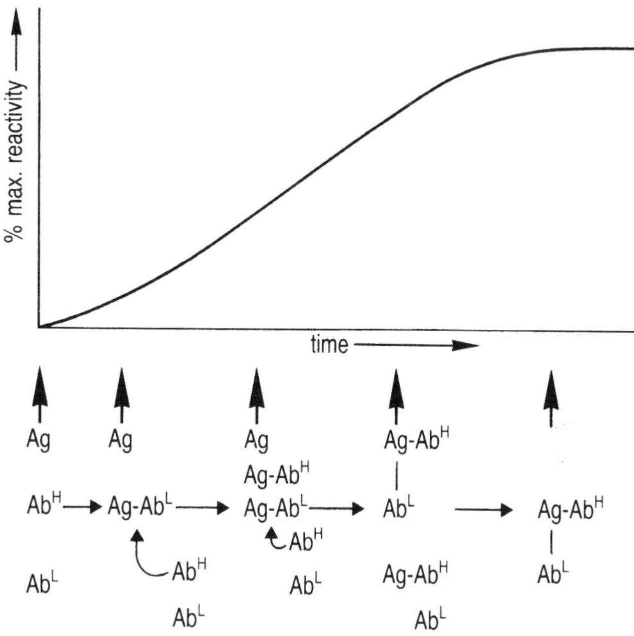

Fig. 1.25. An idealised situation involving two antibody populations, one of high affinity (Ab^H) and one of low affinity (Ab^L) to show how high affinity and low affinity antibodies interact during the reaction with antigen (Ag). (From McCullough (39).)

subsequently enhancing the binding of that low affinity antibody. The result is an antiserum avidity reflective more of the high affinity antibody, irrespective of the relative molarities of high and low affinity molecules.

Avidities, cross-reactivities, and specificities of antisera are complicated phenomena owing to the numerous antibody activities present. MAb do not have these drawbacks. Indeed, the characteristics of MAb need not necessarily reflect the characteristics of an autologous antiserum (obtained from the animal whose spleen was used for hybridoma and MAb production). If derived from an animal producing an antiserum of avidity influenced as shown in Fig. 1.25, the majority of MAb will be of lower affinity than that of the antiserum.

1.5.2. *Affinity of the immune response and the relevance to memory*

The B lymphocytes which are ultimately responsible for the generation of the antibody-secreting plasma cells carry antigen-specific receptors of similar paratope and affinity to the subsequently produced antibody (1, 2, 4) (Table 1.14). Cells with low affinity receptors can be stimulated more rapidly than cells with high affinity receptors in an immune

Table 1.14. *Serum concentrations of the different immunoglobulin classes*

Immunoglobulin	Concentration in serum μg/ml
IgG	8000–16 000
IgA	1500–4000
IgM	500–2000
IgD	3–400
IgE	0.1–0.5

response, because fewer bonds, and consequently fewer events of change in free energy, are required (see also below regarding receptor density on B lymphocytes). However, the stimulation of highest affinity receptors will subsequently be more effective with respect to increasing the specificity of the reaction for the inducing antigen, owing to the interaction of receptors with epitopes being more stable and more effective at producing the cross-linking of receptors required for B lymphocyte activation. Stimulation and re-stimulation of the immune system result in an increase in the affinity of the response. Consider the priming of the immune system (first encouter with an antigen). The unstimulated or virgin immune system 'specific' for a particular epitope is of relatively low affinity. After stimulation, memory cells are produced which are of higher affinity (44). With each stimulation, more and higher affinity memory cells are generated owing to somatic re-arrangements and deletions in the V_H and V_L genes. That is, under genetic control the immune response is continually attempting to 'fine-tune' the recognition of antigenic determinants which it has encountered (1, 4, 44). There is, of course, the concomitant generation of low affinity (or lower affinity) memory cells. This increase in affinity can be seen alongside an alteration in the isotype of the B cell receptor. The virgin cell population carry antigen receptors of the IgM isotype. Initially, memory cells will also carry IgM-like receptors, but gradually cells appear with both IgM-like and IgD-like receptors (Fig. 1.26) (44, 45). After further stimulations, memory cells appear bearing both IgD and IgG-like receptors, or IgD-like receptors alone, and eventually some memory cells may carry only IgG-like receptors (44, 45). The affinity of these receptors increases as shown in Fig. 1.26, but at the same time, the density of the receptors decreases (44, 45). The most rapid stimulation should be with the B cells bearing a high density of receptors, and hence having the lowest affinity. Thus low affinity antibody will be generated before high affinity antibody in an immune response. But the stability of the reaction between the B cell

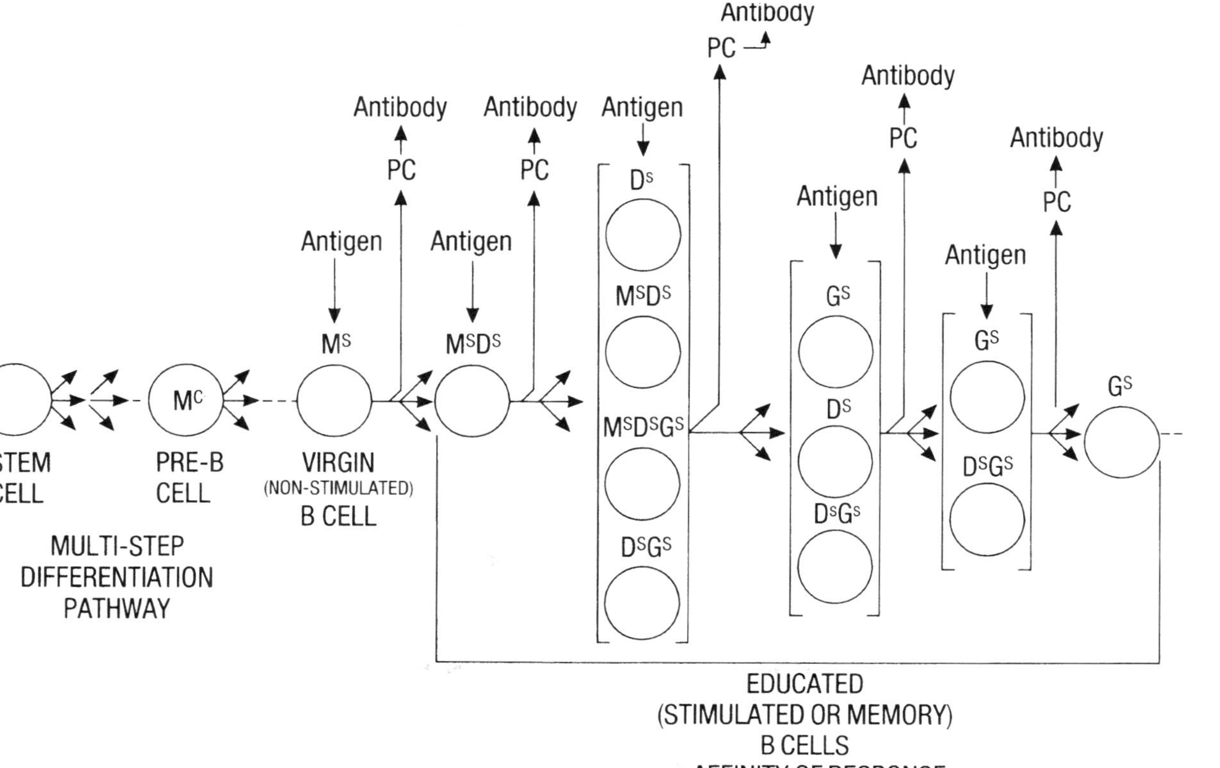

Fig. 1.26. Development of the IgM, IgD and IgG antigen receptors on B lymphocytes, and the relationship to education and affin ty of response. M^c, cytoplasmic IgM (monomeric); M^s, D^s, G^s, surface IgM (monomeric), IgD and IgG respectively; PC, plasma cells.

receptors and antigen is greater with the cells bearing 'high affinity' receptors. Consequently, these can become the more efficiently stimulated cells. Thus, if the immune system has been stimulated only once or twice, the majority of antibody-producing hybridomas derived will secrete low affinity antibody. Conversely, multiple re-stimulations of the immune system will give rise to a mixed population of antibodies, which will be reflected in the derived MAb having a wide range of affinities.

Antibody of the highest affinity is not always desirable. For immunoadsorbent columns, antibody of a relatively intermediate or even low affinity is most appropriate (see §6.3). Conversely, high affinity MAb and highly specific MAb are required for prophylaxis and diagnosis respectively (see §§6.5 and 6.2).

Antisera can therefore vary greatly in avidity and specificity for a particular antigen, as can MAb derived from fusions using autologous spleens. These MAb will not ncessarily represent the antibody population of that autologous antiserum. Nor need there be any immediate relationship between the affinities or specificities of the MAb and those of the autologous antiserum. The immune system is designed to present the most effective defence mechanisms possible to protect the body against foreign substances (antigens). Manipulation of the immune responses can preferentially stimulate one compartment, such as memory or a delayed-type hypersensitivity response. Sections 1.4.2–1.4.9 dealt with these various compartments, but those which are of most relevance to current hybridoma technological procedures are the antigen-specific B lymphocyte reactions. The T_h or T_s lymphocytes are of less relevance owing to the smaller quantity of work on T cell hybridomas and the greater difficulty in detecting T_h or T_s factors (the products of B cell hybridomas, MAb, are easily detected by a number of assay procedures; see §4.1). The production of Id-bearing or anti-Id MAb relies on established techniques developed for the production of MAb against antigens such as viruses, bacteria, protozoa, defined chemicals, leukocytes, etc. These established techniques have relied on the stimulation of antigen-specific B lymphocytes (memory cells in a previously immunised animal) to proliferate and differentiate into the antibody response. This differentiation was introduced in §§1.4.3 and 1.4.6, and will now be explained in more detail to comprehend which cells are the 'ideal' fusion partner for myeloma cells.

1.6. **Antibody response**

The object of hybridoma technology is to generate antibody-secreting hybridoma cells. This relies on the successful fusion between a myeloma cell and a stimulated (and probably differentiating) antigen-specific B lymphocyte (B lymphoblast). However, this blastogenic response of the

B lymphocyte results in a heterogeneous population of precursors to the major antibody-secreting cell in the body (the plasma cell). But which cell is the 'ideal' fusion partner for the myeloma cell? To answer this question requires a more detailed understanding of the B lymphocyte blastogenic response, under the three major headings of: (i) the cellular interactions of the blastogenic response from a morphological and physiological point of view; (ii) the lymphocyte receptors which control the blastogenic response and the functional nature of the secreted antibody (paratope specificity); and (iii) the relative capacity of the different B cell lymphoblasts to produce antibody, before one can decide which cell(s) is the probable ideal for the production of an antibody-secreting hybridoma.

1.6.1. *Cellular interaction*

The stimulation of the antibody response is effected through antigen-specific B lymphocytes reacting via their Ig-like surface receptors with antigen, in the presence of macrophages and, in the majority of cases, T_h lymphocytes (§§1.4.3–1.4.6). The first noticeable effect of this stimulation is the 'capping' of the Ig-like antigen-specific receptors: the receptors migrate to one pole of the cell. This can be visualised *in vitro* using immunofluorescent staining of the receptors. An FITC-conjugated IgG against the Ig-like receptor (for example, if one wished to stain the receptors of mouse B cells, one would use FITC–anti-mouse Ig) is incubated with the cells at 37°C. This results in 'capping' since the anti-Ig has the same effect on the Ig-like receptor as the appropriate antigen. Fig. 1.27 shows the result. If the cells are incubated with the FITC–anti-Ig at 4°C or in the presence of NaN_3, the cells show a diffuse staining over

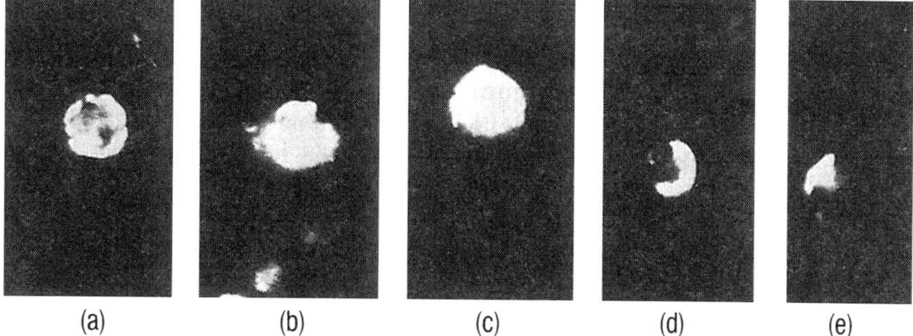

Fig. 1.27. The capping of mouse lymphocyte receptors after stimulation of B lymphocytes. (*a*)–(*c*) Immunofluorescent staining of receptors before and at time of stimulation; (*d*)–(*e*) gradual movement of the receptors to one pole of the cell with time. The receptors were stained with FITC-conjugated anti-mouse immunoglobulins for 45 min at 37°C (69).

the cell surface. This staining under higher magnification appears more globular, since the B cell cannot metabolise at 4°C or in the presence of NaN_3, and thus 'capping' is prevented. With cells which can metabolise, and hence 'cap', the immunofluorescent staining is confined to one pole of the cell (46). If the reaction is permitted to continue, this surface staining disappears because the receptors become internalised (4). Eventually, the receptors are regenerated except when the 'capping' is stimulated by a TD antigen in the presence of T_h cells. (In the absence of T_h cells, the regeneration process occurs.) With T_h cell help, the capped B cells will differentiate into the antibody-producing plasma cells (Fig. 1.28). It should be re-emphasised that capping will only occur following cross-linking of the B cell antigen-specific receptors (4). Using FITC conjugated to whole molecules, to $F(ab')_2$ fragments or to Fab fragments of antibody specific for the Ig-like receptor, only the whole antibody or the $F(ab')_2$ can induce capping. This is because the whole molecule or its $F(ab')_2$ moiety, but not the Fab, can cross-link receptors on the B cell (Fig. 1.28). This differentiation or blastogenic pathway results in a number of morphologically different lymphoblasts, each with different antibody-secretion potential. The original (before stimulation) small lymphocyte secretes little if any antibody; 80–90% of the Ig molecules produced by these lymphocytes remain cell-associated as either antigen receptors on the cell surface or intracytoplasmic monomeric IgM. After the onset of differentiation of the stimulated B cell, there is an increase in cell size followed by a gradual decrease concomitant with an increasing secretion of antibody. The consequence of this differentiation is the terminal plasma cell (*c.* 1.5–2 times the size of the resting small lymphocyte). The lymphoblast precursors of the plasma cell are well described elsewhere (2). Suffice it to say that the plasma cell secretes by far the highest concentration of antibody per cell. There is also an accumulation of antibody molecules in crystal lattices (Russell bodies) which are released on the death of the plasma cell. All the precursors of the plasma cell secrete antibody, the quantities increasing from the haemocytoblast through plasmacytoblast to immature plasma cell. The antibody-synthesising machinery of these cells is obviously active, in contrast to the resting B cell, and such cells should make the best candidates for the production of antibody-secreting hybridomas. This subject will be dealt with further in §1.6.3.

1.6.2. *Lymphocyte receptors and antibody secretion*

B lymphocytes, like T lymphocytes, carry a mixture of cell surface antigens which are characteristic of the B cell population as a whole or of the B cell at a particular stage of maturity. The Lyb proteins will differentiate mature from immature B cells, and subsets of cells which may differ

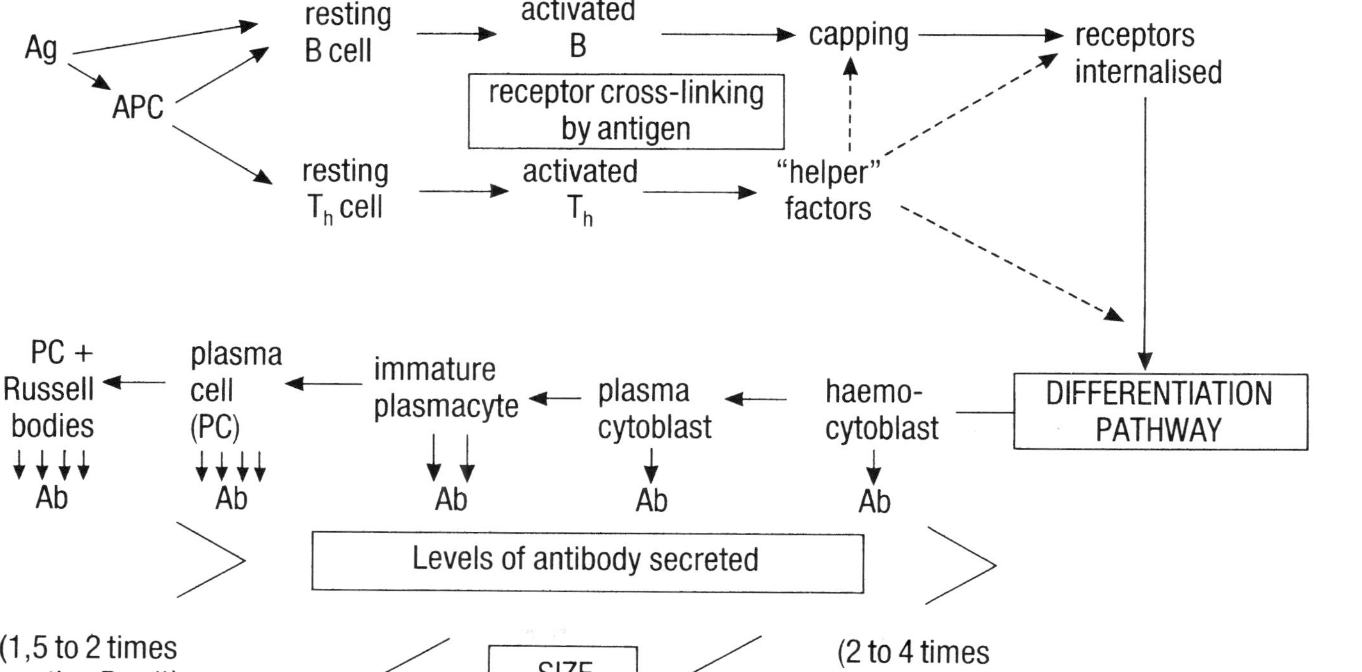

Fig. 1.28. Activation of B lymphocytes by antigen, and the differentiation pathway to the antibody-secreting cells. The plasma cells secrete the greatest quantity of antibody.

in the requirement for responsiveness. The details of these surface proteins on B and T cells and their relationship to maturity and function have been reviewed extensively by Mackenzie & Potter (47). The Ig-like antigen receptors on the surface of the immunologically mature (immunocompetent) B cell have been introduced in §§1.4.3 and 1.4.6. Before the B cells become immunocompetent they carry no Ig-like receptors but do have cytoplasmic monomeric IgM. This distinguishes them as 'pre-B cells'. The precursors of these, which possess no detectable Ig molecules, have to be differentiated by the other surface protein markers they carry (47).

With the immunocompetent B cell, the isotype of this antigen receptor determines the state of maturity with respect to the specific response (encounter) against that antigen. With immunologically virgin (before antigen encounter) B cells, these receptors are monomeric IgM. After stimulation, and with repeated stimulation, genetic rearrangements result in the appearance of receptors of IgD and, eventually, IgG isotype (see §§1.3, 1.4.6, 1.4.9 and 1.5.2). Two of these isotypes are often represented among the receptors of a single B cell, but each receptor will be a single isotype.

Another result of antigen stimulation of the specific B cell is a change in the isotype of the *secreted* antibody. This usually takes the form of IgM (pentameric) to IgG or IgM to IgA, and is also explained by genetic rearrangements of the genes for the constant region (C_μ, C_δ, C_γ, C_ϵ, C_α) (see Fig. 1.29) of the heavy chain of the antibody. As can be seen in Fig. 1.29, the cell can splice out gene sequences and thus switch from an IgM (C_μ) secretor to an IgG (C_γ) or IgA (C_α) secretor, but not vice versa (Fig. 1.30). However, the isotypic determinants are not necessarily identical between antigen receptor and subsequently secreted antibody. For example, the majority of memory B cells carry IgD-like receptors (either alone or in conjunction with receptors of IgM or IgG isotype) but the majority of plasma cells arising from memory lymphocytes secrete IgG. With virgin B cells on the occasion of first encounter with antigen, both the receptors and subsequently secreted antibody are of the IgM isotype; but the receptor is monomeric (7*S*) IgM while the secreted antibody is pentameric (19*S*). The receptor and secreted antibody can also differ in some allotypic and idiotypic determinants. (It has been proposed that some of the idiotopic determinants of IgM-like antigen receptors on B cells are unique to those receptors (29).) The one major area of identity between the Ig-like antigen receptor and the secreted antibody, which is relevant to hybridoma technology, is the paratope. The closeness between the two molecules at this 'idiotope' is reflected by the receptor and secreted antibody having identical affinities for the antigen. There are other idiotopes which are common to secreted and receptor Ig. Since certain idiotypic and allotypic determinants are genetically linked (29) some allotypes will also be in common.

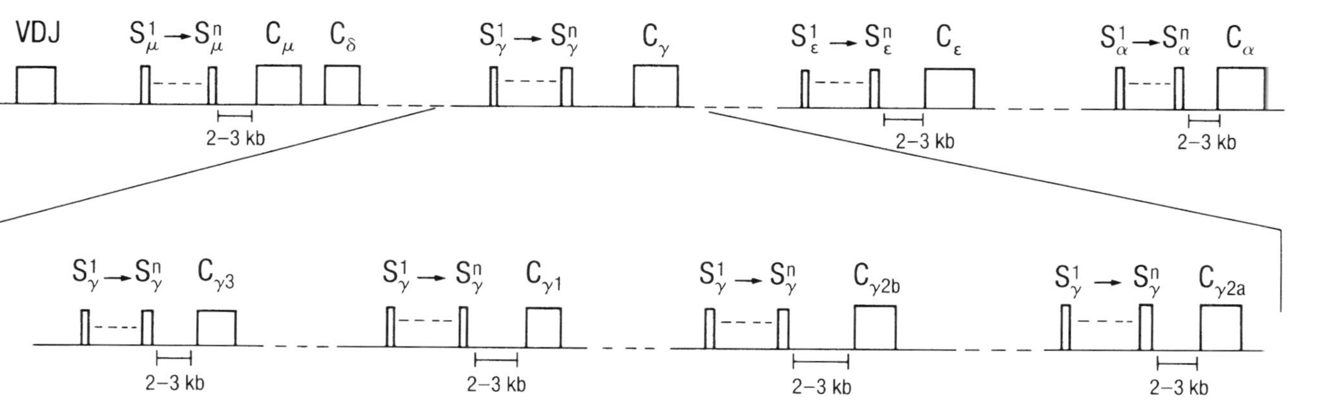

Fig. 1.29. The gene arrangements for the heavy chains of mouse immunoglobulins, showing the switch regions which permit class switching (inter-gene splicing and gene rearrangement). $S^1 \rightarrow S^n$, switch regions composed of multiple copies of short repeated elements.

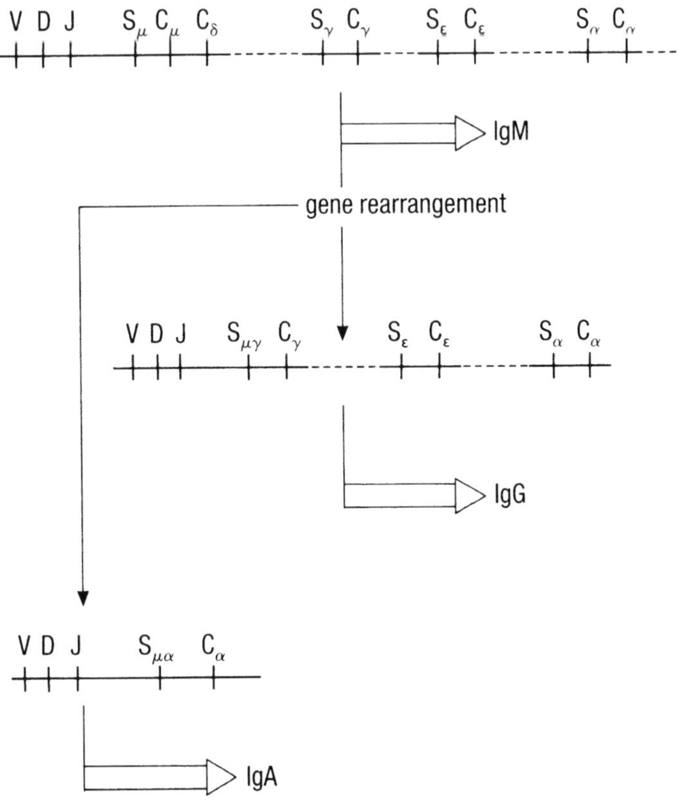

Fig. 1.30. The function of the switch regions (S) during the inter-gene splicings and rearrangements which result in a B cell switching from producing antibody of the IgM isotype to antibody of the IgG or IgA isotype.

1.6.3. *Antibody production and its relevance to the generation of hybridomas*

As mentioned above, the plasma cell is the major antibody-producing lymphocyte but is a terminal cell; hence this particular B lymphocyte differentiation pathway is a terminal one. For this reason, the plasma cell is of little use in the generation of hybridoma cultures, probably because it is too differentiated with its chromosomes already committed to death. Thus, the plasma cell will probably form unstable hybridomas when fused with myeloma cells (see §§2.3.1 and 2.5.6). In a hybrid generated using plasma cells and myeloma cells the plasma cell chromosomes will probably cease to function correctly after a short period of time. At this time the hybrid may regain certain myeloma cell characteristics, the most relevant one being aminopterin sensitivity. Aminopterin is an inhibitor of the synthesis of the nucleotide building blocks of DNA and RNA. The myeloma cells used in hybridoma technology are selected for sensitivity to this drug (see §2.3.2). Mammalian lymphocytes, on the other hand, have an alternative synthesis pathway which can bypass the aminopterin 'block'. Plasma cells will possess this aminopterin resistance, but once these chromosomes cease to function they cease to confer aminopterin resistance on any hybridoma which contains them. This cessation of plasma cell chromosome function in a hybridoma may result from a loss of plasma cell gene translation (and hence loss of the enzyme required to bypass the aminopterin block) or a loss of plasma cell chromosome replication. In the latter case the hybridoma cell and myeloma cell chromosomes would divide but the plasma cell chromosomes would not. Thus one daughter cell would become aminopterin-sensitive, whereas the other would continue the process. In such a culture, only one cell would ever survive in the presence of aminopterin, and as such would be unlikely to survive for long without the growth supplements normally provided by other cells.

The precursors of the plasma cell (Fig. 1.28), which can also secrete a low level of antibody (compared with the plasma cell), would appear to be better fusion partners for the production of stable antibody-secreting hybridoma cells. These plasma cell precursors are committed to antibody production, unlike the resting B lymphocyte parent in which much of the antibody-synthesising machinery is under genetic repression. Stahli *et al.* (48) have shown that blast cells 2–3 times the size of the resting B lymphocytes are the more efficient at yielding antibody-secreting hybridomas. As shown in Fig. 1.31, the haemocytoblast is the largest cell in the series, followed by the plasmacytoblast, then the immature plasma cell, the plasma cell and finally (the smallest cell in the series) the resting B lymphocyte (called a 'small lymphocyte'). It would appear from the work of Stahli *et al.* (48) that the haemocytoblast and plasmacytoblast may be the best candidates for the 'ideal fusion partner', the cell which after fusion with a myeloma cell will generate stable antibody-secreting hybridomas. This is not to say that other cells in the series (excluding the plasma cell) will not be useful in the generation of antibody-secreting hybridomas. Even the resting B lymphocyte may be used, since there is evidence that the myeloma cell chromosomes may influence the function of the splenocyte chromosomes in a hybridoma (38, 49). This aspect of hybridoma technology will be discussed in §2.5.6.

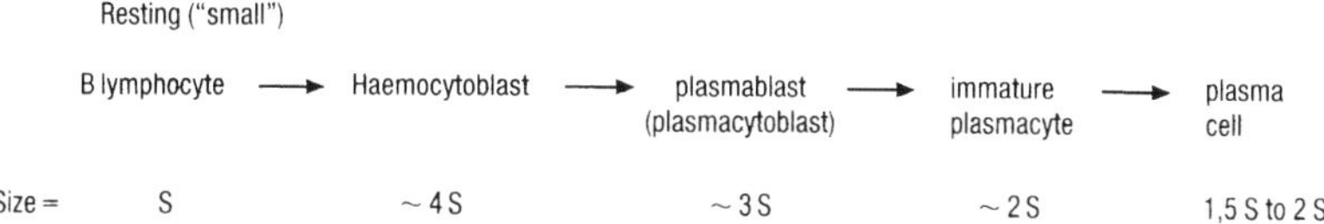

Fig. 1.31. The relative sizes of the resting (unstimulated) B lymphocyte, and the various plasma cell precursors arising from the differentiation of the B lymphocyte following antigen stimulation.

The function of the antigen-specific humoral immune system is to generate antibodies specific for determinants on the stimulating antigen. These antibodies will vary in their paratopes, and hence against which epitopes they will react. The antibodies will also vary in their isotype or class, and these Ig classes are relevant to both the status and function of the immune system.

1.6.4. *The relevance of antibody classes to the immune response*

The Ig molecules found in the body fluids can be divided into IgM, IgG, IgA, IgD and IgE (in decreasing order of serum concentration) (see Table 1.14). The class of antibody which may be of interest in hybridoma technology depends on which compartment of the humoral immune system is to be investigated. IgM and IgG are the most important serum immunoglobulins, IgA the most important with respect to the body secretions (although IgG is also found in certain body secretions) and IgE is associated with various aspects of immediate-type hypersensitivity (allergy) (Table 1.15) and eosinophil-dependent ADCC against parasites. The main interest in the IgD class concerns the role of the receptors on the B lymphocytes which are of this subclass.

Some of the biological and chemical properties of the Ig classes are shown in Table 1.5. The different subclasses can be separated by their functional and physical characteristics. Electrophoretic tests such as polyacrylamide gel electrophoresis (PAGE) or isoelectric focusing (IEF) will separate each isotype, as does the ability to fix complement (C′). The latter characterisation will relate to the role of the antibody in passive protection (see §6.5) because not all isotypes fix C′. It should be noted, however, that MAb are notoriously poor in classical C′ fixation tests (CFT), and a better assay is the indirect CFT in which the C′ cascade is activated by an anti-mouse IgG reacting with the MAb (Fig. 1.32). This does not mean that the MAb itself cannot fix C′, simply that the density of C′ mediated cell membrane damage is too low to effect lysis (the cell can repair the damage; see below). Those IgG isotypes of the mouse which have been shown to be capable of fixing C′ will still fix C′ as MAb. With viruses it is often the alternative, as opposed to the classical, pathway of C′ which is activated (Fig. 1.33). The function of both pathways is to concentrate the activated third component of C′ (C3b) on the surface of the virus or cell (infected, bacterial, protozoal, tumour). This efficiently stimulates immune defence functions, e.g. C′-enhanced ADCC reactions and opsonisation, and probably further alters the conformation of the antigen with which the antibody reacted. K.C. McCullough & J.R. Crowther (unpublished results) have demonstrated an enhanced neutralisation by C′ when using polyvalent guinea pig IgG or mouse monoclonal IgG against FMDV (see also references 39 and

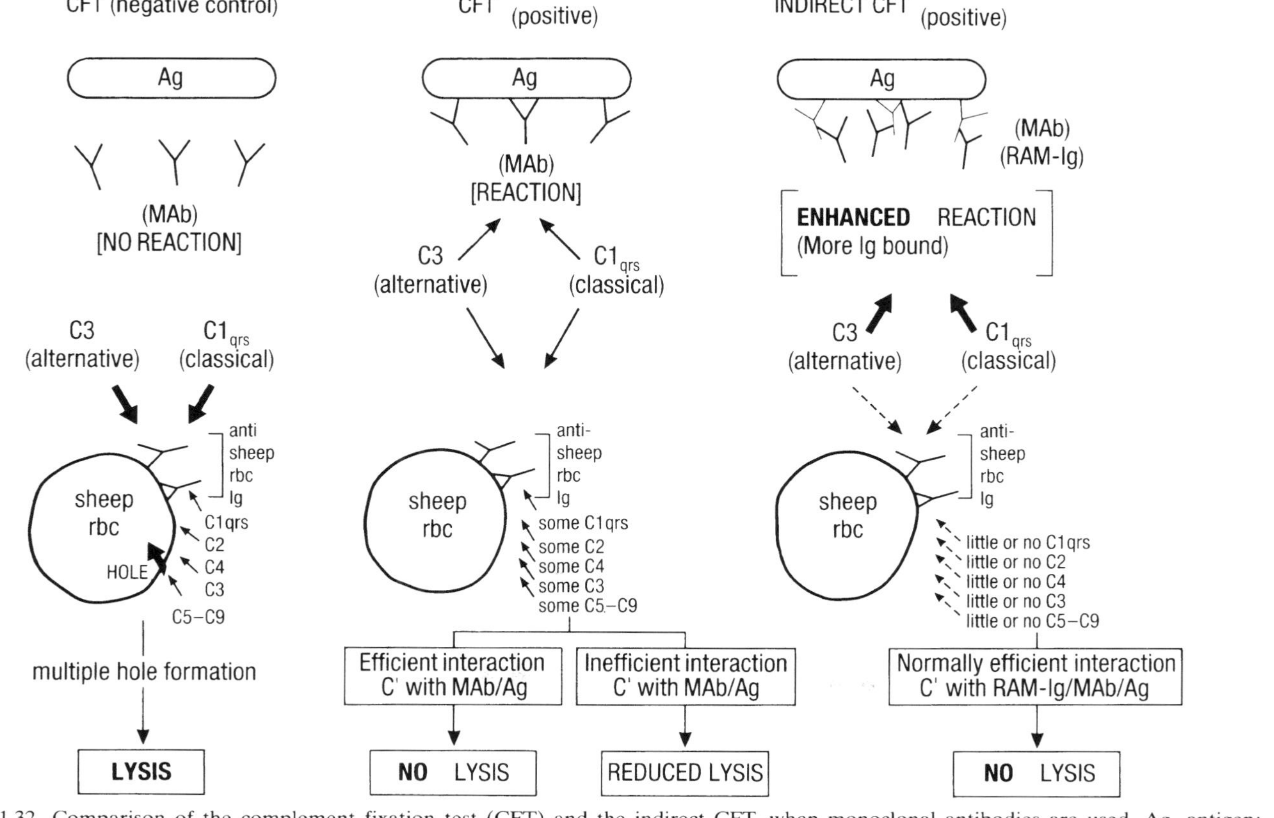

Fig. 1.32. Comparison of the complement fixation test (CFT) and the indirect CFT, when monoclonal antibodies are used. Ag, antigen; RAM-Ig, rabbit anti-mouse immunoglobulins; C1qrs, C2, C4, C3, C5–C9, the complement components; sheep rbc, sheep erythrocytes; C′, complement.

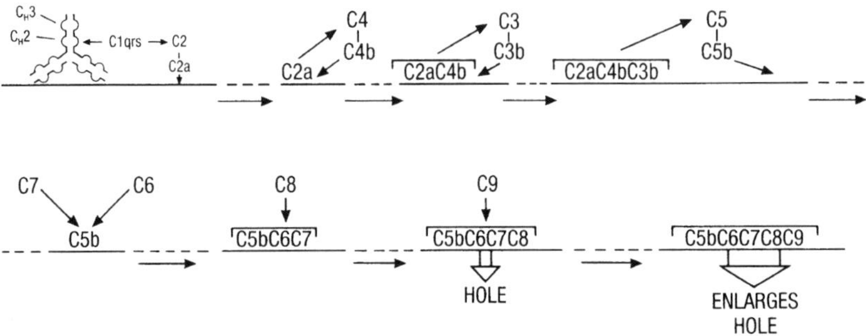

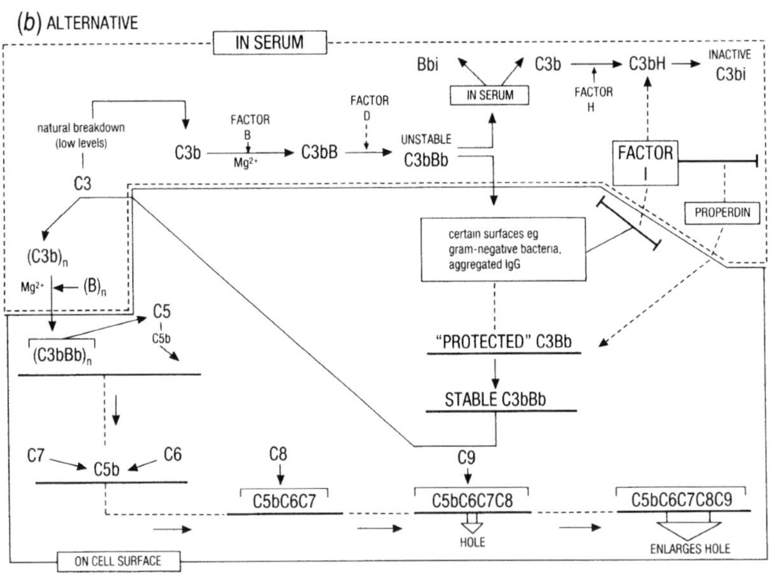

Fig. 1.33. Comparison of how the classical pathway (*a*) and the alternative pathway (*b*) of complement result in deposition of complement components on the membranes of certain viruses, virus-infected cells, bacteria and other parasites, leading to the production of holes in the membrane. ⊢—⊣ identifies the factors or events which will compete with Factor I inactivation of C3b (when complexed with factor H).

40). The concentration of C3b onto the surface of the virus or cell also activates the remainder of the C′ cascade. Whether or not this activation will result in cell lysis can best be explained by considering the situation with viruses and virus-infected cells.

The activation of the full cascade results in membrane attack where the C5–C9 complex has attached (1, 2, 4). This will effect irreversible damage to either the envelope of enveloped viruses or the plasma membrane of virus-infected cells in which viral proteins or infection-associated proteins have been inserted (50). When dealing with MAb, however, complement-effected lysis or membrane damage may not occur if the antibody reacts with an epitope near the extremity of prominent surface projections on the virus. In such a situation, the activated C4b, C3b or C5b may lose its ability to bind to the membrane before it can diffuse from the site of activation to the membrane (51); the binding site of C4b, C3b or C5b remains active for only a fraction of a second (half-life <0.1 s). Furthermore, MAb may not bind to epitopes which are close enough to facilitate the required density of complement-mediated damage to effect lysis. If this density of complement-mediated membrane damage is too low, the cell can recover and repair such damage. Finally, MAb may fail to activate complement if the ratio of antibody to antigen is too low to overcome the natural inhibitory factors present in serum (51).

1.6.5. *Antibody isotype distribution in body fluids*

The dominant isotype of serum antibody, and presumably of MAb resulting from hybridoma technology, varies with time after immunisation with the antigen. Initially, IgM is preferentially stimulated, reaching a maximal response within 10 days of the primary inoculation. In contrast, IgG will not reach peak production until after 14–30 days (whether it is produced at all depends on the nature of the antigen). IgG production is most efficiently stimulated using an anamnestic response (antigen stimulation of immunologically educated or memory lymphocytes). The synthesis of IgA is similarly time-dependent to the synthesis of IgG except that the former has a much greater rate of turnover (Table 1.5). It should be noted that the half-life and rates of turnover for IgG shown in Table 1.5 are in normal serum, but during an active immunological response the rate of turnover increases, since the rate (the ratio between the synthesis of new IgG molecules and the catabolism of old) is directly related to the concentration of IgG. The rate of catabolism of IgA (and also IgM, IgD and IgE) is not related to Ig concentration. IgA is also the predominant Ig in body secretions (colostrum, parotid saliva, tears and mucous secretions of the upper and lower respiratory tracts and into the lumen of the small intestine) and may be of greater relevance to the response against pathogens at these sites than is IgG, which is the major Ig in sera. However, IgA, which in sera is usually in its 7*S* monomeric form, is secreted as an 11*S* dimer; the two molecules are linked by a carbohydrate moiety called the transfer piece. With hybridoma technology a monoclonal IgA antibody would be monomeric since the 'transfer piece' (also called 'secretory piece') is produced by epithelial cells in the glands responsible for the production and secretion onto mucosal surfaces of the dimeric IgA.

Physico-chemical characterisation of such monoclonal IgA should be approached cautiously because of the apparent readiness of monomeric IgA to polymerise; IgA myelomas (myelomas are transformed plasma cells which consistently secrete a structurally and electrophoretically homogeneous or monoclonal Ig molecule) will secrete 9*S*, 11*S*, 13*S* or occasionally higher polymers of IgA.

The Ig classes also differ from one another in the time course of production after antigenic stimulation. Fig. 1.34 shows the development of IgM- and IgG-secreting plasma cells in a primary and anamnestic response, and the development of IgE in an anaphylactic response. The IgM and IgG are detected by lysis of antigen-coated rbc; IgE production is measured by histamine release or the production of typical immune-type hypersensitivity inflammation (52). A single antigen may induce IgM, IgG and IgA. The relative proportion of cells secreting IgM compared with IgG or IgA will depend on the immunological education of the animal (early after a primary response the majority population of plasma cells will secrete IgM, whereas in an anamnestic response the major populations will secrete IgG; see also §§1.4.5, 1.6.2 and Table 1.13). IgA production is dependent on the antigen, and on whether or not Ig is required in the body secretions. For hybridoma technology, this time-dependence of antibody development is useful if a particular isotype of MAb is required. The route of inoculation can also facilitate this process, especially with respect to IgA (see §2.5.2).

The induction of cells producing IgM (19*S*) and IgG (7*S*) in spleens most often uses immunisation protocols by the intraperitoneal or intravenous route (typical of those in use with hybridoma technology; see §2.5.2). For IgE production, an allergen must be used (see §1.6.6) and the animals must be sensitised and boosted intradermally.

1.6.6. *Antibody-mediated anaphylactic reaction*

IgE is found in many anaphylactic reactions. The antibody is also termed reaginic or cytophilic antibody owing to its readiness to be bound by certain tissue cells. Of these IgE-binding cells, the mast cells are of greatest relevance. The IgE molecule effects the typical inflammatory response of anaphylaxis by reacting with the F_c receptor either on these mast cells in the body tissues or on basophilic and eosinophilic polymorphonuclear leukocytes. It appears that the IgE can bind to the F_c receptors without being complexed with the antigen for which the IgE is specific. However, only when antigen has reacted with the IgE (whether

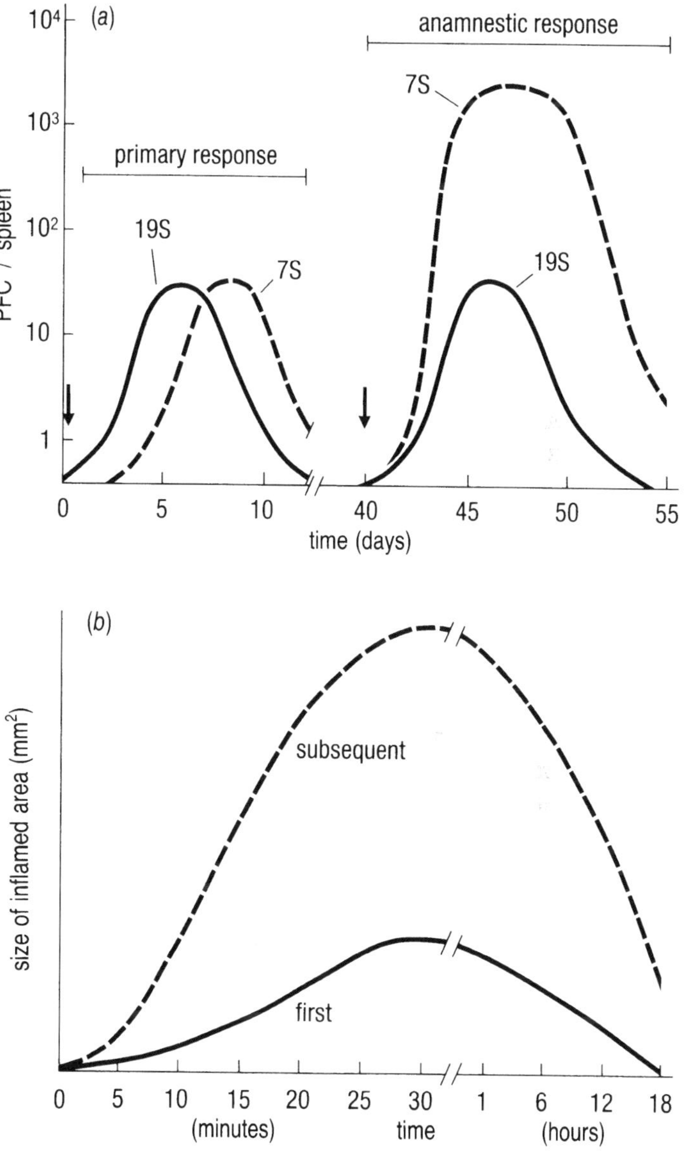

Fig. 1.34. (*a*) Development of the cells which produce IgM and IgG in primary and anamnestic (secondary) responses. Solid lines, 19*S* antibody (IgM) producing cells; broken lines, 7*S* (IgG) producing cells; PFC, plaque-forming cell assay (see Chapter 4). (*b*) Development of an IgE response during an immediate-type (type I) anaphylactic response, either on first encounter with the allergen (solid lines) or as a subsequent encounter (broken lines).

before or after binding to the receptor is unclear) will the mast cells be activated by that bound IgE. The activation may be similar to that required of IgG binding to macrophages for phagocytosis: IgG can bind to F_c receptors specific for IgG isotypes on mononuclear phagocytes and granulocytes, but is rapidly eluted by free IgG molecules; when that IgG has complexed with antigen, the bond with the F_c receptor is more stable and permits two antibody molecules reacting with the same antigen molecule to form a bridge (cross-link) between F_c receptors on the one cell, stimulating the phagocytic process (53). The mast cells upon activation release pharmacologically active agents, such as histamine and serotonin, which cause capillary dilation or vasodilation (hence the localised inflammation), vasoconstriction, increased capillary permeability and muscle contraction (hence the localised muscular pain associated with many allergic reactions). To test if the immunised animal will produce an anaphylactic response after antigen challenge, the animal can be inoculated intradermally in a small area of the skin with antigen in Evans' blue dye. If an immediate-type hypersentitive reaction (antibody-mediated, in constrast to delayed-type, which is T cell mediated; see §1.4.8) occurs, the dye will identify the inflammation around the site of inoculation by colouring the area blue. It should be noted that high levels of circulating antigen-specific IgG (such as within 5–14 days of boosting an already hyperimmune animal) may also give a localised hypersensitive reaction; see discussion of the Arthus reaction, below. Thus, to determine that the anaphylactic response is due to IgE, the presence of high levels of antigen-specific serum IgG should be excluded.

Conventional antigen, such as viruses, bacteria, protozoa and other parasites, and many proteins, will induce the immune system to synthesise IgM followed by IgG and/or IgA. Only those antigens known as allergens (Table 1.15) preferentially induce IgE. However, antigen not classified as allergen can induce certain subclasses of IgG which can act as reaginic antibody. The γ_1 subclasses of guinea pigs and mice can, under appropriate conditions, appear reaginic. Such cytophilic IgG (binds to mast cells) is effective as such for a very short period of time (half-life 24 h). In contrast, IgE will persist at the site of allergen inoculation for many days. The dominant reaginic antibody is indeed IgE, which, unlike cytophilic IgG, is primarily reaginic. It also plays a dominant role, being the most important opsonising antibody in parasite infections.

Anaphylaxis due to reaginic antibody (IgE or IgG) should not be confused with the Arthus reaction, which is also a severe inflammatory response. This latter reaction is not due to IgE, but due to antigen–antibody aggregates forming within the capillary vessel walls of an animal with moderate to high levels of circulating antibody. When specific antigen is re-introduced, it forms complexes with the antibody and these

Table 1.15. *Examples of antigens and allergens which will induce IgE as the major effector immunoglobulin isotype*

IgE-inducing antigens	Allergens[1]
Schistosomula; helminths; *Trichinella*	pollens (particularly of the grasses); certain food additives, particularly colouring and flavouring (for particular individuals); insect venoms (variation in effectiveness as allergens depending on the individual); certain antibiotics (certain individuals – fortunately few in number – can be sensitive to some of the commonly used antibiotics such as penicillin)

Note:
[1] Excess doses of allergens can result in a severe anaphylactic (hypersensitive or allergic) reaction termed anaphylactic shock, which can be fatal.

can become trapped within capillaries. The antibody responsible is primarily IgG, and the inflammation is caused by an influx of phagocytic cells into the area to attack the complexes by a variety of means, which include the release of inflammatory substances.

1.6.7. *The humoral immune response: summary*

The stimulation of the immune response will generate T_h cells, T_s cell and B cell lymphoblasts. The time after antigen administration (immunisation) at which such cells should be harvested for hybridoma production is variable (see §§2.5.2 and 2.5.6 for B cells, and §2.7.1 for T_h and T_s cells). With the appropriate cellular interactions (e.g. antigen-specific B lymphocytes, T_h lymphocytes, APC and macrophages for TD antigens) the appropriate blastogenic response will be stimulated. In the case of B cells, this involves a heterogeneous population of lymphoblasts, which can be differentiated morphologically and on the basis of their cell surface markers and antibody productivity. These cell surface markers also relate to the maturity of that particular immune response (the number of times the cells have been stimulated by antigen) and can give some information about the probable affinity of subsequently produced antibody. The B cell lymphoblasts terminate in the plasma cell, which is probably of little importance in the generation of antibody-secreting hybridomas. Of greater importance are the haemocytoblasts and plasmacytoblasts, although the other lymphoblasts and the precursor 'resting' B cell may also prove effective to a certain degree. The consequence of stimulating B cell blastogenesis, and generating antibody-secreting hybridomas, is to produce antibody of varying antigen reactivity and of different isotypes. Many of these isotypes have subtle influences on the immune response, whereas others perform specific functions; for example, IgE is associated with many of the hypersensitivity reactions known as allergy.

Using the mechanisms of lymphocyte stimulation, and the procedures of hybridoma technology, MAb can be produced. But what exactly are MAb? Having described how the immune system functions it is now possible to explain the concept of the 'monoclonal antibody'.

1.7. Monoclonal antibodies (MAb)

A single clone of activated B lymphocytes will, under the appropriate conditions of APC–T_h cell help, produce a homogeneous population of antibody molecules. The duration of this secretion is short, owing to the short half-life of the plasma cell. In order to immortalise this production, the technology of hybridoma generation is used. A hybridoma cell is derived from fusion of a myeloma cell with a single B lymphocyte–lymphoblast. Each B lymphocyte is derived from a clone which bears receptors homogeneous in their paratope, and differentiates into lymphoblasts which will secrete an antibody population which is also homogeneous for that paratope. Thus, each hybridoma cell will also originate from a single clone, and produce a culture in which the antibody will be a homogeneous population: antibody with the same paratope (antigen-binding site) and therefore monoclonal.

'Monoclonal antibody' is not a strictly correct term for describing the antibody derived by hybridoma technology. It is not the antibody molecules which are cloned and hence monoclone (a single clone), but the cells which secrete them. Thus, the cells should be given the term monoclonal (monoclonal hybridoma) and the antibody produced by them should be termed monospecific. However, to avoid confusion, the convention of 'monoclonal antibody' will be used below.

Cross-reactivity between related paratopes and with related epitopes depends on the affinity of the antigen–antibody reaction (see §1.5). This applies equally to MAb (§1.5.1). However, the avidity of an antiserum (or polyclonal antibody preparation) is a result of a complement of different affinities possessed by the different antibody molecules present. The affinity of MAb is often less than that of the autologous antiserum (see §1.5.1). This may be explained by combinations of antibodies interacting to form a more stable (higher affinity) antigen–antibody complex than would have occurred had each antibody been used alone (see Fig. 1.25). In addition, humoral factors such as C′ may interact with and increase the stability (affinity) of antigen–antibody complexes *in vivo* or in antiserum. Finally, antibody of higher affinity in an antiserum will compete for epitopes more efficiently than those of lower affinities and thus a minor population of high affinity antibody could dominate (see §1.5.1). A further complication arises when dealing with complex antigens such as bacteria, viruses, protozoa and other cells. Some antibody molecules (Ab′) may react with a high affinity only after conformational alterations have been induced in the antigen by a second antibody (Ab″). In the absence of such an alteration, the Ab′ molecules may show weak (low affinity) or no reaction with the antigen (39). McCullough *et al.* (54) have identified MAb which will react to a higher affinity with FMDV antigen complexed with specific IgG than with free antigen or antigen physically treated to expose more internal epitopes (adsorbed to a solid phase PVC plate).

So, when MAb are produced, they often show gross differences from the autologous antiserum. But why not simply culture B lymphocytes or antigen-stimulated lymphoblasts *in vitro*? Why produce hybridoma cell lines secreting MAb? Click & co-workers (55, 56), in the early 1970s, were able to culture B lymphocyte colonies *in vitro*, for the study of biological and biochemical properties of the B cells. Problems arose when continuous production of antibody was attempted. Sections 1.4.6, 1.6.1 and 1.6.3 demonstrate that stimulation of B cells into antibody production results in the generation of short-lived terminal cells: the plasma cells. Hence continuous production over a long period *in vitro* of stimulated B cell cultures would be difficult. Furthermore, lymphoblasts have stricter growth requirements *in vitro* than resting lymphocytes. Conversely, hybridoma cells are long lived (adapted to growth) *in vitro*, even when secreting antibody, and their growth requirements are simple relative to those of B lymphocytes and lymphoblasts. This is effected by the myeloma cell chromosomes in the hybrid cells. It was the myeloma cell which was adapted (readily, since it was a tumour cell) to growth *in vitro*. Table 1.16 summarises the differences between hybridoma cultures and B lymphocyte–lymphoblast cultures. The table highlights the advantages of using hybridoma cultures for the generation of antibody *in vitro*. These different areas of hybridoma technology will be dealt with in detail in Chapters 2–4.

1.8. Summary

A substantial knowledge of the functioning of the mammalian immune system has developed over the past 100 years. Recently, the ‘compartmentalisation’ of the immune response has been studied, and interactions between different cells responsible for phagocytosis, presenting of antigen for the stimulation of antigen-specific cells, antibody production, antibody-dependent leukocyte cytotoxicity, antibody-independent lymphocyte cytotoxicity and hypersensitivity reactions characterised. This knowledge permitted the development of *in vitro* culture techniques for the maintenance of antigen-specific B lymphocytes and

Table 1.16. *Differences between hybridoma and B lymphocyte–lymphoblast cultures*

Hybridoma cultures	B cell cultures
Produced from fusions between lymphocytes and tissue-culture-adapted myeloma cells	Manipulations, such as those required for the preparation of lymphocytes before fusion in hybridoma production, are not required
Only a small number of cells survive (maximum of 10 in every 10^6 lymphocytes) the fusion and selection protocols	The majority of lymphocytes can survive the initial preparation if the correct media are used, because the adverse conditions of fusion are not used
A very basic culture medium can be used once the hybridoma cells have been isolated	Highly enriched and specialised media have to be used
Hybridomas can be cultured for years	B lymphocytes can normally be cultured for only 2–6 weeks
Antibody-secreting hybridomas are few because of the small numbers of hybridomas produced	Antibody-secreting lymphoblasts are a small percentage of the culture, but their number per unit volume is greater than the number of hybridomas
Antibody-secreting hybridomas can be cultured for years	Lymphoblasts can be cultured for a maximum of only a few days
Antibody-secreting hybridomas can be cloned to give a homogeneous population of antibody	Lymphoblasts cannot be easily cloned, if at all
Large quantities (mg to g) of homogeneous antibody can be produced from hybridomas, and repeated productions used	Very small amounts (ng to μg) quantities) of antibody can be produced from lymphocyte cultures, and then only once; probably not homogeneous

T lymphocytes, and the induction of the humoral factors (antibody, T_hF, T_sF) specified by these cells. The *in vitro* culturing requirements were, however, rather specialised, and stimulated B lymphocytes could generate antibody for only a short period of time. This prompted the development of techniques for immortalising the antibody-producing capacity of stimulated B lymphocytes (lymphoblasts): the techniques of hybridoma technology, which can also be used to immortalise T_h and T_s lymphocytes. Since the techniques are similar for both B cell hybridoma and T cell hybridoma production, reference will be made to the B cell system in the main, although §2.7.1 will concentrate more on T cell hybridomas.

Chapter 2 will introduce the concept of the technology and progress through the procedures used to generate antibody-secreting hybridomas. Chapter 3 will highlight the different factors and culture conditions which affect hybridoma production, and discuss the value of 'feeder layers'. Chapter 4 will describe methods for detecting and selecting antibody-secreting hybridomas, and the cloning procedures used to isolate the monoclonal antibody-producing cells. Chapter 5 will deal with MAb production; Chapter 6 will describe the various fields in which MAb have been and are currently being used.

2 Making hybridomas (hybridoma technology)

Chapter 1 described the interactions and communications which occur during an immune response against non-self material (antigen). From this, it can be seen how hybrid cell lines could be produced which would secrete antibody reactive against a particular antigen. In this chapter, the requirements for the production of such hybrid cell lines – hybridomas – will be explained. The two major factors involved are the use of a tissue-culture-adapted lymphoblastoid cell line (myeloma cell line) and antigen-stimulated (*in vivo* or *in vitro*) lymphocytes. The characteristics and production of myeloma cells will be described; details of how these cells play a major role both in the production of hybridomas, through chemical-induced fusion with the antigen-stimulated lymphocytes, and in subsequent stabilisation of the hybrid cells *in vitro* will be presented. Procedural requirements for generating antigen-stimulated lymphocytes which are to be used in hybridoma production will be explained; and §2.6 will present a practical guide to the preparation of the myeloma cells and lymphocytes, fusion to produce hybridomas and selection of myeloma cell-lymphocyte hybrid cells. Since this book is concerned with antibody-secreting hybridomas, most of the details will be concerned with these; but reference will be made to other types of lymphocyte-derived hybrid cell lines, in particular in §2.7.

2.1. Basic requirements

The basic constituents of any hybridoma or hybrid cell line are the parent cells required for its formation. With the immune B cell hybridomas (which secrete antibody) these parents are splenocytes from the appropriate animal immunised with the antigen of choice, and tissue-culture-adapted myeloma cells (1–6). (The splenocytes are the lymphocyte population from the spleen of these immunised animals.)The animal is termed 'appropriate' if the splenocytes readily fuse with myeloma cells to form stable hybridomas. This usually requires the splenocytes to be genetically closely related to the origin of the myeloma cell. The closer this relationship, the more stable (with regard to chromosome loss) will be the hybridoma. This topic will be dealt with in more detail in §2.5.8. Table 2.1. shows the animals to date from which splenocytes have been obtained and successfully used to produce hybridomas.

Table 2.1. *Examples of animal species from which lymphocytes have been taken to generate hybridomas*

Animal		Source of lymphocytes
mouse	(most commonly used strain: Balb/c)	spleen, lymph nodes
rat	(most commonly used strains: DA, AO, Lewis)	spleen, lymph nodes
human		peripheral blood
cattle		peripheral blood, lymph nodes
sheep		lymph nodes
rabbits		lymph nodes, spleen

Having isolated the splenocytes from an immunised animal, why generate hybridoma cell lines? The reason lies in the *in vitro* biological characteristics of splenocytes and myeloma cells. In a hybridoma, the myeloma cell chromosomes confer culture stability and longevity *in vitro* on the splenocyte. Splenocytes have a short life span *in vitro*, normally less than two weeks, although they can be cultured for up to six weeks by using specifically enriched media (7). Thus, hybridomas carrying myeloma cell genes will have an indefinite life span. Accepting the need for hybridoma cultures, and having selected the two parents (the fusion partners), the splenocytes and myeloma cells must now be successfully fused and the subsequently generated hybridomas selected from the unfused splenocytes and myeloma cells. The fusion procedure will be dealt with in §§2.3.1 and 2.6.2; the selective procedures will be described in §§2.3.2 and 2.6.3. Sections 2.3 and 2.5 will also explain (i) why certain types of hybridoma are more successfully produced, (ii) which lymphocytes preferentially fuse with myeloma cells, (iii) what the expected characteristics of hybridoma antibody may be, and (iv) what influence this has on the properties of the antibody. The procedural requirements for successful immunisation of the animal sources of the splenocytes will also be discussed. Stepwise detailed descriptions will be given in §2.6 for the removal and preparation of the immune lymphocytes, fusion of lymphocytes with myeloma cells to generate hybridomas, and selection of those hybridomas from the unfused splenocytes and myeloma cells. The chapter will end with a brief overview of the state of the art with respect to which types of hybridoma cell lines have been generated, and to what purpose they or their products have been put.

Firstly, to facilitate a better understanding of why hybridomas can be generated and what their properties are, a description of the myeloma cell will be presented.

2.2. The myeloma cell

2.2.1 *Definition*

A myeloma cell is classically defined as a neoplastic plasma cell in myelomatosis (in humans, mice and possibly other animal species) producing a structurally and electrophoretically homogeneous (monoclonal) paraprotein (8). The reason for the latter statement – production of a homogeneous paraprotein – is that induction of the myeloma cell results from the transformation of a clone (derived from a single cell and hence a homogeneous population) of plasma cells. Paraprotein is defined immunologically as immunoglobulin (Ig) derived from an abnormally proliferating clone of neoplastic cells. Hence, a myeloma cell is a transformed plasma cell derived from a clone of plasma cells. Unlike normal non-transformed plasma cells, which die after approximately 48 h, the myeloma cell has the life span of a tumour cell (the life of the animal body which harbours it) and like most transformed cells can readily adapt to *in vitro* growth.

2.2.2. *Myeloma cell induction*

The most common method of inducing myeloma cells is by inoculating animals with a mineral oil such as paraffin oil (Table 2.2). One of the reasons for the common use of Balb/c mice in hybridoma technology and the fact that most mouse myeloma cells used are of Balb/c mouse origin is that these mice are especially susceptible to myeloma cell induction.

The normal route of inoculation of the myeloma cell inducer is intraperitoneal. Table 2.2 shows the different compounds which have been used successfully to induce myeloma cell production *in vivo*. The review by Potter (9) describes and discusses these techniques in more detail.

2.2.3. *Detection*

Myeloma cell production (neoplastic proliferation of plasma cells), or myelomatosis as it is clinically defined, can be detected by:

Table 2.2. *Methods used for the induction of myelomas in Balb/c mice*

(i)	Implantation of Millipore diffusion chambers (17 to 21 mm diam.) intraperitoneally
(ii)	Implantation of rough-edged plexiglass (Lucite) borings (1–21 mm diam.) intraperitoneally
(iii)	Intraperitoneal injection of 'staphylococcal adjuvant': one part heat-killed *Staphylococcus aureas* + one part incomplete Freund's adjuvant (8.5 parts Bayol F and 1.5 parts Arlacel A (mannide monooleate)).
(iv)	Three 0.5 ml injections intraperitoneally, spaced 2 months apart, of the mineral oils Bayol F, Drakeol 6VR, Primol D or any other USP grade white mineral oil.
(v)	As in (iv) but using the purified saturated hydrocarbons pristane (2, 6, 10, 14-tetramethyl pentadecane), phytane (2, 6, 10, 14-tetramethyl hexadecane), or 7*n*-hexyloctadecane.

(a) The presence of lymphoblastosis, i.e. an abnormally high rate of B lymphocyte replication (blastogenesis). Since myelomatosis can most often occur in the bone marrow, this method of detection is not always reliable.

(b) The detection of large amounts of homogeneous (monoclonal) Ig. Since the myeloma cell is a clone of transformed plasma cells, both the myeloma cell and its paraprotein product are monoclonal. Thus, the myeloma protein will be homogeneous for isotypic, allotypic and idiotypic determinants, and can easily be detected in the sera of patients or animals suffering from myelomatosis. Electrophoresis, especially the crossed immunoelectrophoretic procedures, will present the myeloma cell Ig as a dominant peak or pattern of bands (Fig. 2.1). This is a fairly reliable method for detecting myelomatosis and hence myeloma cell induction.

(c) The detection of Bence–Jones proteins. This is probably the best-known method for detecting myelomatosis, and is due to the structure of the myeloma protein (Ig). As with any plasma cell, the myeloma cell will, through somatic variation during its selection, secrete either IgA, IgD, IgE, IgM or one of the subclasses of IgG (γ_1, γ_2, γ_3, γ_4 in man; γ_1, γ_2 in guinea pig; γ_1, γ_2 in rabbits; γ_1, γ_{2a}, γ_{2b}, γ_3 in mice; γ_1, γ_{2a}, γ_{2b} in rats). These isotypic differences of the Ig molecules are conferred by the heavy chains of the molecule. The light chains of the Ig are much less diverse, having only two types – κ and λ – which are unrelated to the antibody isotype; that is, all Ig isotypes can have either κ or λ light chains. Hence, detection of light chains is relatively

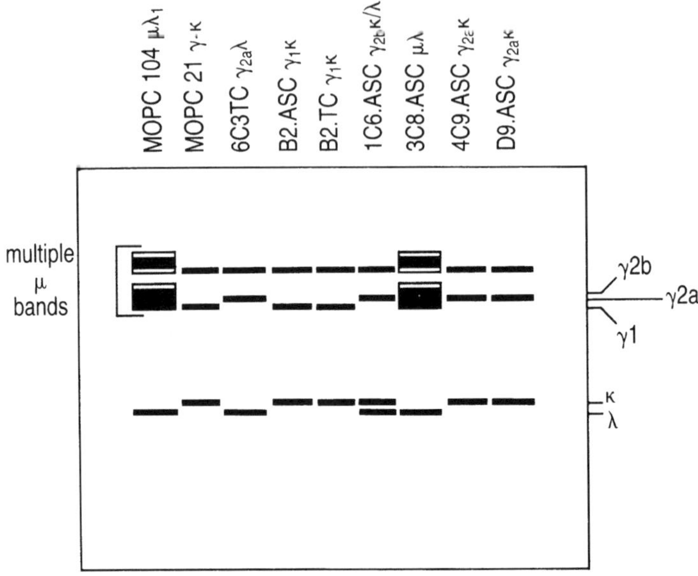

Fig. 2.1. Polyacrylamide gel electrophoresis of myeloma (MOPC) immunoglobulins using 7.5% (w/v) polyacrylamide and the buffer system of Laemmli (23), after denaturing the MOPC proteins with 2-mercaptoethanol and SDS.

more straightforward. In the urine of patients suffering from myelomatosis the light chains of the myeloma protein are found in a dimerised form M_r 40 000) called the Bence–Jones protein (Table 2.3). They can be precipitated by heating at 60 °C and re-dissolved after further heating to 90 °C. The detection of Bence–Jones proteins is probably the most reliable method for determining myelomatosis.

2.2.4. *Characteristics*

Myeloma cells are identical to plasma cells (differentiated, terminal cell of the B lymphocyte series) in all but their longevity and culture stability. (Table 2.4). In contrast to the plasma cell, myeloma cells will grow *in vitro* without a specifically enriched culture medium, and can be subcultured, theoretically, indefinitely. In practice, there are certain requirements for successful myeloma cell culture. Like any lymphocyte cell line, myeloma cells grow as suspension cells, best in slightly acid to neutral conditions (pH 6.8–7.2) but poorly in slightly alkaline conditions (pH > 7.8). Although the cells grow in suspension, if a culture is incubated in a flask without agitation (static culture), the cells settle to the bottom of the flask. Unlike tissue culture-adapted epithelial and fibroblastic cells (e.g. HEp_2, HeLa, Vero, BSC-1, AGMK, Lu106, BHK, L and 3T3

Table 2.3. *Characterisation of Bence–Jones proteins useful to the detection of myelomatosis*

Immunoglobulin determinants	k or λ light chains
Location	urine
Structure	dimerized light chains
Relative molecular mass (M_r)	40 000
Physico-chemistry	precipitated at 60 °C redissolved at 90 °C

Table 2.4. *Biological comparisons between myeloma cells and plasma cells*

Myeloma cells	Plasma cells
transformed plasma cells	normal plasma cells (stimulated B cell–lymphoblast)
long life span: months to years	short life span: days
can be easily adapted to culture *in vitro*	cannot be adapted to culture *in vitro*
for maintenance *in vitro*, can use several conventional tissue culture media	for maintenance *in vitro*, require specialised media
can be subcultured indefinitely	can be cultured for only a few days

cells), which attach to the surface upon which they are growing and form an adherent monolayer, myeloma cells attach loosely to their growing surface. Adherent cell cultures are normally resuspended for subculture (passage) by enzymic treatment and the use of chelating agents. Myeloma cells are resuspended by gently agitating the culture medium: rotating the flask in which the cells are growing, or forcing medium over the cells with a pipette.

There are certain myeloma cell lines, such as P3.X63.Ag8.653 (NS653) mouse myeloma cells, and the SP2/0 murine hybridoma line often referred to as a myeloma cell, which are more adherent than others and thus require more vigorous agitation to resuspend them. The rat myeloma cell line Y3-Ag.1.2.3 is also relatively adherent.

These technical 'difficulties' with NS653, SP2/0 and Y3-Ag.1.2.3 cell lines can be overcome by using spinner cultures, in which the cells are kept in suspension by mechanical agitation, such as that given by a bar magnet and stirrer (provided the correct environmental conditions are supplied). These conditions and the different means of producing spinner cultures will be discussed in Chapter 3 (§3.5) and Chapter 5 (§5.3).

Unlike most 'tissue culture' cell lines, myeloma cells must be kept in an *exponential* phase of growth. Failure to do this will result in either loss of the myeloma cell culture, or poor generation of antibody-secreting hybridomas. In order to achieve the desired results, myeloma cells are generally cultured within the cell density limits of 1×10^4 cells/ml to 6×10^5 cells/ml (depending on the composition of the culture medium). Similar conditions apply to the culturing of hybridoma cells (§3.8.2). However, there is a finite time span over which both myeloma cells and hybridomas can be successfully maintained in culture. Owing to natural variation, a myeloma cell culture can alter its properties, and a hybridoma culture can acquire a reduced efficiency for secreting antibody, or even stop secreting antibody. The P3-NS/1-Ag 4.1 (NS1) myeloma cell line synthesises but does not secrete a κ light chain. After continuous culture over several months, natural genetic variation selects for the dominance of an NS0 cell line, which neither synthesises nor secretes any Ig chains. Some NS0 lines are less efficient than NS1 at generating stable antibody-secreting hybridomas after fusion with immune splenocytes, but recent cloning yielded an NSO myeloma cell line which is one of the most efficient at generating hybridomas. Undesirable somatic mutation can be overcome by (i) storing an adequate number of aliquots of cells during early subcultures, and (ii) recloning the cell line periodically (every 3–6 months) to reselect cells with the desired properties.

The growth of myeloma cells is also influenced by the composition of the culture medium and other environmental factors, but these topics will be dealt with in detail in §§3.5 and 3.6.

2.3. The production of hybridomas from myeloma cells

2.3.1. *Fusion between splenocytes and myeloma cells*

Treatment of a mixture of splenocytes from an immunised animal (see §2.5.2) and myeloma cells with a cell-fusing agent such as PEG (see §2.6.2) will generate a culture containing unfused myeloma cells, unfused splenocytes, hybridomas of myeloma cells and splenocytes (heterokaryons), and hybridomas of either splenocytes with splenocytes or myeloma cells with myeloma cells (homokaryons) (Fig. 2.2). The splenocyte homokaryon hybrids and unfused splenocytes grow slowly and die within 1–6 weeks depending on the physiology of each splenocyte (the further each has differentiated towards the terminal plasma cell, the shorter its expected life *in vitro*) and the composition of the growth

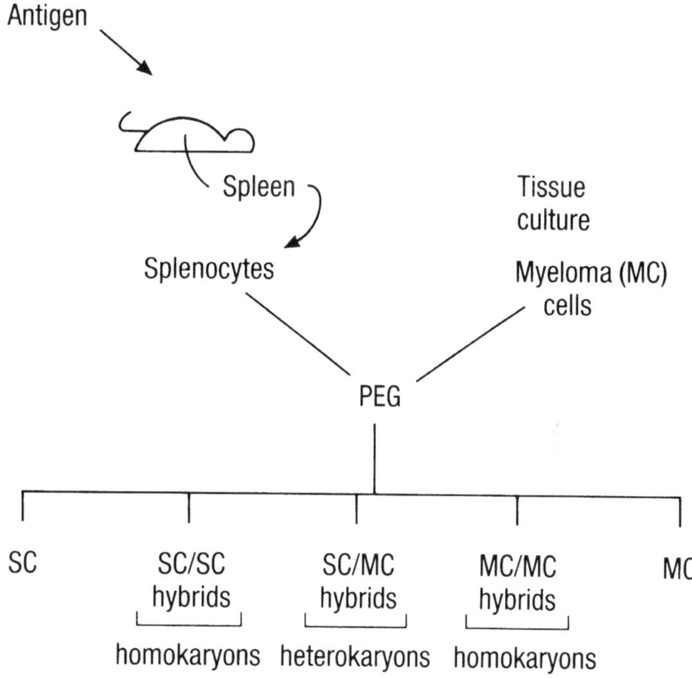

Fig. 2.2. The different cell types which can arise out of fusions between splenocytes (SC) and myeloma cells (MC).

medium (see §3.5). Conversely, heterokaryon hybridomas of myeloma cells and splenocytes should have the indefinite life expectancy of the original myeloma cell. However, longevity does not necessarily follow the generation of such hybridomas by cell fusion. The fusion procedure causes the resultant hybridomas to enter a 'low growth rate phase' during which time a physiological stabilisation occurs with respect to cell integrity and chromosome complement. That is, the gross characteristics of most hybridomas are determined within the first week or two after fusion. The cell division (controlled by the myeloma cell chromosomes which divide in synchrony with the cell) and splenocyte chromosome division must synchronise to establish a stable hybridoma. Without this synchrony, the splenocyte chromosomes will be 'shed', resulting in an antibody-non-producing cell line (Fig. 2.3). More subtle intragene stabilisations must also occur, since splenocyte gene functions as opposed to complete chromosomes can also be lost. Most hybridomas stabilise within the first two to four weeks after fusion, although some hybridoma lines can take months to stabilise and others never do so, having to be re-cloned periodically to isolate the cells carrying the desired gene functions (see Chapter 4 for cloning procedures). After, or sometimes during, this

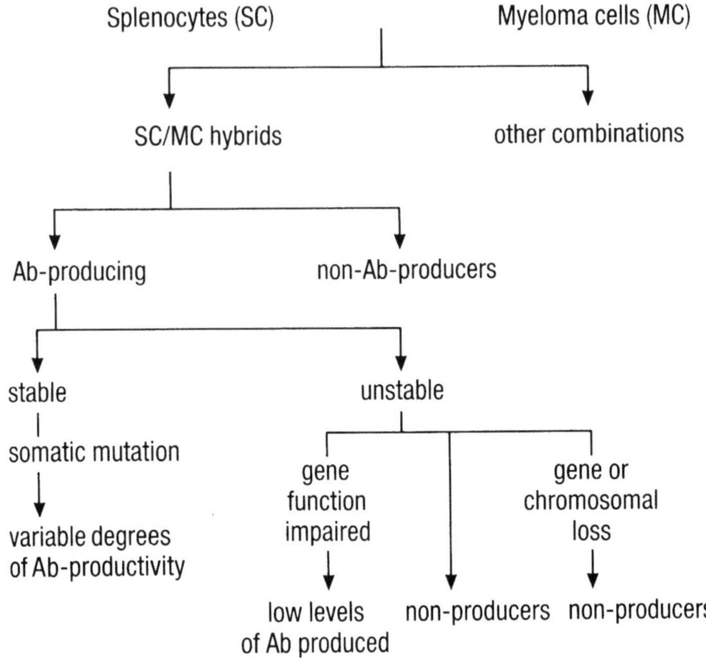

Fig. 2.3. How asynchronous division, genetic recombination and other mechanisms of impairment of gene function can yield hybridomas which are non-producers of antibody from parent hybridomas which were Ab-producers.

period of stabilisation, the hybridoma cells begin growing more rapidly. The overall outcome is the generation of cultures containing a mixture of hybridomas: some may secrete antibody while others will not. Whether the genetic alterations occur during the first two weeks after fusion or continue for another four weeks, after this time most hybridomas will be relatively stable, with only a low rate of genetic variation (somatic mutation) as the cell line is cultured. Such variation can be seen by a reduction in antibody production by the culture, and can be overcome by regular cloning and selection of the highest-producing clones of cells (see Chapters 3 and 4). The reduction in antibody productivity may be noticed after a matter of weeks or months, or may not be seen until after a long time in culture. No two hybridoma cell lines will necessarily show the same characteristics, and it is therefore difficult to make generalisations.

These considerations are of the utmost importance when cloning stabilised hybridoma cultures after fusion. These hybridomas are a heterogeneous mixture of myeloma cell–splenocyte hybrids since there are several B lymphocytes–lymphoblasts of different morphology and antibody-secreting properties which could fuse with the myeloma cell.

It has been proposed (10) that myeloma cells will fuse preferentially with these cells of the B lymphocyte lineage (see §2.5.6), and the ideal hybrid, with respect to antibody production and *in vitro* culture stability, appears to be between a myeloma cell and one of the precursors of the plasma cell but not the plasma cell itself (see §2.5.6). Hence, there will be a variable degree of stability in antibody productivity (and in the antibody production itself) among the different hybrids of a fusion mixture. Some of the hybridomas which will not secrete antibody, e.g. a hybrid of a myeloma cell with a resting B lymphocyte (see §2.5.6), would be similar to those hybridomas which lost their capacity to synthesise antibody through 'chromosomal loss'.

Non-producing hybridomas often have a higher growth rate than, and should subsequently outgrow, the antibody-producing hybridomas. This may take 2–10 weeks or more after fusion (depending on the initial ratio of non-producing to producing hybridomas and the antibody-producing stability of the latter). Hence, the antibody-secreting hybridomas should be cloned away from the non-producers as soon as the newly formed hybridomas have adapted to *in vitro* culture (see §§3.8, 4.2 and 4.3).

There is, however, a more immediate threat to the success of obtaining antibody-producing hybridomas after fusion. Unfused myeloma cells will have a higher growth rate than hybridomas after the fusion; they are affected much less (physically, physiologically or biochemically) by this fusion procedure than are the splenocytes or hybridomas. They are also in a much higher density than hybridomas (Fig. 2.4), most often of the order of $10^4 : 1$ (myeloma cell : hybridoma) although this can vary from $10^6 : 1$ to $10^4 : 1$. Within a few days, the culture arising from a fusion would be overgrown with myeloma cells and soon die through lack of nutrients and high levels of acidic, toxic metabolites. It is therefore imperative that these unfused myeloma cells be removed from the culture after fusion. This cannot be achieved directly, so a selective procedure is used which kills unfused myeloma cells within a matter of hours, but is ineffective against splenocytes and myeloma cell–splenocyte hybrids.

2.3.2. *Selective procedures*

In order that a selective procedure can be used, fusions are performed using myeloma cells (mouse, rat, human or any other species one may be using) which are deficient in the enzyme hypoxanthine phosphoguanidine ribosyl transferase (HPGRT). This enzyme is an essential component of the alternative (hypoxanthine shunt) pathway in the nucleoside synthesis for DNA production.

Should the major nucleoside synthesis pathway be blocked, $HPGRT^-$ myeloma cells cannot make use of hypoxanthine and the alternative pathway. The drug which is used to block this major pathway is aminopte-

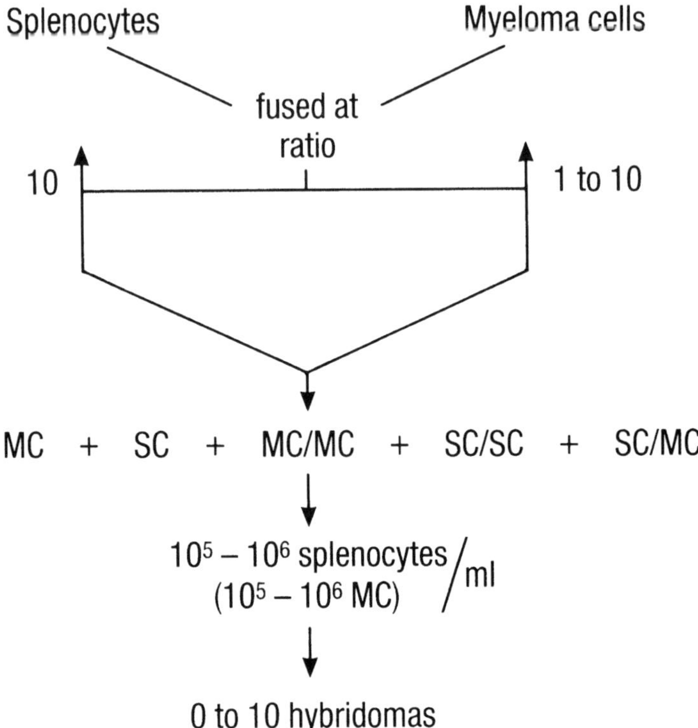

Fig. 2.4. Variations in the fusion ratio between splenocytes (SC) and myeloma cells (MC), the plating density of the fusion mixture, and the number of hybridomas generated.

rin. There is, of course, the possibility that a small proportion of myeloma cells in a culture will undergo a somatic mutation resulting in reversion of aminopterin sensitivity. In addition, some nucleoside biosynthesis can occur through the use of thymidine. Hence, a second enzyme deficiency can be induced in the myeloma cells: that of thymidine kinase (TK), the major enzyme for the conversion of thymidine to TMP.

The inclusion of aminopterin in culture media after fusion will kill any unfused myeloma cell, and myeloma cell–myeloma cell hybrids. Since splenocytes will possess both HPGRT and TK, they will be resistant to aminopterin toxicity, providing hypoxanthine and thymidine are supplied in the culture medium. Consequently, the splenocyte chromosomes will confer aminopterin resistance, and the capacity to use exogenous thymidine, on splenocyte–myeloma cell hybridomas.

Using this 'selective medium' – termed HAT (Table 2.5) – splenocyte–myeloma cell hybrids can be selected from the fusion products. But will this medium select against all myeloma cells? The answer is 'No'.

Table 2.5. *The selective media used in hybridoma technology*

Conditioned medium	Medium from 72 h old culture of myeloma cells in RPMI 1640 medium or DMEM or GMEM containing 10% (v/v) foetal calf serum, 2 mM glutamine, 25 mM HEPES, 5.5% (w/v) $NaHCO_3$ and antibiotics; centrifuged 1200 rpm, 5 min; filtered through 0.2 μm sterilizing filter
HAT medium	RPMI 1640 medium or DMEM or GMEM containing 50% (v/v) conditioned medium (to which had been added 10% (v/v) foetal calf serum and 2mM glutamine), 10% (v/v) foetal calf serum or 5% (v/v) foetal calf serum + 5% (v/v) horse serum, 2 mm glutamine, 25mM HEPES, 5.5% (w/v) $NaHCO_3$, 125 units/ml benzylpenicillin, 187 units/ml streptomycin sulphate, 1×10^{-4}M hypoxanthine[1], 4×10^{-7}M aminopterin[2] and 1.6×10^{-5}M thymidine[1]
HT medium (for young cultures)	as HAT medium, but without aminopterin
HT medium (for cultures weaned off feeder layers)	as HAT medium, but without the aminopterin and the 50% conditioned medium
Additional (not obligatory) supplements	10mM sodium pyruvate, 5×10^{-5}M 2-mercaptoethanol, 1 μg/ml *E.coli* B lipopolysaccharide, non-essential amino acids

Note:

[1] The hypoxanthine and thymidine are added to the medium from a 50 × concentrated stock (2 ml of stock to every 100 ml of medium). The stock is prepared as follows, or purchased ready-made:

136 mg hypoxanthine + 100 ml distilled H_2O;
Heat to 70 °C and hold at 70 °C for 10 minutes with stirring;
Continue to stir until the hypoxanthine has dissolved;
Cool to room temperature;
Add 38.75 mg thymidine;
Make up to 200 ml with distilled H_2O;
Sterilise by filtration through a 0.2 μm filter;
Store in 20 μl aliquots at −20 °C.

[2] The aminopterin (the solid should be stored desiccated at −20 °C) is added to the medium from a 1000 × concentrated stock (100 μl of stock to every 100 ml of medium). The stock is prepared as follows, or purchased as '50 ×' stock:

17.6 mg aminopterin + 10 ml 0.1 M NaOH;
Stir until dissolved;
Make up to 100 ml with distilled H_2O;
Sterilise by filtration through a 0.2 μm filter;
Store in 1 ml aliquots at −20 °C.

Myeloma cells do not normally lack HPGRT or TK and must be mutated before use in hybridoma technology. The myeloma cell lines currently used for generating hybridomas have undergone this mutation (1, 3, 11).

How were HPGRT$^-$ myeloma cell lines selected? After transformation of the plasma cells (myelomatosis) had been detected in the animal of choice, the myeloma cells were isolated and grown in an *in vitro* lymphocyte culture medium such as RPMI 1640, F8 or Click's medium. Once established to these *in vitro* conditions, the cells could be cloned and selected in the presence of 6-azaguanine or 5-thiouracil. Only cells which had become HPGRT$^-$ would be resistant to these nucleotide analogues, and thus sensitive to aminopterin.

TK deficiency is selected by growth in the presence of bromodeoxyuridine (a thymidine analogue). Such HPGRT$^-$TK$^-$ myeloma cells will grow well in tissue culture provided neither aminopterin nor toxic concentrations of thymidine are present in the medium.

After fusion, the selective killing of unfused myeloma cells or myeloma cell–myeloma cell hybrids by aminopterin is rapid, with few, if any, myeloma cells remaining viable after 24 h. The cultures are still monitored, however, in HAT medium for up to 14 days, because chromosomal loss, which is most likely within the first 2–3 weeks after fusion, can result in myeloma cell–splenocyte hybrids losing aminopterin resistance. This would occur if the splenocyte chromosome(s) shed from the hybrid carried the gene responsible for HPGRT synthesis. Thus, the continued presence of aminopterin in the medium for 14 days may eliminate some of these unwanted hybrids. After 14 days, cultures are then fed with HT medium. Half of the old HAT medium is replaced by HT medium; re-feeding with such 'half volumes' is performed every 2–3 days and during subculture for up to 14 days (Fig. 2.5). Although the aminopterin may have been removed from the cultures by the first two or three feedings, the cells will have already pinocytosed the drug and so hypoxanthine and thymidine must remain in the medium until these intracytoplasmic factories of drug are metabolised. The rate of this metabolism will vary greatly between cultures, being related to the growth rate of the cells. Hence, it is advisable to feed with HT medium and re-feed until one can be confident that no toxic traces of aminopterin remain in the cells of the culture.

2.4. **Myeloma cells available**

The various myeloma cells which are currently available and have been used successfully to produce hybridomas are shown in Table 2.6. The X63 cell line synthesises and secretes heavy and light chains; the NS1 cells synthesise but do not secrete a light (κ-specificity) chain. Other mouse myeloma cells neither secrete nor synthesise Ig chains. The secreting properties of the other available myeloma cells are shown in the table. These secretions (or lack of them) have certain implications in hybridoma technology. Hybrids produced using the X63 myeloma cell

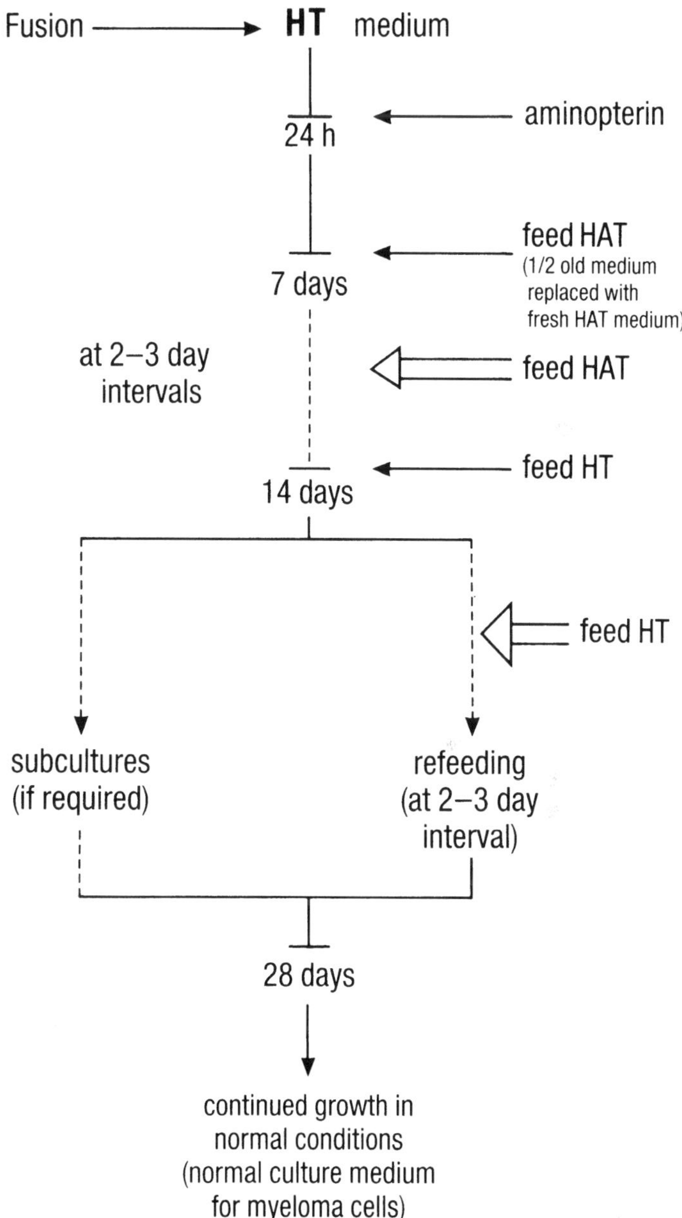

Fig. 2.5. Feeding regime for cells after fusion (see Table 2.5 for explanation of HT and HAT medium).

Table 2.6. *Some of the most commonly used myeloma cell lines for hybridoma production*

Myeloma cell[1]	Animal source	Immunoglobulin chains secreted
P3-X63-Ag8 (X63)	mouse[2]	γ_1, κ
P3-NS/1-Ag 4.1 (NS1)	mouse	κ (synthesised, not secreted).
P3-X63-Ag8.653 (NS653)	mouse	none
SP2/0-Ag.14 (SP2 or SP2/0)[3]	mouse	none
NSO/u (NSO)	mouse	none
Fox/NY	mouse	none
Y3-Ag 1.2.3 (Y3)	rat	κ (synthesised, not secreted)
YB2/3.0Ag20 (YB2)	rat	none
GM 1500 6TG-A11	human	γ_2, κ
GM 1500 6TG-A12	human	γ_2, κ

Note:
[1] Abbreviated form in brackets.
[2] All mouse myeloma cell lines originate from the Balb/c mouse myeloma cell line X63, except the SP2 cells.
[3] The SP2 cell line was derived from a hybridoma which became altered such that it had myeloma cell characteristics; it is often referred to as a myeloma cell line.

line, which have the genetic loci responsible for the antibody heavy and light chains of the splenocyte, also have the genetic loci for the different heavy and light chains of the myeloma cell. (When the myeloma cell antibody chains are combined to form the myeloma cell Ig, this Ig is a termed MOPC protein.) Fig. 2.6 shows the theoretical genotypic and phenotypic (with respect to antigenic reactivity of the synthesised antibody) random distribution of antibody secretion by such hybrids. This distribution depends on the compatibility of the individual light chains (shown as L and κ in the figure) for the individual heavy chains (shown as H and γ) and of the different heavy chains (splenocyte 'H' and myeloma 'γ') to form stable whole Ig molecules through the requisite number of disulphide bridges. The situation is further complicated by the possibility that the hybridoma will synthesise two Ig molecules or Ig chains (heavy and/or light) as opposed to a hybrid molecule (Fig. 2.7). Concentrate for the moment on the relatively straightforward situation in which all Ig chains can recombine as shown in Fig. 2.6. Cumulating the results gives a ratio of 17 hybridomas secreting antigen-reactive antibody to 19 hybridomas secreting non-reactive antibody; of these 17

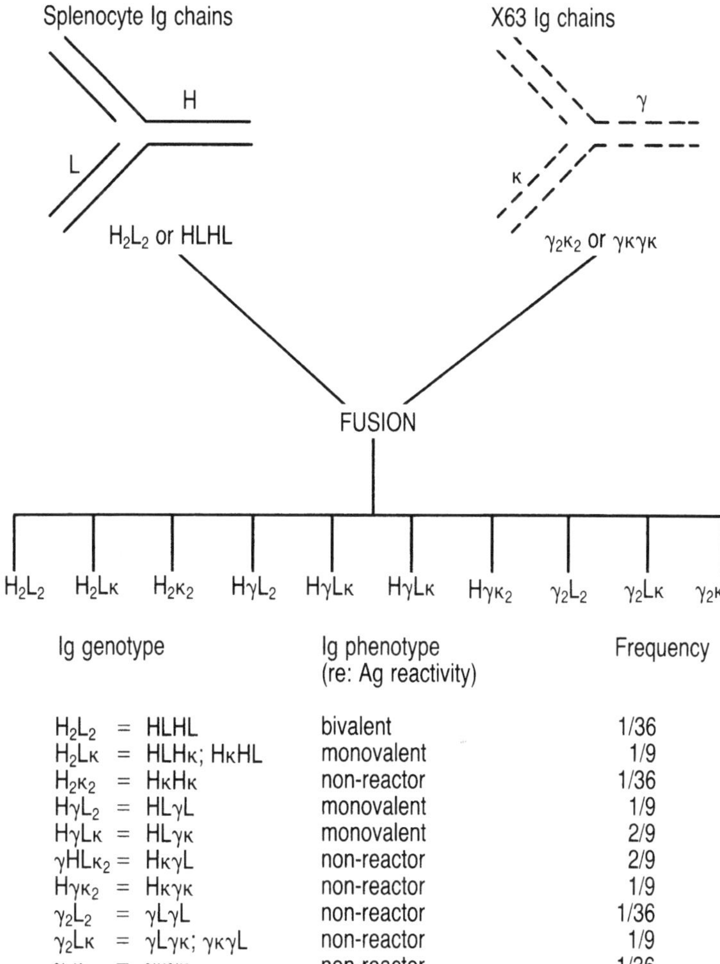

Ig genotype	Ig phenotype (re: Ag reactivity)	Frequency
H_2L_2 = HLHL	bivalent	1/36
$H_2L\kappa$ = HLHκ; HκHL	monovalent	1/9
$H_2\kappa_2$ = HκHκ	non-reactor	1/36
$H\gamma L_2$ = HLγL	monovalent	1/9
$H\gamma L\kappa$ = HLγκ	monovalent	2/9
$\gamma HL\kappa_2$ = HκγL	non-reactor	2/9
$H\gamma\kappa_2$ = Hκγκ	non-reactor	1/9
γ_2L_2 = γLγL	non-reactor	1/36
$\gamma_2L\kappa$ = γLγκ; γκγL	non-reactor	1/9
$\gamma_2\kappa_2$ = γκγκ	non-reactor	1/36

Fig. 2.6. Genotypic and phenotypic distribution of antibody secretion from hybridomas between X63 myeloma cells (MC) and antibody-secreting splenocytes (SC). H, splenocyte immunoglobulin heavy chain; L, splenocyte immunoglobulin light chain; γ, myeloma cell immunoglobulin (MOPC) heavy chain; κ, MOPC light chain.

only 1 will secret bivalent antibody, i.e. antibody with 2 paratopes per molecule (see Fig. 2.8).

The situation with hybridomas using NS1 myeloma cell chromosomes is simpler, because the κ light chain synthesised by NS1 genes can only be secreted in recombinant antibody molecules.

HLHκ	HκHκ
(monovalent)	(non-reactor)

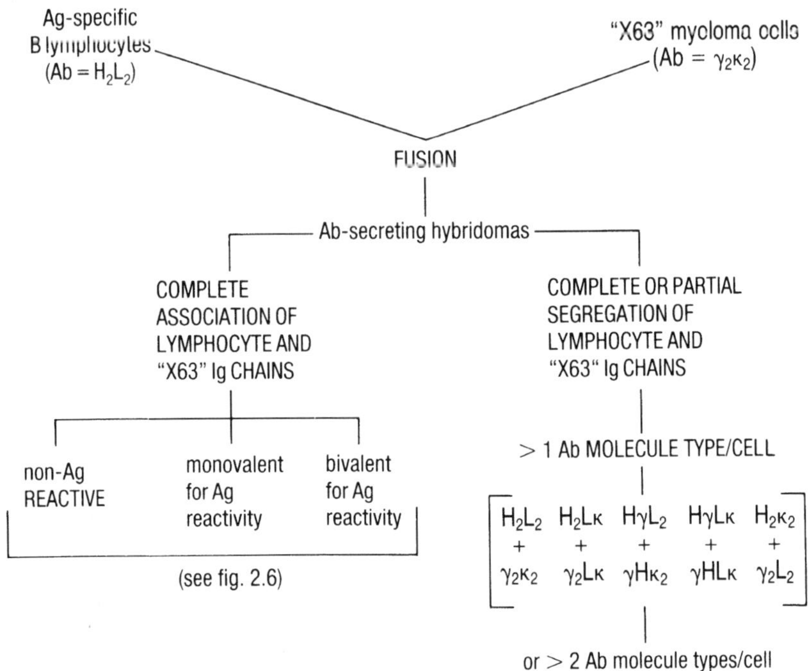

Fig. 2.7. Depending on the myeloma cell line, and the secretory properties of the splenocyte, a hybridoma can be generated which will produce two different antibody molecules.

When non-synthesisers NS653, SP2/0, NS0 and YB2 myeloma cells are used, no such recombinant antibody molecules are secreted by the resultant hybridomas.

So what is the relevance of this? Not all hybridomas will be between myeloma cells and splenocytes with specificity for the antigen under investigation. If the number of such desired hybridomas is reduced because the synthesised antibody product is non-reactive owing to recombination, then the efficiency of the technology is also reduced. Furthermore, if the antibody is required for a specific purpose, then monovalency may abrogate the usefulness of that antibody in certain immunological tests. Examples of this are to be found with certain cytotoxicity and haemagglutination tests (see §4.1) and certain mechanisms of virus neutralisation (12, 13).

Hence, the desired hybridoma would appear to be between a non-synthesising myeloma cell, and syngeneic splenocytes. But there are other considerations to be made (Table 2.7). McCullough *et al.* (14) have shown that fusions using NS1 cells were more successful at generating anti-FMDV antibody-secreting hybridomas than when X63, NS653 or

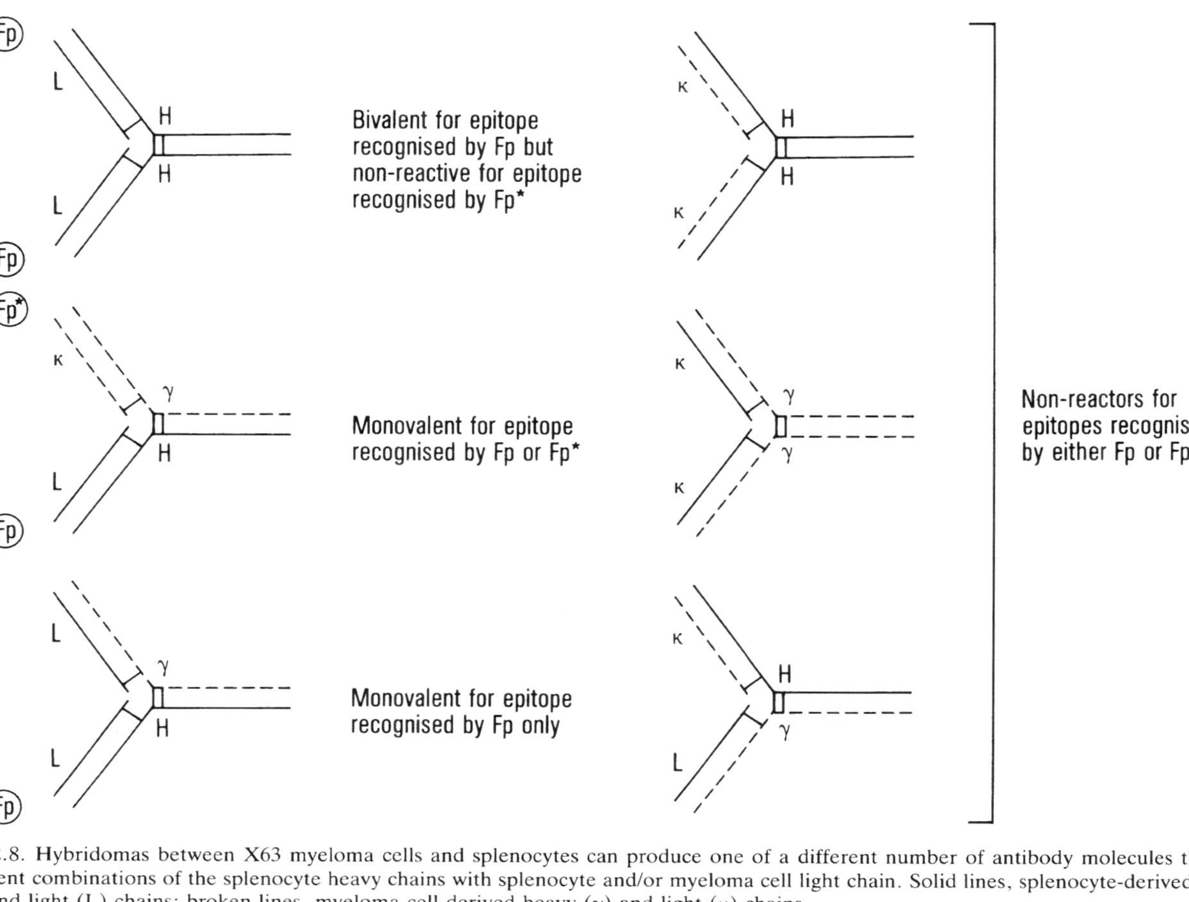

Fig. 2.8. Hybridomas between X63 myeloma cells and splenocytes can produce one of a different number of antibody molecules through different combinations of the splenocyte heavy chains with splenocyte and/or myeloma cell light chain. Solid lines, splenocyte-derived heavy (H) and light (L) chains; broken lines, myeloma cell-derived heavy (γ) and light (κ) chains.

Table 2.7. *Efficacy of different myeloma cells at generating hybridomas*

Lymphocyte source	Myeloma cell	Percentage efficiency[1]
Balb/c mouse	X63	11–26
	NS1	51–100
	NS653	57–88
	SP2	53–100
	NSO[2]	28–68
	Y3	55–100
	YB2	32–59
Lewis rat	NS1	0–35
	Y3	57–100
	YB2	51–83

Note:
[1] Efficiency: percentage of wells giving hybridoma cells which could be cultured, out of the total number of wells seeded.
[2] Recent NSO lines have proved to be amongst the most efficient myeloma cells at generating hybridomas.

SP2/0 cells were used. Fazekas de St Groth & Scheidegger (15) obtained similar results when comparing NS1 and SP2/0 cells in fusions. Milstein (16) has shown that syngeneic fusions using NS1 cells were more successful than those using NS0 or NS653 cells with respect to Ig secretions, although recent NSO lines have proved to be very efficient. Syngeneic fusions using the Y3 and YB2 rat myeloma cell lines were the most successful, but a surprising result was that fusions between the Y3 line and *mouse* splenocytes were also very efficient. Fusions between YB2 cells and mouse splenocytes were only moderately successful, and NS1 × *rat* splenocyte fusions were the least successful.

Thus, the efficient generation of antibody-secreting hybridomas relies on the choice of the correct myeloma cell line and use of the most effective selection procedures. There are, however, other considerations concerning the induction of the immune splenocytes, preparation of these for fusion, and procedural requirements for that fusion.

2.5. Generation of hybridoma cell lines

The controlling factors for the successful generation of hybridomas can be broadly divided into (i) immunisation protocols, (ii) isolation and preparation of immune splenocytes, (iii) choice of myeloma cell, (iv) fusion and selection of hybridomas, and (v) types of hybridoma line which can potentially be generated. Since this is generally the routine followed when generating hybridomas, these topics will be described in this order.

2.5.1. *Choice of animal for immunisation*

In order that immune splenocytes which will fuse with available myeloma cell lines can be stimulated, the animal used for immunisation must be carefully chosen. Syngeneic fusion partners, i.e. Balb/c mouse myeloma cells with Balb/c mouse splenocytes, etc., should theoretically be the most suitable. However, Milstein (16) has shown that the rat Y3 myeloma cell × mouse splenocyte fusion was an exception to this rule. When species non-relatedness is increased, for example by using human or rabbit splenocyte × mouse myeloma cell fusions, the success of such fusions is generally very low. This is due to a genetic instability in the hybrids: the rapid loss of splenocyte chromosomes on continuous culture. A recent modification of established methods (Fig 2.9) has increased the efficiency of such xenogeneic fusions (heterohybridoma production) to achieve up to 20% efficiency. This compares with 40–90% efficiency in syngeneic fusions (14, 16).

2.5.2. *Choice of immunisation protocol*

Having chosen the animal to immunise, the immunisation protocol must now be carefully selected. The first consideration is which route of inoculation should be used. This probably varies for different antigens, and a survey of the literature highlights the diversity in this area. Intraperitoneal, subcutaneous, intramuscular, intravenous, intradermal, intranasal and intraorbital (into the eye socket) routes have all been used. There is no general protocol which can suit all needs except that the final inoculation (3–4 days before removal of the spleens) should be intravenous. The reason for this is that intravenous injection of an antigen will preferentially stimulate the spleen. Although intravenous injections prior to the final inoculation will also stimulate the spleen preferentially, other lymphoid organs soon become involved. Similarly, other routes of inoculation will preferentially stimulate the draining lymph nodes, with subsequent stimulation of the spleen. This second phase of lymphoid organ stimulation is due to the antigen which has escaped from or by-passed the draining lymphoid organ. In addition, some of the stimulated lymphocytes will leave their organ of origin, and colonise other lymphoid organs. Since this subsequent stimulation takes longer to reach maximal lymphoblastosis than the initial response, a final intravenous inoculation is required to activate the spleen, if that organ is required for hybridoma generation. The relatively short delay (3–4 days) before removing the spleen is the time taken for a maximal lymphoblastogenic response.

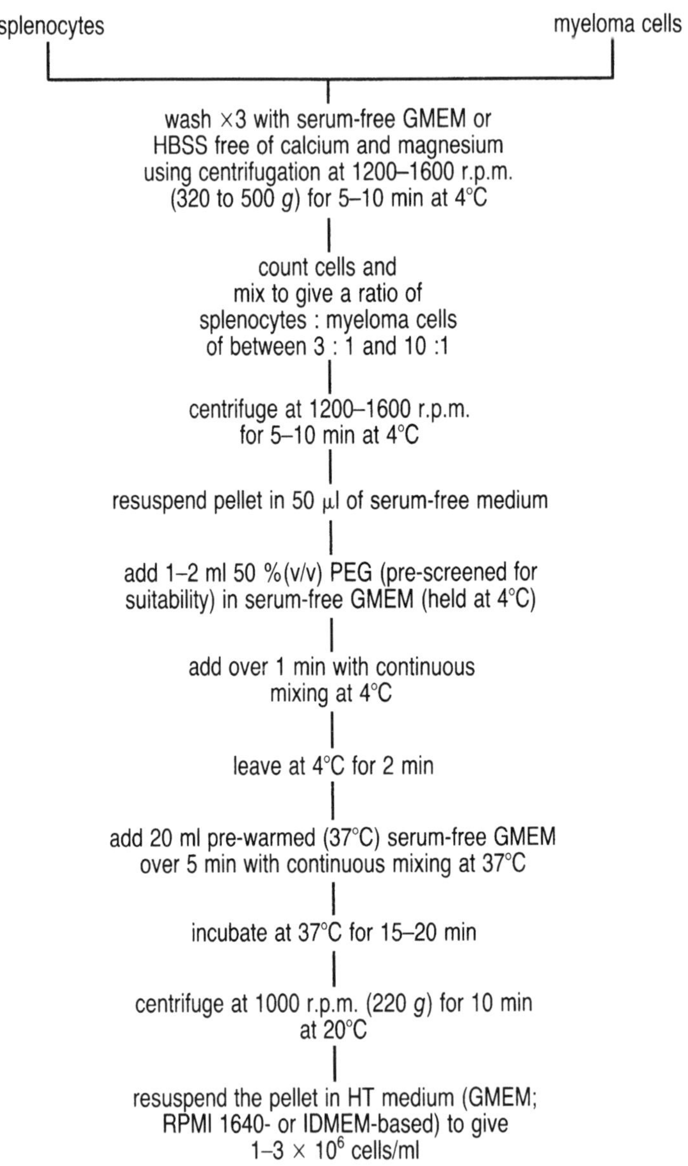

Fig. 2.9. Optimum method for the fusion of cells with polyethylene glycol (PEG).

Conversely, if lymph nodes are required as opposed to spleens, then other routes for the final inoculation should be chosen, e.g. intraperitoneal when the mesenteric and submaxillary nodes are required (Table 2.8), intradermal into the hind foot pad for the inguinal nodes. This topic of the final inoculation will be discussed further in §2.5.4.

Table 2.8. *The different routes of inoculating animals with antigen which has resulted in the subsequent generation of hybridomas, and the lymphoid organs which are preferentially stimulated*[1]

Route	Lymphoid organ stimulated
intravenous (iv)	spleen
intraperitoneal (ip)	mesenteric and submaxillary lymph nodes (also the spleen in rats)
intramuscular (im)	the draining lymph nodes (also the spleen in rats)
intradermal (id) (hind footpad)	inguinal and popliteal lymph nodes
intrasplenic[2]	spleen

Note:
[1] Although certain lymphoid organs will be preferentially stimulated, immunological memory to the antigen injected will be communicated to the other lymphoid organs; hence, ip inoculation followed, after one month, by iv inoculation will give a good memory response in the spleen of mice.
[2] This method was recently described by Spitz *et al.* (24), and from this report, the procedure has greatest application for the final boosting 3 days before removal of the spleen. Spitz *et al.* (24) surgically opened the peritoneal cavity to inoculate the spleen; it is also possible to inject the spleen without surgically opening the mouse (T.U. Obi and K.C. McCullough, unpublished data): after shaving the left side of the anaesthetised mouse, and applying 70% (v/v) methanol in water to sterilise the skin, it is possible to see the spleen through the skin and inoculate accordingly. A successful inoculation is seen by a very small amount of red-brown liquid which appears at the site of inoculation through the skin, immediately on removal of the needle.

Intranasal inoculations have been used when studying respiratory infections such as influenza virus, or the induction of IgA. The final inoculation would again have to be intravenous (if splenocytes were to be used as fusion partners). Intramuscular inoculation will stimulate both lymph nodes and spleen, subcutaneous and intradermal will pref-

Table 2.9. *Examples of different immunisation protocols used for different antigens*

Nature of immunogen	Dose of antigen	Number of inoculations	Frequency	Characterisation of MAb
potent immunogen[1] (e.g. lymphocytes)	10^6–10^7 cells or 1–10 μg	2–4	monthly or fortnightly	high titre, moderate to high affinity
moderate immunogen[1]	10–100 μg	2–4	monthly or fortnightly	moderate to high titre and affinity
weak immunogen[1] (i)	20–400 μg	2–4 then 2–3	monthly every 2–3 months	moderate titre, high affinity
(ii)	10–50 μg then 200–400 μg	2 then 4	monthly daily	moderate titre, moderate affinity
(iii)	10–100 μg	2 then 4 then rest then boost	monthly 10-day intervals 1–2 months	moderate titre, moderate to high affinity

Note:

[1] The use of the intrasplenic inoculation three days before removal of the spleens (24) can produce a more effective splenic immune response than may have been otherwise obtained. Thus, lower concentrations of antigen or cells can be used for such an immunisation.

erentially stimulate T lymphocytes, and intraorbital seems rather drastic; intravenous should suffice.

Generally, the route of inoculation is not as important as the immunisation protocol, excepting, of course, the final inoculation which must be chosen to stimulate the lymphoid organ of choice. The number and frequency of immunisations of the recipient animal can have a significant effect on the immune response; some antigens require more frequent inoculations and higher doses than others to generate enough immune splenocytes to facilitate efficient hybridoma production. The experiences of many workers has been summarised in Table 2.9. This shows the varied requirements when using antigens of different potency. Other protocols may be used, but these may generate smaller numbers of immune splenocytes which will produce antibody of lower affinity.

The general rule is that the higher the affinity required, the more 2–3 month rests should be given between inoculations. These rest periods may be reduced to 1 month early in the immunisation programme (since the intensity of the immune response can subside within 1–3 weeks). In a more immunologically-experienced animal, however, when the intensity of an immune response may take months to fall to a relatively low 'resting' level, the time between inoculations must be increased. Animals which receive these multi-boost immunisation programmes are said to be hyperimmunised.

One point should be raised about Table 2.9. When describing the derived MAb as being high affinity, this is the major proportion of the derived MAb, and the affinity is relative to other MAb and not to any antiserum. An explanation of this can be found in Chapter 1. The affinity of any selection of such derived MAb can vary considerably both between experiments and within experiments owing to the variable affinities present in different antisera. The relative proportions of MAb with a particular affinity depend on the antigen used for immunisation, the immunisation protocol and the individual animal used. No two mice will generate identical immune responses. In fact, the individual responses can vary considerably both qualitatively (specificity and affinity) and quantitatively (the relative proportions of MAb with certain specificities and affinities). Hence, two fusions using mice given the same immunisation programme may generate very different populations of MAb.

The consequence of using different immunisation schedules on the success of hybridoma production will be discussed in Chapter 3 (§3.1) and examples will be given of how particular schedules are chosen for particular antigens.

2.5.3. *Choice of immunopotentiating agents*

These factors are used to enhance a particular immune response, and among this group are the agents known as adjuvants. The choice of adjuvant depends largely on the choice of antigen. For an efficient stimulation of the immune system, an antigen probably requires 'presentation' by accessory cells (Table 2.10): the antigen-processing cells (see §1.4.4). Amongst these cells are the mononuclear phagocytes. Hence a pyrogenic substance which would stimulate the influx of phagocytes to the site of antigen inoculation should enhance this presenting phenomenon and thus prove an effective adjuvant. An example of such a pyrogenic substance is the extract of tubercle bacillus (the muramyl dipeptide sold commercially as adjuvant peptide) in Freund's complete adjuvant. Conversely, small protein antigens – the so-called 'soluble antigens' – such as adenovirus fibre antigens are poorly 'presented' when in a monomeric form, but if aggregated become more potent immunogens. In such cases, an adjuvant which would aggregate, precipitate or otherwise make the antigen more particulate would prove useful. Exam-

Table 2.10. *The different cells which have been associated with antibody production* [1]

Cell	Leukocyte type	Function
B	lymphocyte	produce antibody and memory
T_h	T lymphocyte	produce factors required for the growth and differentiation of B lymphocytes
accessory cell (antigen-presenting or APC)	macrophage, dendritic cell, Langerhans cell, astrocyte, follicular dendritic cell	present (probably after some degree of processing) antigen to the T_h lymphocyte, and probably also the B lymphocytes; also to produce factors which assist the growth and stimulation of B and T lymphocytes

Note:
[1] T_h and B lymphocytes are involved with one or maybe two types of antigen-presenting cell.

ples of such adjuvants are aluminium hydroxide, saponin and potassium alum. A list of adjuvants and their usefulness is shown in Table 2.11.

2.5.4. *The final inoculation*

Before proceeding to the next section, elaboration of this all-important final inoculation step should be made. As with the route of immunisation, the time interval of three days between the final inoculation and splenectomy is chosen to provide optimal stimulation of lymphocytes. In an anamnestic response, the resting memory B lymphocytes are rapidly induced by the stimulating antigen to differentiate into the antibody-producing plasma cells (Fig. 2.10). This is reflected in the specific antibody levels of serum which will peak at 6–8 days after inoculation. This plasma cell induction is maximal at 4–6 days after inoculation (Fig. 2.11). However, as already mentioned in §2.3.1, it is not the plasma cells but their precursors which provide the best fusion partners and the response of these cells should peak before that of the plasma cell, i.e. before 4–6 days post-inoculation. An example of when this occurs has been provided by work on diphtheria toxoid (17). With a secondary (memory) response to diphtheria toxoid injected into a rabbit's foot pad, antibody-containing cells (haemocytoblast, plasmablast and immature plasma cells, the

Table 2.11. *Adjuvants in current use*[1]

Group	Activity	Adjuvant
muramyl peptides	probably through the direct activation of macrophage and T lymphocyte functions although there is also an apparent direct enhancement of the B lymphocyte response	Freund's complete MDP MDP-derivatives: Nor MDP MDP (D-D) MDPA MDP (Ser) MDP (Abu) Murabutide Pol-PAP-MDP L18-MDP B30-MDP BH48-MDP 6-*o*-mycoloyl-MDP Quinonyl-MDP-66 MDP-Lys (L18) MTP-PE Triglymic LTP FK 156
nucleic acid derivatives	Activation of cytotoxic macrophages and NK cells; direct induction of anti-viral and immunomodulating interferons	polyribonucleotides inosiplex (isoprinosine or methisoprinol) hypoxanthine derivatives: NPT15392 NPT16416 PCF guanosine derivatives adenine derivatives pyrimidinones
sulphur containing compounds	Possibly through the induction of immunomodulating thymic hormone-like factors	levamisole sodium diethyldithiocarbamate cimetidine thiabendazole imidazothiazole derivatives 2-mercaptoethanol 2-mercaptopropionylglycine *N*-2-mercapto-2-methylpropanoyl-L-cysteine D-penicillamine

Table 2.11. *(cont.)*

Group	Activity	Adjuvant
polymers, heterocyclic and aromatic compounds	Pyrans and aziridines act on T lymphocytes and macrophages; dextran sulphate acts on Tand B lymphocytes; tilorone increases humoral responses	pyran copolymers (MVEs) NED 137 (ethylene–maleic anhydride copolymers) dextran sulphate pluronic polyols (polymers of polyoxyethylene and polyoxypropylene) aziridine derivatives: imexon azimexon tilorone
amine-containing adjuvants	Probably through the activation of macrophages, and possibly also in the induction of interferon	DDA CP-20, 961 (Avridine) CP-46, 665 CCA (Lobenzarit)
lipid-containing adjuvants	Activate macrophages, and also have an effect on granulocytes, NK cells and B lymphocytes	alykyl-lysophospholipids lipid A analogues retinoids
recombinant lymphokines and monokines	Activate or enhance the stimulation of macrophages, granulocytes, T lymphocytes, or B lymphocytes, depending on the material used.	recombinant interferons recombinant interleukins recombinant TNFs

Source:
[1] Reviewed by Arlette Adams (25).

plasma cell precursors) may be seen in germinal centres as early as 30 h (Fig. 2.12), with hundreds of these *immature* plasma cells being detected by the third day. (This is in contrast to the 5–15 cells seen at this time during a primary response.) The response progresses to a peak of *mature* plasma cell production after 5–6 days, and then rapidly declines, presumably owing to neutralisation of the antigenicity of the toxoid by circulating antibody and the opsonisation phenomena, and the short (8–12 h) life span of plasma cells. Hence the three days rest period between the final inoculation and the splenectomy is used to permit the plasma cell precursor response to reach its maximal level.

2.5.5. *Removal of immune cells*

Animals (usually mice or rats) which have been immunised with the desired antigen of choice are test bled from the tail for the presence of high

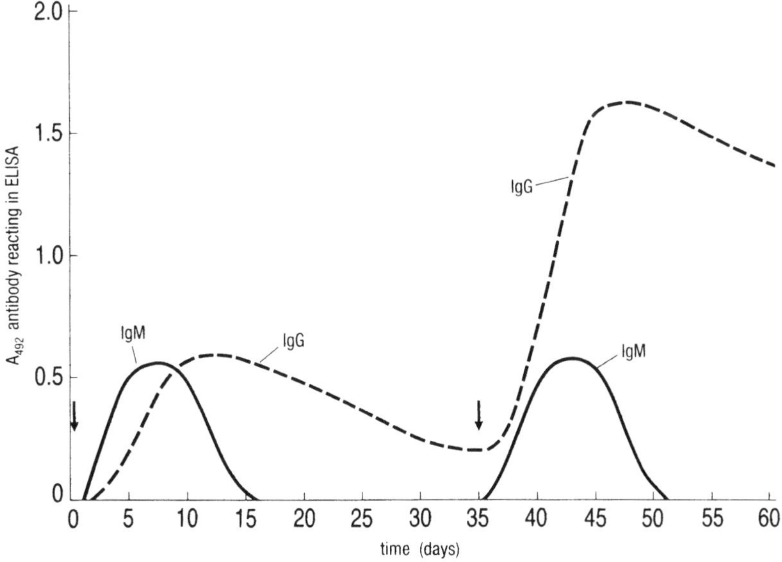

Fig. 2.10. Production *in vivo* of IgM (solid lines) and IgG (broken lines) during a primary response and secondary (anamnestic) response against antigen. The arrows indicate the times of inoculation with antigen.

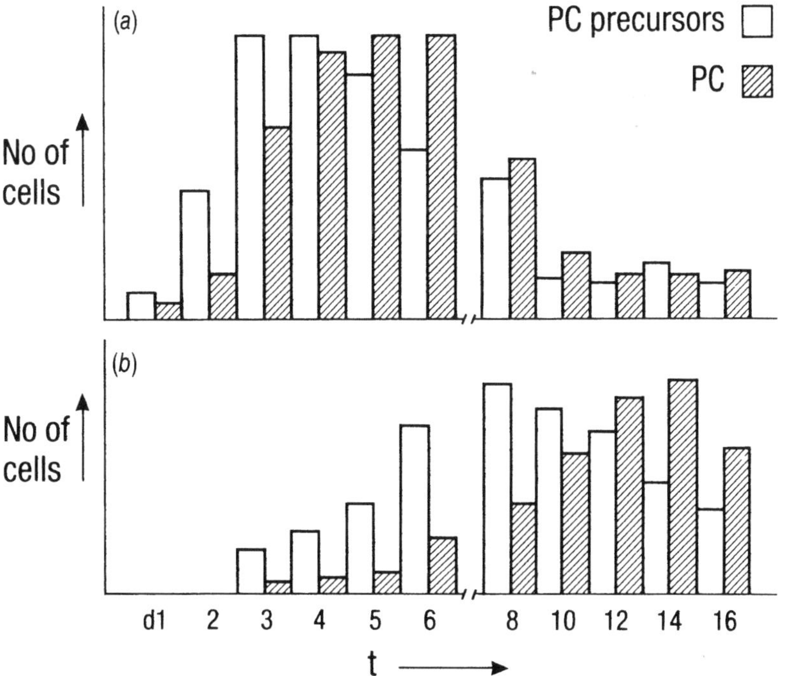

Fig. 2.11. Kinetics of production of plasma cells (PC) and PC precursors in guinea pigs during a primary (*b*) and a secondary (*a*) response against diphtheria toxin.

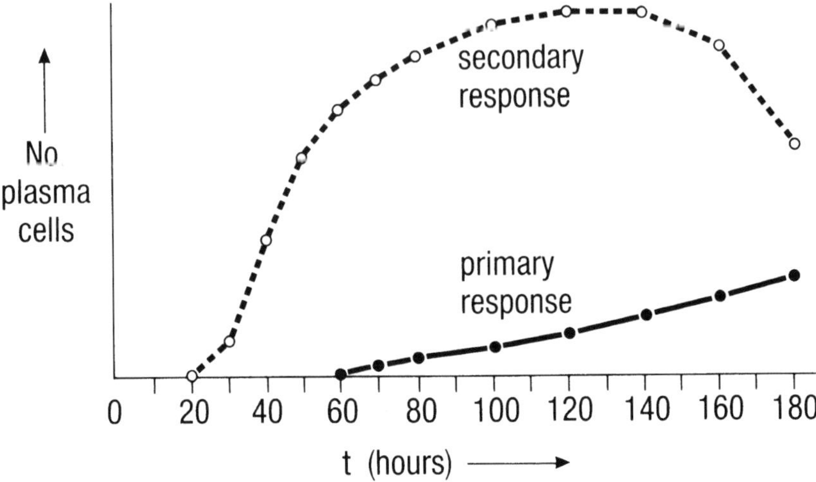

Fig. 2.12. Relative production of plasma cells with time in the draining lymph nodes after injection of antigen in a primary response (closed circles) or a secondary response (open circles).

levels of circulating antigen-specific antibody, usually 7–8 days after a booster immunisation. If the desired result is obtained, the animals are rested until the antibody response reaches a constant level (usually 14–28 days after the booster, although a subsequent immune response of higher affinity will be obtained if rested for 2–3 months) and then given their final immunisation as detailed in §2.5.2. After three days, the spleen or draining lymph nodes (draining the site of inoculation) are removed, *immediately* after killing the animal. The organ is cleaned of connective tissue, and disrupted by passing through a fine-gauge sieve or gently grinding in a loosely fitting Griffiths' tube.

Spleens are the most commonly used source of lymphocyte fusion partner. However, the spleen, unlike the lymph node, is also a 'depository' for erythrocytes and these must be removed from the splenocyte preparation (Fig. 2.13). This is achieved either by lysing with 0.83% (w/v) aqueous solution of NH_4Cl or 1:10 dilution of a balanced salt solution, or by density separation on Ficoll–Hypaque (18). This latter method is often applied when lymph nodes are used, since the erythrocytes to be lysed are only those contained within the blood vessels of the organ. Of the remaining cells, the lymphocytes are the dominant population, and it is with these that the myeloma cells preferentially fuse, as outlined in Table 2.12.

2.5.6. *Which lymphocytes produce the best hybridoma?*

Within the B lymphocyte population are the B cell blasts with variable degrees of antibody synthesis and secretion, the plasma cell being the

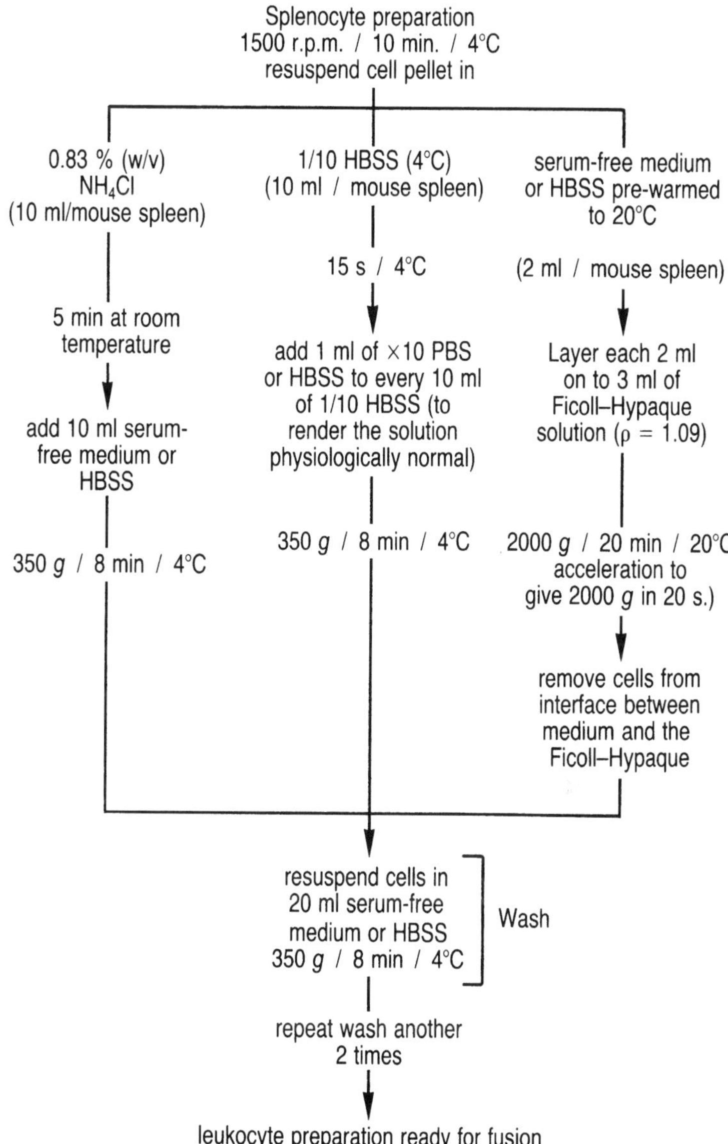

Fig. 2.13. Different methods for the removal of erythrocytes from a splenocyte preparation. HBSS, Hank's balanced salt solution.

most active producer of Ig. It therefore follows that a hybridoma of myeloma cell with plasma cell should be the most active Ig-producing hybridoma. However, it appears that these are not successful fusions, perhaps owing to the phenotype of the plasma cell: a terminal cell with a life span of only 8–12 h. The other B cell blasts are not terminal cells and hence fusions between these and myeloma cells should prove more

Table 2.12. *Probably fusion partners in hybridoma production*

Splenocytes	Fusion with myeloma cells (MC) to produce stable hybrids
phagocytes	unlikely
PMN	unlikely
DC	unlikely
epithelial cells	unlikely
T lymphocytes	low probability
B lymphocytes	high probability

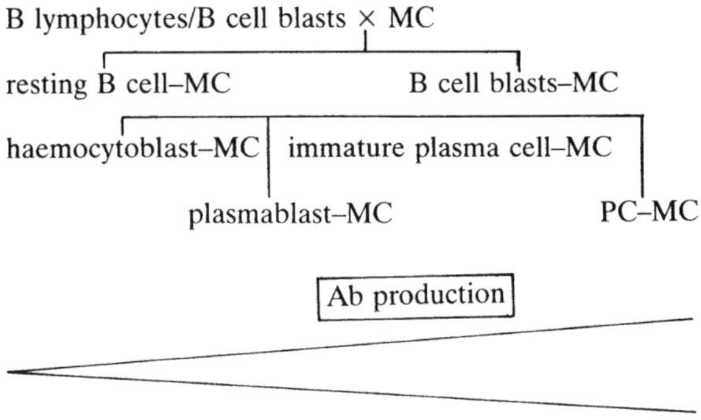

B lymphocytes/B cell blasts × MC

resting B cell–MC | B cell blasts–MC

haemocytoblast–MC | immature plasma cell–MC

plasmablast–MC | PC–MC

Ab production

stable. Considering the relative degree to which these blasts produce antibody, it might be expected that hybridomas would reflect this, with the antibody synthesis increasing from myeloma cell–haemocytoblast hybrids to myeloma cell–immature plasma cell hybrids, and myeloma cell–resting B lymphocyte hybrids being non-productive. The situation does not appear to be as straightforward as this. Milstein (16) described the situation in which a larger percentage of Ig-secreting hybridomas than expected can be produced from a fusion. Table 2.13 highlights this point by comparing immune splenocytes and hybridomas derived from such splenocytes in their Ig-secreting potential. The solution to this anomaly may rest with the myeloma cell. Milstein suggests that the myeloma cell chromosomes may de-repress the antibody-synthesising and secreting genes of the resting B lymphocyte in hybridomas of these two cells. Furthermore, it is possible that with hybrids of, for example, myeloma cells and haemocytoblasts, the myeloma cell chromosomes may enhance the normally low secretory potential of the haemocytoblast genes. This unexpectedly high frequency of efficient antibody-producing hybridomas still requires further clarification, but the relevant point with respect to

Table 2.13. *Comparison of the number of plasma cells (antibody-secreting cells) produced after an immunisation of Balb/c mice, with the number of antibody-secreting hybridomas generated with those lymphocytes*

Source of cells	Immunoglobulin specificity	% cells secreting immunoglobulin
spleen lymphocytes	antigen-specific	1
hybridomas	antigen-specific	10
spleen lymphocytes	all specificities	5
hybridomas	all specificities	25–90[1]

Note:
[1] Depending on the source of spleen cells and line of myeloma cells used.

hybridoma technology is that there is indeed a larger percentage of antibody-synthesising (and also of 'high-producing') hybridomas than can be expected from splenocyte analyses.

2.5.7. *From splenocyte to hybridoma: the alternative methods*

The majority of fusion procedures use monocellular preparations of *in vivo* stimulated splenocytes fused with myeloma cells in suspension. There are also variations on this theme (Fig. 2.14). Spleen fragments can be used after *in vitro* stimulation (19), as can *in vitro* stimulated monocellular suspensions of splenocytes; in addition to this, the fusion may be performed on a supporting matrix. Although *in vitro* stimulated splenocytes are infrequently used for generating B cell hybridomas, they are essential for the production of T cell hybridomas. Splenocytes are isolated from an immune spleen and treated *in vitro* with the polyclonal T cell mitogens phytohaemagglutinin or concanavalin A (for T cell hybridomas), the polyclonal B cell mitogens lipopolysaccharide or pokeweed mitogen (for B cell hybridomas) or the antigen of choice (for B or T cell hybridomas). Fig. 2.14 shows how these *in vitro* stimulations of splenocytes can be used for the production of hybridomas.

Alternatives to fusion in suspension have been reported by Buttin *et al.* (20). Briefly, immune lymphoid cells are prepared as for fusion in suspension (see §2.6.1), mixed with myeloma cells in serum-free medium and centrifuged on to a filter disc using a filtering centrifuge tube. The filter, carrying the cell mixture, is dipped into 45% (w/v) PEG 6000 in

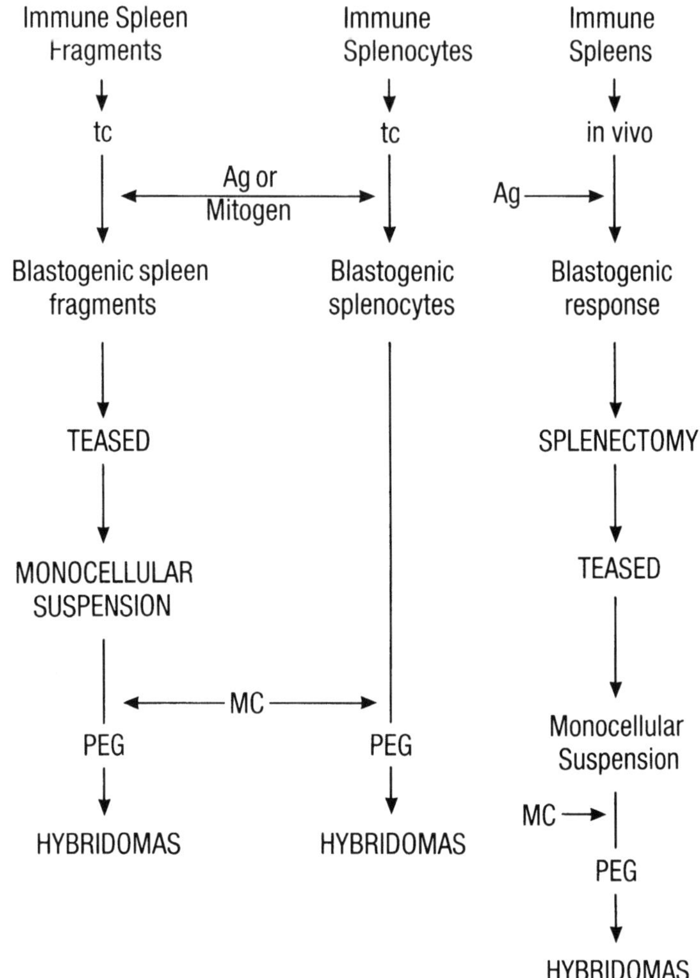

Fig. 2.14. Different methods of generating hybridomas from immune spleen fragments or immune splenocytes *in vitro* (tc, tissue culture) or immune spleens *in vivo*. Ag, antigen; MC, myeloma cells; PEG, polyethylene glycol.

serum-free medium, and then transferred to a Petri dish and incubated in serum-containing medium for 24 h at 37°C. The cells are washed from the filter and dispersed in multi-well plates; after a further 24 h incubation, hybrids are selected (HAT medium; see §§2.3.2 and 2.6.3).

The most popular method of generating B cell hybridomas utilises monocellular suspensions of splenocytes mixed with myeloma cells: the fusion is effected in suspension (21). This is the procedure which will subsequently be concentrated on; but before proceeding, consider the choice of myeloma cells. This becomes most relevant when considering the histocompatible relatedness of myeloma cells and splenocytes, since this is irrevocably associated with the success of the fusion and the relative efficiency of generating antibody-secreting hybridomas.

2.5.8. *Choice of myeloma cells*

The histocompatible relatedness of myeloma cells and splenocytes apparently has a gross influence on the stability of subsequently generated hybridomas. This histocompatibility refers to the antigenic determinants on the surface of cells which, when those cells are injected into a recipient animal not carrying such determinants on its cell surfaces, will induce an immune response. Among the inbred strains of mice in use with hybridoma technology, there are certain determinants common between some strains but not others. For instance, Balb/c mouse lymphocytes carry an H-2K determinant (b) which is distinct from the H-2K determinant (k) of C3H/HeJ and C57/Bl6 mice, whereas both Balb/c and C3H/HeJ carry a common determinant coded for by the IA region of the H-2 histocompatibility complex (IA^d) which is distinct from the IA^k of C57/Bl6 mice. The mouse myeloma cells in current use are mostly of Balb/c mouse origin. Hence, it could be imagined that owing to phenotypic, and ultimately genotypic, variation in the expression of lymphocyte determinants by the cells of different inbred strains of mice, the most efficient fusions (stable hybridomas) with these mouse myeloma cells would use Balb/c mouse lymphoid cells. But this is not so. Most fusions between the mouse myeloma cells and splenocytes from any strain of mouse, or even rats, are of fairly equivalent efficiencies. In fact, some of the most efficient fusions reported used mouse lymphoid cells and the rat Y3 myeloma cell line (see §2.4).

Generally speaking, syngeneic, allogeneic and xenogeneic fusions between closely related species (rat–mouse) are successful, producing stable hybridomas easily. Only when distantly related animal species are used (rabbit–mouse, sheep–mouse, human–mouse) are difficulties encountered, although with manipulation of the environmental conditions limited successes have been reported (4–6).

Therefore, the histocompatible relatedness of myeloma cell and lymphocyte only has a noticeable influence on the success of a fusion procedure when there are gross differences between the two cells. This instability in distantly related or unrelated xenogeneic fusions (heterohybridomas) may be due to the differences in the surface antigens of the cells, creating an unfavourable environment for successful fusion. Alternatively phenotypic parameters may not favour accommodation of the double set of chromosomes. Or the differences in the chromosomes themselves (genotypic parameters: which genes are functioning and controlling the environment of the cell?) may have the dominant influence. Apparently, these genotypic parameters may indeed have the greatest influence.

2.5.9. *The proposed genetic requirements for hybridoma stability*

Studies on the stability, or instability, of heterohybridomas have shown that failure to establish a stable antibody-secreting hybridoma is linked to the functioning of the lymphoid cell chromosomes in the presence of those of the myeloma cell. Instability is often accompanied by 'repression' of antibody synthesis or 'shedding' of the lymphoid cell chromosome. That is, the instability is related to impairment of the translation or replication of the lymphoid cell genes.

Milstein (16) proposed that myeloma cell chromosomes may 'switch on' the antibody-synthesising potential of resting B cell chromosomes in a hybridoma. In a heterohybridoma, the myeloma cell chromosomes may be inefficient or totally ineffective at regulating the lymphoid cell chromosomes. Furthermore, the replication of the lymphoid cell DNA, which relies on the cooperation of the myeloma cell genes since it is these which ultimately control the *in vitro* properties of the hybridoma, may be out of synchrony with the replication of the hybridoma cell. This may be caused by an unfavourable cellular environment produced and controlled by the myeloma cell genes. The most common cause for instability of heterohybridomas does appear to be loss of portions of, or complete, lymphoid cell chromosomes, especially those responsible for antibody synthesis and/or secretion.

2.5.10. *The use of genetically related myeloma cells and splenocytes*

With the syngeneic, allogeneic and closely related xenogeneic fusions (mouse–mouse, rat–rat, and rat–mouse), mismatched histocompatibility still has an influential role, but not on stability of the hybridoma. The success of the fusion is relatively independent of histocompatibility mismatch between these myeloma cells and splenocytes. On the contrary, problems may be encountered when ascites tumours of the hybridomas are required.

Using spleen cell donors syngeneic to the myeloma cell permits resultant hybridomas to be cultured as ascites fluids in syngeneic recipient animals. With allogeneic fusions, e.g. C57/Bl.10 mouse spleens fused with the Balb/c myeloma cells, the resultant hybridomas cannot be readily cultured in either C57/Bl.10 or Balb/c mice. The immune system of either mouse would recognise determinants on the hybridoma cell specified by the allogeneic genes as foreign, and hence reject the hybridoma. Ascites tumour induction by the hybridomas from allogeneic fusions may be overcome by using F_1 progeny of crosses between Balb/c (myeloma cell source) and the mouse strain of the splenocyte source. This reduces the efficiency with which the non-Balb/c mouse determinants on the hybridoma are recognised as foreign. But there is an additional problem.

Since the myeloma cell is a transformed (tumour) cell, the immune system of even the syngeneic Balb/c mouse would recognise the tumour-associated antigens of the myeloma cell as foreign, and again reject the hybridoma. For this reason, a minimum number of hybridoma cells must be used – usually more than 10^5 cells (see §4.5) – to overcome the immune system's tumour surveillance rejection and thus grow to produce an ascites tumour.

There are, of course, other possible solutions to these problems (Table 2.14). Firstly, nu/nu (nude) mice may be used for ascites tumour production. This strain of mouse has a congenital immunological defect, part of which is an inability to destroy tumour cells or reject tissue grafts (which in essence is what inoculation of hybridoma cells is). A second alternative solution relies on the fact that destruction and hence rejection of inoculated hybridoma cells requires activated and functional DTH and cytotoxic T lymphocytes. Whole-body irradiation (800 rads) of mice destroys most lymphocyte subpopulations (only T_h cells can be somewhat resistant). Hydrocortisone (10^{-5}M) treatment will also destroy all but the T_h subset of T lymphocytes, while thymectomy of mice can have a similar effect to these irradiation or hydrocortisone treatments. The effectiveness of thymectomy is because the thymus is the source of all immunocompetent T lymphocytes in the body, although some final differentiation and adaptation will occur outside the thymus. Removal of this organ at birth (neonatal thymectomy) impairs all immune responses which rely on T lymphocytes. With increasing age of the animal, thymectomy has reduced influence on immune responses. In fact, adult thymectomy (or even thymectomy at a few weeks after birth) has little effect since most T cells are long-lived and their effectiveness wanes gradually (over several months). There is, however, a population of short-lived T lymphocytes which are susceptible to adult thymectomy. It has been proposed from recent work on adult rat 'thymectomy' through a tin-rich diet that CTL are amongst this population of short-lived T lymphocytes (it has yet to be determined whether such animals are defective in their ability to reject tumours). If adult thymectomy could be used, this would prove more favourable than neonatal thymectomy because of the wasting disease (loss of weight, ruffled fur, oedema, diarrhoea and death) which develops within a few weeks or months of the latter operation. These alternative procedures using T cell-deficient animals would be the only method of propagating rat–mouse, rabbit–mouse, bovine–mouse, human–mouse, etc. heterohybridomas as ascites tumours.

Having determined the components required for a successful fusion, the technical procedures for producing and selecting hybridomas will now be described in more detail. The procedures for preparation of lymphocytes, fusing with myeloma cells to generate hybridomas, and

Table 2.14. *Different methods for the production of ascites tumours in mice and rats*

Source of hybridoma[1]	Method
(a) Balb/c:Balb/c	4 week-old male Balb/c + 0.5 ml Pristane intraperitoneally per mouse; leave 2 weeks, then 3×10^5 to 3×10^6 hybridoma cells in 1 ml serum-free medium interperitoneally per mouse; ascites develop in 7–14 days[2]
(b) other mouse strain: Balb/c	(i) As above under (a) (ii) use F_1 progeny of the two strains of mice, and repeat as above under (a)
(c) Balb/c or any mouse strain:Balb/c; rat:mouse; rat:rat	(i) use nu/nu mice as above under (a) (possible to reduce number of hybridomas to 10^3–10^4 cells/mouse) (ii) pre-treat mice with cyclophosphamide or 10^{-5}M hydrocortisone, then proceed as under (a) (iii) use neonatally thymectomised mice, and proceed as under (a) (iv) pretreat mice with cyclosporin A, and proceed as under (a)
(d) rat:rat	(i) if syngeneic combination, use the procedure of (a) but with syngeneic rats (ii) if allogeneic combinations, use F_1 progeny of the two strains of rat, and the procedure of (a); or use the procedures of (c)

Note:
[1] Lymphocyte source: myeloma cell origin
[2] Based on the method of Brodeur *et al.* (26) which has proven to be most effective.

the selection of those hybridomas will be described in a stepwise fashion. This 'recipe' will follow the individual steps of hybridoma technology in a consecutive manner, much as would be done experimentally. Hence, the next three sections should be considered as an experimental manual for generating hybridomas.

2.6. A practical guide to generating hybridoma cell lines

2.6.1. *Preparation of lymphocytes*

(i) Kill mice by cervical dislocation 3 days after final booster immunisation.
(ii) Lay a mouse on its right-hand side on paper towelling on a dissection board.

(iii) Soak left-hand side (now uppermost) with 70% (v/v) methanol in water.

(iv) Using sterile instruments lift skin in midregion of left-hand side and make a small incision.

(v) Pull the skin apart exposing the peritoneum, through which can be seen the spleen (dark red organ 0.5–1.0 cm wide by 1.5–3.0 cm long in most strains of mice) lying along the posterior and dorsal sides of the stomach.

(vi) Swab peritoneum with 70% (v/v) methanol. Using fresh sterile instruments, make an incision in the peritoneum over the spleen wide enough to remove it (about 4–5 cm). Lift the spleen with the forceps, and trim off the white connective tissue which will free it and permit removal. Place the spleen in 5 ml serum-free RPMI 1640 medium or DMEM on ice.

(vii) The spleen is disrupted by (a) teasing apart with 21-gauge needles; (b) grinding through a fine mesh stainless steel grid (sterilised by autoclaving) and washing through 5 times with 1 ml cold medium; (c) gentle grinding (2–3 'half circumference' turns of the plunger) in the 5 ml of medium in a Griffith's tube.

(viii) Transfer the suspension to a centrifuge tube. Leave on ice for 5 min and remove the cell suspension from the larger spleen fragments which have now settled to the bottom of the tube.

(ix) Centrifuge the cell suspension at 250 *g* for 5 min.

(x) Remove and discard the supernatant and resuspend the cells firstly in 1 ml of 0.83% (w/v) NH_4Cl in water (sterilised by filtration through a 0.2 μm filter) and then make up to 10 ml with NH_4Cl. Leave on ice for 5 min. This lyses the red blood cells. An alternative is to layer the cells (resuspended in medium) onto Histopaque 1088 (Sigma) and centrifuge at 400 *g* for 30 min. The red blood cells migrate to the lower third of the gradient and the lymphocytes and monocytes will be found at the interface between the medium and the Histopaque.

(xi) Add 10 ml per spleen of cold serum-free medium to the lymphocytes (either in the NH_4Cl or their fraction of the Histopaque gradient). Centrifuge at 250 *g* (350 *g* for Histopaque fractions) for 10 min.

(xii) Remove and discard the supernatant and wash the cells (resuspend in 1 ml *serum free* medium, make up to 10 ml with this medium and centrifuge at 250 *g* for 10 min) three times. It is important to remove serum protein from both myeloma and lymphoid cells since it is the interaction of serum with polyethylene glycol-treated cells which stimulates completion of intermembrane fusion.

It should also be noted that the myeloma cells must be actively growing. To achieve this, the cells are subcultured to give a density of 2–3 × 10^5 cells/ml on the day before the fusion, when they are again subcultured to a density of 1 × 10^5 cells/ml (usually a 1 : 2 split will suffice). After a further 24 h at 37 °C the cells will be ready for fusion.

2.6.2. *Fusion*

(i) Count lymphoid and myeloma cells in a haemocytometer counting chamber. (Viability of the lymphoid cells can vary between 50% to 90%, but should be more than 80% under normal circumstances. The viability of the myeloma cells *must* be greater than 90%.)

(ii) Mix lymphoid cells with the myeloma cells at a ratio of 5 lymphoid cells : 1 myeloma cell (although ratios can vary from 10 : 1 to 1 : 1; see §3.4) in serum-free medium in a sterile 20–50 ml conical centrifuge tube and centrifuge at 250 *g* for 5 min.

(iii) Remove all but 50–100 μl of the supernatant (simply pour off the medium; this will leave about 100 μl in the tube) and gently resuspend the cells in this by tapping the bottom of the tube with the fingers.

(iv) Liquify polyethylene glycol by heating to 100 °C in a boiling water bath (several batches of different sources and molecular masses should be tested for the batch yielding the most efficient fusion, or purchase the PEG 'tissue culture reagent' from Sigma, no. P2906; the influence of the source of PEG on successful fusion will be dealt with in more detail in Chapter 3 (§3.3)). While held at a temperature of over 70 °C, dispense the liquid in 1.5 ml aliquots in 5 ml glass bottles. These aliquots may be sterilised by autoclaving at 15 lbf/in^2* for 15 min but this is found to be unnecessary if the aliquot dispensing is performed aseptically; some recent unpublished work (N. Pringle of UCL; R.N. Butcher & K.C. McCullough) suggests that autoclaving can be detrimental to the efficacy and non-toxicity of PEG in the subsequent fusion procedure. These PEG aliquots are stored at 4 °C.

(v) When required, heat an aliquot of the now solid PEG, again using a boiling water bath. Remove the liquid PEG from the water bath and add an equal volume of pre-warmed (37 °C) serum-free medium *immediately* with rapid vigorous mixing to prevent the PEG from re-solidifying. Place this in a 37 °C water bath. When the splenocyte–myeloma cell pellet is ready – see (iii) – 1 ml of the 50% (v/v) PEG in serum-free medium may be added *slowly* (dropwise) over 1 min at 37 °C with constant

* 1 lbf/in^2 ≈ 703 kg/m^2.

shaking. This is regarded as the classical procedure. Recent modifications have proven the following to be more effective: after mixing the PEG and medium, cool this 50% (v/v) PEG in an ice-bath; add 1–2 ml slowly to the splenocyte/myeloma cell mixture over 1 min with constant shaking in the ice-bath.

(vi) In the classical procedure, the reaction mixture is left for another minute at 37 °C, and then 10 ml serum-free medium is added over 5 min at 37 °C with constant shaking. Again recent modifications have proven the following to be more effective: hold the reaction mixture in the ice-bath for 1–2 min, then add 20 ml pre-warmed (37 °C) serum-free medium over 5 min *at 37 °C* with constant shaking. Leave the mixture at 37 °C for 15–20 min. The reasons for these alterations in the classical procedure are (a) PEG (and DMSO, which is often used as a 10% v/v supplement to the 50% v/v PEG) is least toxic at 4 °C; (b) PEG at 4 °C most efficiently induces membrane bridging and communication over a 2–3 minute period; (c) warming to 37 °C with concomitant dilution in serum-free medium promotes the progression of intercytoplasmic bridging towards completion, which is about 80–90% complete within 15–20 minutes, and 100% complete by 4 h (4 h is too long to leave these cells under these conditions to obtain successful hybridoma production). For a more extensive explanation, see the review by Westerwoudt (21).

(vii) Centrifuge the reaction mixture at 200 *g* for 10 min. The supernatant medium is then removed and the cells re-suspended in a volume of RPMI 1640 medium or DMEM containing 10% (v/v) foetal calf serum, hypoxanthine and thymidine (HT medium) to give 10^6 splenocytes/ml and 10^6–10^5 myeloma cells/ml (the number of myeloma cells depends on the fusion ratio). The presence of the serum induces completion of the fusion between adjacent PEG-treated cells. The reasons for this are still poorly understood, but it appears that the procedures (v) and (vi) result in intercytoplasmic communication between cells without complete exchange of cytoplasmic proteins. The completion of this exchange occurs after serum is added, resulting in the cytoplasmic mixing which produces single cells with two nuclei from two cells. On cell division, the nuclear membranes break down for chromosomal replication, and it is at this point that the chromosome mixing occurs. Should this be an inefficient process, or should the division of the two nuclei be out of synchrony, then the hybridomas will be regarded as unstable (suffering from 'chromosomal loss').

It should be noted that although PEG is now the fusing agent of choice, the original fusing agent was inactivated Sendai virus. There are several groups of viruses, one of which is the Paramyxoviridae, which induce intercellular fusion in infected cells. Sendai virus is a paramyxovirus, and another characteristic of such viruses is that of 'fusion from without'. If a high ratio of virus particles to cells is used, the cells are induced to fuse. This is a purely chemical reaction since virus viability is not required. Hence, inactivated Sendai virus was used to induce cell fusion in the early days of hybridoma technology. However, some cells could not be fused because they lacked receptors for the Sendai virus fusion protein. This fusion agent has now been superseded by PEG.

Having fused the splenocytes with the myeloma cells, selection of hybrid cells is now required. Since splenocytes which have not fused with myeloma cells have a relatively short finite life *in vitro*, the selection procedures concentrate on removing myeloma cells which have not fused with splenocytes.

2.6.3. *Selection of hybridomas* (Fig. 2.15)

(i) After resuspending the PEG-treated cell mixture in HTmedium, plate 1 ml of the fused cells into each well of 6 × 4 well plates (14) in which 2–10 × 10^4 syngeneic macrophages or 2 ×10^4 mitomycin C-treated 3T3/B (3T3/A31) cells have been cultured for 3–5 days (see §§3.7.3 and 3.7.5).

(ii) After incubation for 24 h at 37 °C in a humidified atmosphere, add 100 μl of × 10 concentration of aminopterin (ten times that which will be in the medium feeding the cells in the wells) in HT medium to each well (1 ml). This final concentration of aminopterin will kill unfused myeloma cells within a few hours.

(iii) Incubate the cultures at 37 °C for 7 days. During this time, the majority of unfused splenocytes will die, although a large proportion may survive for 2 or 3 weeks. The longest time span for longevity of B lymphocytes *in vitro* is 6 weeks. It is only the B lymphocytes which are of relevance here, since these might secrete antibody which would give a false impression of the antibody productivity of a culture. Thus, the presence of splenocyte-derived antibody in the culture fluid of recently generated hybridomas can pose a problem. IgG has a half-life of 15–20 days, with that of IgM and IgA being 5–6 days. Hence, the splenocyte antibody must be removed to permit a more accurate detection of hybridoma-secreted antibody. In addition, the few growing hybridomas per millilitre of fusion mixture (usually in the range of 3–10 for different fusion partners under optimal conditions) are very sensitive to environmental conditions. All media must therefore be maintained at pH 6.8–7.2, and the cultures left undisturbed for 7 days. The culture medium pH should not become too acidic in this time.

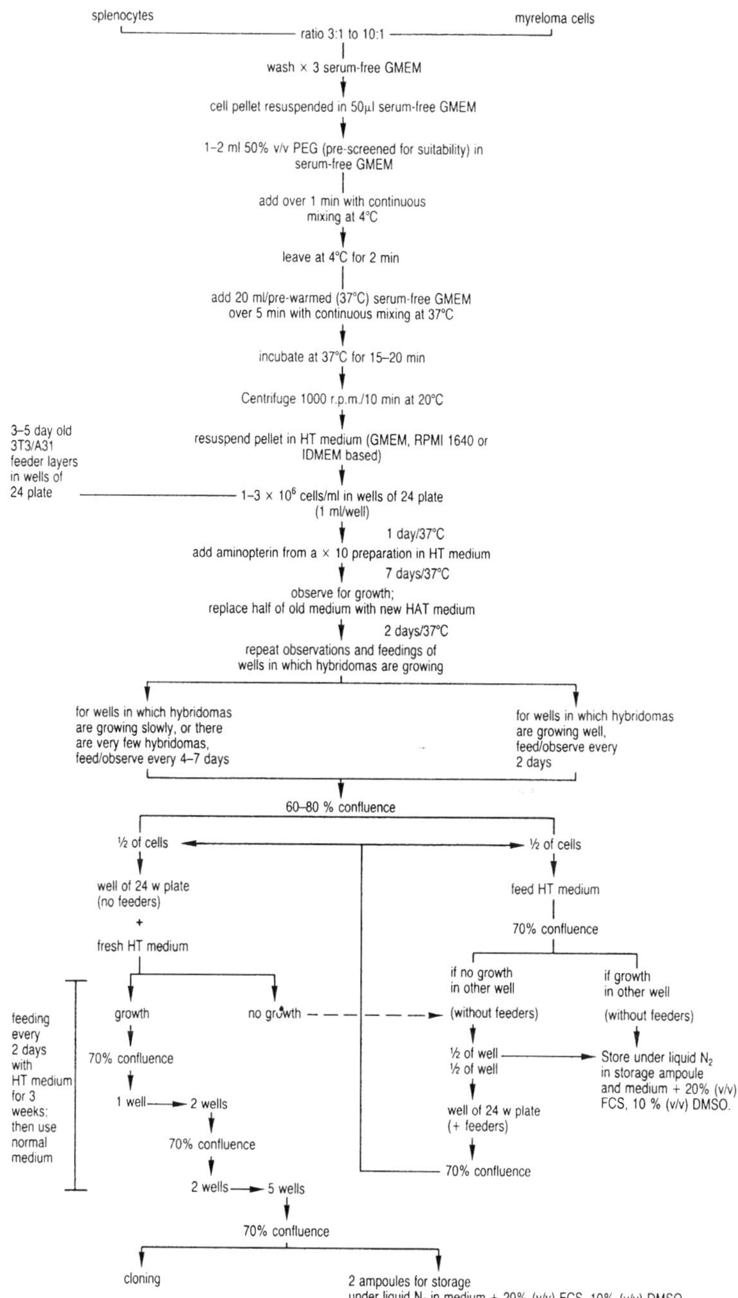

Fig. 2.15. Flow diagram of the selection of hybridomas after fusion. MC, myeloma cells; PEG, polyethylene glycol; 24W/3T3 (feeders), 24-well plates (6 × 4 wells) with feeder layers of 3T3/A31 cells; 1 : 2, dilution factor for the cells (1 well to 2 wells or ½ well to 1 well); N_2, liquid nitrogen storage.

(iv) At 7 days, replace half the medium with fresh HAT medium. This has a dual function. It dilutes the splenocyte antibody and stimulates more vigorous growth of the hybridomas (probably through the removal of toxic metabolites and replacing 'spent' serum factors and glutamine, the activity of which is considerably reduced after 3–4 days at 37 °C).

(v) Perform further feedings as described in (iv), normally every 2–3 days until the hybridoma cells require subculture. This is best achieved when the cells cover 70% of the growing surface. The first subculture is effected by resuspending the cells and transferring half of this suspension to another well of a 6 × 4 well (24 w) plate and feeding both wells with half of the original volume of fresh HAT medium or HT medium. Through such feedings and subcultures using the HT medium, aminopterin will be removed from the medium. Hence, enough changes with HT medium (normally 7–10) are performed to ensure this, and then the cells are given one further subculture in HT medium to ensure that no intracytoplasmic aminopterin remains.

(vii) If that first subculture mentioned in (v) is unsuccessful, culture the remaining cells on the feeder layers in the 'masterplates' (plates seeded with the original fusion mixture) until they again cover 70% of the growing surface. Subculture again, but this time plate half of the cells into wells of 6 × 4 well plates containing fresh feeder layers. When these cells grow to cover 70% of the growing surface, subculture into wells without feeder layers as described under (v). If these cells (without feeders) again fail to grow, repeat the procedure with feeder layers, using the healthiest-looking cultures, until they will grow without feeder cells. Hybridoma cells must be capable of growing without feeder layers to ensure success with cloning these cells and recovery from liquid nitrogen storage, when feeder cells are again used (hybridoma cells which can grow in the absence of feeder layers will get the full benefit of the feeders in the cloning or recovery from liquid nitrogen procedures).

(viii) When the cells can be passaged without feeder layers, give one further subculture and store in liquid nitrogen or clone (see §§4.2 and 4.3). A typical routine is shown in Fig. 2.15. This is an ideal, rapid and efficient routine of subculture, but there are variations which will be dealt with in §3.8.

(ix) There is one other parameter which must be considered: the production of specific antibody. Among the fusion products will be hybridomas which are non-producers, poor (and probably unstable) producers, producers of antibody which is not reactive against the antigen of choice, and the stable antigen-specific antibody producers. Therefore, screen cultures 10–14 days after fusion (when splenocyte antibody has been diluted by two feedings) for the presence of antigen-specific antibody (see §4.1).

(x) Discard non-producing cultures. Those producing low levels of antibody (taking into account the number of hybridoma cells present) are also discarded since such low levels of antibody often reflect residual splenocyte antibody, unstable hybridomas, or a very low percentage of antibody-secreting hybridomas which would very soon be overgrown by the non-producing cells.

(xi) Select those cultures secreting at least moderate amounts of antibody (usually to a titre of $\frac{1}{20}$ by ELISA for a culture in which the cells cover about 25% of the growing surface) for continued passage.

(xii) After the first two passages, test these cultures again for specific antibody. Those cultures secreting the highest titres of antibody are usually the most stable, contain relatively large proportions of antibody-secreting cells and are therefore the best choice for successful cloning.

One final point which should be made about the unfused splenocytes which can be found in hybridoma cultures. The undesirability of unfused B lymphocytes in these cultures has been mentioned, but the short life span of these cells *in vitro* solves that problem. T lymphocytes and monocytes can, on the other hand, have greater longevity *in vitro*. This can prove advantageous since these cells may continue to provide growth factors. There are the 'general growth-promoting substances' which can be provided by both lymphocyte–monocyte cultures and endothelial–fibroblast cells. In addition there are the more specific substances: B cell growth and maturation factors (BCGF, BCMF), T cell growth factor (TCGF or interleukin 2; will help the helpers, so to speak) and other lymphokines and monokines. Hence, the presence of contaminating T lymphocytes and monocytes is usually beneficial to the success of the hybridoma cultures. The same can be said of the contaminating cells in the peritoneal washings of mice, which are used as sources of the macrophage feeder layers. These contaminating cells are mainly T lymphocytes and monocytes. For this reason, the peritoneal exudate feeder layers are not washed vigorously to remove non-adherent cells. (Although they are a mixture of lymphocytes, macrophages and monocytes, they are often referred to as macrophage feeder layers. More accurately they should be termed PEC feeders.)

2.7. Types of hybridoma cell line

This chapter has so far dealt exclusively with hybridomas of B lymphocytes and myeloma cells. These are the major fusion products when splenocytes and myeloma cells are used. Viable hybrids of T lymphocytes with myeloma cells are apparently more rare, probably reflecting the closer ancestry of myeloma cells with B lymphocytes. Thus, the T lymphocytes should display greater genotypic and phenotypic differences from myeloma cells than should the B lymphocytes. These factors may influence the efficiency of fusion and/or the stability of the hybrids. In addition, the detection of the antibody produced by B cell–myeloma cell hybrids is relatively easy compared with the detection of hybridoma products specified by T lymphocyte chromosomes. These T cell products are the helper and suppressor factors which are detected through their ability to help or suppress an antigen-driven B lymphocyte response *in vitro* (see §§1.4.5 and 1.4.6) or the cytotoxic mechanisms of cytotoxic T lymphocytes (CTL or T_c).

Despite these greater difficulties in detecting T lymphocyte products, there are methods for producing T cell hybridomas equivalent to the B cell–myeloma cell hybrid. Just as the myeloma cells are lymphoblastoid (transformed lymphocyte) B cells – the myeloma cell being a transformed plasma cell – there are lymphoblastoid T cell lines available, which can be used efficiently to produce T cell hybridomas. The methodology for the generation of these has certain differences from that for B cell hybridomas, although the T cell hybridoma procedures could be applied to both systems. The major difference lies in the induction of cycles of T cell blastogenesis before attempted hybridoma generation, and it is this procedure which is central to the success of T cell hybridoma production. An example of the methodology is shown in Fig. 2.16.

2.7.1. *Generation of T cell hybridomas*

Immune lymphocytes and accessory cells are isolated and cultured *in vitro* (18). The accessory cells are an obligate requirement, since it is the Ia-bearing macrophages and dendritic cells which will present antigen and/or T cell mitogens such as concanavalin A (Con A) to the T lymphocytes. When using Con A, whole splenocyte populations may be used since only T cells will respond (the resultant stimulated population is referred to as 'Con A blasts'). If antigen is incorporated into the culture medium, the splenocytes must be depleted of B cells (treated with anti-Ig serum and complement (22)) because these would also respond. B cells should be less efficient than T lymphocytes at fusing with T lymphoblastoid cells to yield stable hybridomas, but B cells are removed in order to increase the frequency of T lymphocyte–lymphoblastoid cell fusions. In such B cell depleted cultures both Con A and antigen may be used together to produce a more intense antigen-specific T cell blastogenic response. However, for the production of certain types of T cell hybridoma, Con A is the more desirable of the two reagents. It can stimulate

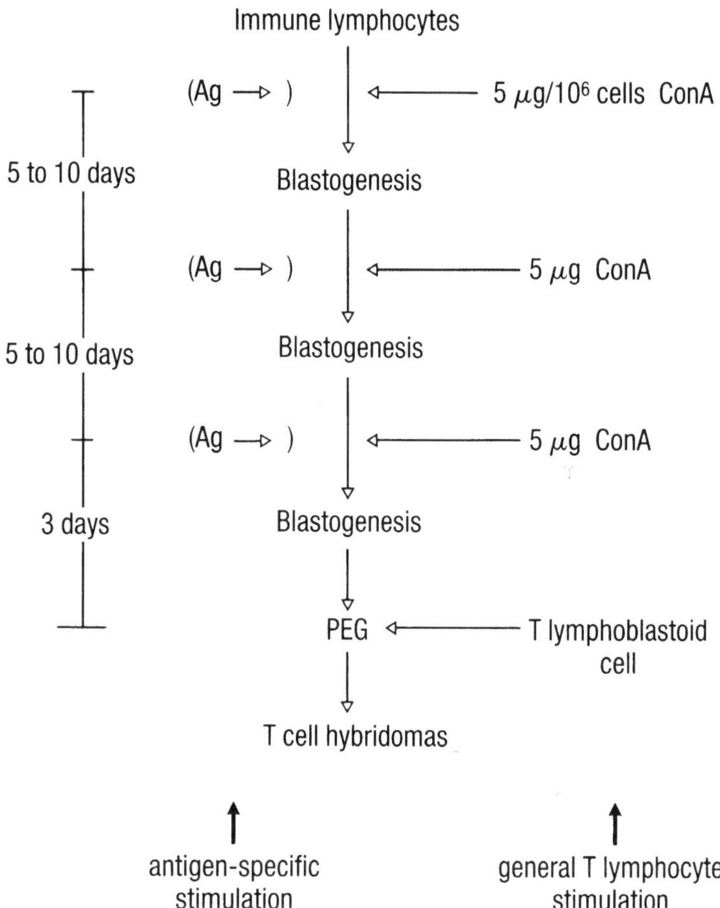

Fig. 2.16. The generation of T cell lymphoblasts *in vitro* for use in fusion with a T lymphoblastoid cell line to produce T cell hybridomas. Ag, antigens; ConA, concanavalin A.

both the non-antigen-specific and antigen-specific T_h and T_s cells, in addition to the antigen-specific T_c and DTH (T_d) cells which would recognise antigen only in association with MHC Class I antigens. In addition, dependent on the dose of antigen used, a preferential stimulation of either helper or suppressor T cell subjects might ensue, a problem also found but more controllable when Con A is used. But the disadvantage with Con A is that it will also stimulate the unwanted populations of T cells, such as those with antigen specifications other than the desired ones. The major advantage of Con A-stimulated cells is that the proportion of resultant hybridomas which secrete cytokines will be higher than with antigen alone; or at least the generation of such hybridomas will be more readily and consistently achieved by using Con A blasts.

T cell hybridomas have, in the main, been generated for the production of monoclonal helper and suppressor factors. The procedure has not been as widely used as with B cell hybridoma production. This is due to a number of considerations. Firstly, there is the difficulty in testing for T cell factors relative to the ease with which antibody produced by B cell hybridomas is detected. Secondly, the generation of hybridomas of functionally active cytotoxic T cell systems (T_c, T_d, NK cell (humans)) has met with little success (or apparently so, to judge from lack of published reports). This may be due to these cells actually destroying the T lymphoblastoid fusion partner, since a function of T_c is the destruction of transformed cells. Finally, and most pertinently, the functionally active B lymphocyte – the antibody-producing cell or plasma cell – is a terminal cell with a life expectancy of 24–72 h. The functionally active T lymphocytes are not terminal cells. When the T_c precursors are stimulated in the presence of T_h cells and T_A (T amplifier) cells, the T_c into which they differentiate are relatively stable and long-lived. In the presence of irradiated spleen cells or interleukin 2 these T_c can be cloned and cultured, sometimes for several months or even years. Thus, T cell hybridomas do not have the obligate requirement or universal applicability which B cell hybridomas have, and where T cell hybridomas can be produced the detection of the factors they produce can often be difficult.

2.8. Summary

The generation of B cell hybridomas, and hence the antibody they produce, is now a well-established routine. One of the basic constituents – the myeloma cells – is readily available for rodent systems, and to a lesser degree for human systems, although myeloma cells from other species may be generated. As opposed to myeloma cells, another lymphoblastoid B cell line – Epstein–Barr virus (EBV)-transformed human B lymphocytes – may be used for generating human homohybridomas (3). Similar lymphoblastoid B cell lines may be generated for other animal species using the appropriate lymphotrophic leukaemia virus.

The other fusion partner, the splenocyte, must be generated for each fusion; of these the B lymphoblast precursors of the plasma cell are probably the most ideal. Efficient induction of antigen-specific B lymphoblasts (immunisation) will vary for different antigens, but the most important factor is that the final inoculation should be given intravenously three days before removal of the immune spleen.

Fusion procedures can also vary. The most widely used is the PEG-induced serum-dependent fusion of monocellular suspensions of immune splenocytes and myeloma cells.

Selection procedures rely on the fact that unfused splenocytes normally die after 2–4 weeks *in vitro*, whereas unfused myeloma cells are destroyed by virtue of their aminopterin sensitivity through the use of selective media containing aminopterin. Splenocytes and splenocyte–myeloma cell hybrids (the hybridomas) are aminopterin-resistant provided hypoxanthine is supplied in the medium, since the presence of splenocyte chromosomes permits the use of hypoxanthine to bypass the aminopterin block of purine–pyrimidine biosynthesis.

A stepwise description of the preparation of cells, fusion and selection of hybridomas is provided in this chapter, but this does not deal adequately with the environmental requirements of hybridomas. Nor does it consider the requirements of cloning, an essential procedure without which the *monoclonal* hybridoma, and hence its so-called 'monoclonal antibody' cannot be obtained. The next three chapters will therefore deal with these questions of environmental requirements and hybridoma cloning in detail.

3 Factors affecting successful hybridoma production

In Chapter 2, the theory of hybridoma generation was described, and the variation in methodology used was discussed. The procedures for the production of hybridomas may differ substantially for different antigens; §2.5.2 showed how the immunisation schedule used for one antigen may not be optimal for another. The use of different myeloma cell lines can also produce different results (see §2.5.8). Thus, the determination of the optimal conditions for generating hybridomas against a particular antigen is central to the success of the technology. Chapter 3 will expand on the discussion of Chapter 2 concerning factors which are influential in the successful generation of hybridomas.

The use of different immunisation protocols for different antigens and how these influence the type of immune response generated was introduced in Chapter 2 (§2.5.2). In this chapter, §3.1 will look at the relative efficacy of different immunisation schedules, and the reasoning behind choosing a particular protocol for a particular antigen. Chapter 2 identified the major influential factors in the fusion event as the myeloma cell, the fusing agent (usually PEG) and the fusion ratio. How the source of myeloma cell, source of PEG and fusion ratio can influence the success of hybridoma production will be discussed in this chapter (§§3.2–3.4), since the physical generation of hybridomas is probably the most important, sensitive and delicate of the *in vitro* steps. For fusion to occur, cell membrane structure must be drastically altered, and thus slight variations in the toxicity of the fusing agent can be detrimental to the success of generating hybridomas. Likewise, the fusion ratio (splenocytes : myeloma cells) must be such as to guarantee fusion between myeloma cells and some antigen-specific lymphocytes.

Once hybridomas have been generated, these cells require relatively strictly defined media owing to the adverse environment in which they find themselves. The culture media must therefore be capable of providing all the necessary factors to permit stabilisation of the hybridoma cell, recovery from the fusion event and eventual adaptation to, and growth under *in vitro* culture conditions. This will be the area covered in §3.5; §3.6 will mention the influence of pH, oxygen tension and the degree of physical stress and movement, which will be discussed in more detail in Chapter 5.

There are other biological criteria for the success of hybridoma technology, namely the provision of growth factors and/or feeder layers. Intrinsically related to the effectiveness of these is the fusion ratio. Too many splenocytes, and the myeloma cells will have a low probability of fusing with the desired lymphocyte. Conversely, too many myeloma cells, and the largest proportion of hybridomas (and hence the more likely to be isolated) will either be non-secretors or produce antibody of undesired characteristics. An excess of myeloma cells will also result in too few unfused splenic monocytes and lymphocytes in a culture to provide adequate growth factors for successful recovery and growth of hybridomas. However, even under optimum conditions of fusion, the number of hybridomas generated is low. It is under such conditions that feeder layers become relevant. After fusion, the concentration of hybridoma cells is too low to yield the required levels of growth factors normally produced when cells of a semi-confluent culture assist one another. These hybridomas are also recovering from the adverse conditions engendered by the fusion procedure. The use of the correct concentration and correct type of feeder layer is intended to overcome these inadequacies in a recently fused myeloma cell – splenocyte mixture; the feeder layer is manipulated to assist the growth of the hybridoma until the latter can support itself. This topic of feeder layers and growth factors will be covered in §3.7.

Once the hybridomas have been established, many of the more difficult manipulations will have been overcome. However, without the correct culturing protocol (§3.8), successful maintenance of the hybridomas is difficult. For example, the densities at which hybridoma cells should grow are strictly defined. Too low a density and the culture fails owing to lack of growth factors. Too high a density, and the viability and ease of passage of the culture decreases rapidly, owing to high competition of nutrients, production of toxic levels of waste metabolites, and self-regulation of growth. The latter results in the reduction of the rate of cell division, producing the stationary phase of a cell replicative cycle. It is most important that this phase should be avoided when culturing hybridomas, because some hybridoma cells do not re-enter an exponential phase, and others can show altered properties (such as antibody non-secretion) after experiencing a stationary phase. Indeed, myeloma cells can show altered properties with respect to their efficiency as fusion partners after they have entered a stationary phase.

These major influences on hybridoma technology will now be described in more detail, with the ultimate goal of facile and rapid generation and maintenance of hybridomas producing antibody of the desired characteristics.

3.1. Efficacy of immunisation

Sections 2.5.1–2.5.3 described the variability of immunisation protocols, and how these can govern the characteristics of the immune response and ultimately the MAb produced through hybridoma technology. The one universal aspect of these immunisation programmes is the use of an intravenous booster inoculation, three days before splenectomy. In §§2.5.2 and 2.5.4, the reasons for this are detailed.

Although certain antigens, such as whole cells, require a particular immunisation route and routine, most protein antigens can be administered by the same route, e.g. intraperitoneally or intravenously for the stimulation of IgG-producing splenic lymphocytes. The efficiency of the immunisation is dependent on the efficacy of the immune system at recognising that injected antigen as foreign and, as a result, stimulating large enough numbers of antigen-specific cells. For hybridoma technology, it is often desirable not only to generate large numbers of antigen-specific cells, but also that these cells should be efficient at recognising antigen (relatively high affinity). Concerning MAb, it is the B lymphocytes which are of direct relevance to hybridoma technology. If the immunisation protocol is inefficient, few antigen-specific B lymphocytes will be generated, and those which are produced are more likely to have receptors of low affinity for the antigen. When hybridomas secreting high concentrations of high affinity (strong binding) antibody are required, a large number of B lymphocytes with receptors of high affinity for antigen are required. The failure of some antigens to generate these hybridomas, with immunisation protocols which are perfectly adequate for other antigens, is often due to the nature of the antigen. For example, when attempts are made to generate anti-idiotope antibody (see §6.6) in syngeneic or allogeneic (with respect to the inducing idiotope-bearing molecule) recipient animals, only a few determinants on the immunising proteins will be recognised as foreign. Hence, much larger concentrations of such proteins than those which bear a large number of 'foreign' determinants are required to effectively stimulate an immune response against them. That is, more of these 'low determinant density' proteins are needed for these determinants to reach immunogenic levels.

The 'solubility' (in an immunological sense) of antigens also influences their efficacy as stimulators of an immune response. The term 'soluble' is used to differentiate certain antigens from those which are described as 'particulate'. For example, small proteins such as bovine gamma globulins can be aggregated by heating. These aggregates are referred to as particulate, while the natural globulins are said to be soluble. The soluble antigen is in fact an antigen of relatively low molecular mass, and the particulate antigen has a higher molecular mass. Generally speaking, the lower the molecular mass (the more 'soluble'), the weaker the protein is as a stimulator of an immune response (it is said to be less antigenic). There are, of course, exceptions such as keyhole limpet haemocyanin, which is an extremely potent antigen (highly antigenic) with a relatively (with respect to other less potent antigens) low molecular mass. Thus, the structure of antigens is also of importance, and this comes to the fore when using small viruses as immunogens (an immunogen is an antigen which stimulates a protective immune response, e.g. against viruses, bacteria, yeast, parasites or toxins).

When a protein or pathogen is found to be a poor antigen or immunogen, three possible solutions have been reported. Two of these deal with low molecular mass or 'soluble' proteins, and the third with small viruses as exemplified by the picornavirus foot-and-mouth disease virus (FMDV).

In the first procedure Stähli *et al.* (1) used a multi-boost immunisation programme with large concentrations of antigens (Table 3.1). These authors showed that human chorionic gonadotrophin (HCG) stimulation of a mouse spleen by the immunisation protocol of earlier reports (priming followed by one or two boosts) was relatively ineffective. Similarly, increasing the dose of antigen given or the number of inoculations did not have a significant influence on the stimulation of the spleens. Conversely, combinations of large doses of antigen with multiple inoculations over a short period of time did induce a relatively high percentage of antigen-reactive lymphocytes in the spleen, as determined by the frequency of antigen-specific antibody-producing hybridomas subsequently generated. An important aspect of the immunisations was the administration of 1 μg antigen three days before the four daily 200–400 μg inoculations. This procedure 'fooled' the immune system into responding through plasma cell production for longer and at higher intensity (less energy devoted to memory production) by increasing the duration of free, 'non-neutralised' (potentially 'harmful') antigen in the circulation. In theory, this procedure could be used for a number of, if not all, antigens. Different concentrations would be required for different antigens, such that the concentrations at which preferential stimulation of suppressor circuits occurs were not attained.

For the second procedure, Russell *et al.* (2) used the soluble protein subunits from adenovirus: fibre antigens, hexon antigens and 'soluble' antigens. When they used the 'common' immunisation programme of a primary injection with one or two booster inoculations beginning four weeks after the primary, the procedure failed to stimulate the spleen sufficiently; hybridomas secreting antibody reactive against these subunit proteins was rarely produced (Table 3.2). To overcome this drawback, the authors precipitated the antigen with alum. This aggregated the proteins and therein lies the success of the procedure. Certain soluble proteins which are poor immunogens, such as bovine gamma globulin

Table 3.1. *Influence of immunisation schedule for human chorionic gonadotrophin on the stimulation of Balb/c mouse spleens and the subsequent generation of hybridomas*[1]

Method	Immunisation schedule	% splenocytes as lymphoblasts	% efficiency at generating hybridomas
(a)	2×50 μg + 1×10 μg over 12 months + 1 μg, day −7; 200 μg, day −4; 400 μg, day −3; 400 μg, day −2; 400 μg, day −1 (splenectomy, day 0)	6.0	41.0
(b)	3×10 μg over 12 months + 1 μg, day −7; 400 μg, day −4 (splenectomy, day 0)	0.9	7.5
(c)	as (b) but 50 μg on day −4	0.4	0.6
(d)	3×10 μg over 12 months + 200 μg, day −4; 400 μg, day −3; 400 μg, day −2; 400 μg, day −1 (splenectomy, day 0)	3.2	18.0
(e)	1×0.5 μg + 1×5 μg + 1×50 μg over 12 months, then as (a)	2.2	15.0

Source: [1] From Stahli *et al.* (1).

(BGG), are more effective immunostimulators when aggregated, for example by heating. This difference may be due to the relative efficacy with which the macrophages and dendritic cells present poorly immunogenic soluble proteins compared with the corresponding aggregated proteins. Without efficient presentation, the B and T lymphocyte compartments will not be effectively stimulated (3).

McCullough *et al.* (4) found that foot-and-mouth disease virus (FMDV) was a relatively poor immunogen compared with larger viruses such as measles virus and vesicular stomatitis virus. This was reflected

Table 3.2. *The influence of alum-precipitation of antigens on the efficacy of the antigen at stimulating lymphoblasts which can be used to generate antigen-specific antibody-secreting hybridomas*[1]

Immunisation	No. of of wells seeded	No. of wells containing hybridomas	% wells containing hybridomas	No. hybridomas secreting antigen-specific antibody	% hybridomas secreting antigen-specific antibody (% of no. of wells seeded)
Soluble antigen (expt I)	450	230	51%	10	(4.3%) (2.2%)
Soluble antigen (expt II)	450	9	2%	1	11.1% (0.2%)
Soluble antigen + alum (expt A)	700	327	47%	92	28.1% (13.1%)
Soluble antigen + alum (expt B)	750	611	81%	94	15.4% (12.5%)
Soluble antigen + alum (expt A)	192 (+ macrophage feeders)	192	100%	45	23.4% (23.4%)
Soluble antigen + alum (expt B)	384 (+ macrophage feeders)	384	100%	138	35.9% (35.9%)

Source: [1] From Russell *et al.* (2).

in the proportion of antigen-secreting cells generated in an immune spleen by FMDV compared with other viruses (Table 3.3). To overcome this, the authors varied the immunisation protocol as shown in Table 3.4, the route of inoculation and the concentration of the antigens. The

Table 3.3. *The relative efficiency of different viral antigens at stimulating antibody-secreting lymphoblasts and the subsequent production of antigen-specific antibody-secreting hybridomas*[1]

Immunogen to prime splenocytes	Efficiency[1] (%)	Titres of antibody[2] produced
FMDV	10–30	low
Measles virus	40–50	high
VSV	40–50	high
Coxsackievirus	30–40	moderate

Notes:
[1] Efficiency is a representative figure of the number of specific antibody-secreting colonies (lymphoblasts or hybridomas, determined using the Jerne plaque-forming cell assay; see §4.1.11) which arose from a fusion programme and could be successfully cultured.
[2] Relative titres from hybridoma cultures or autologous antiserum, determined by ELISA (§4.1.1). It is possible to obtain high titres using FMDV and low titres using VSV, but the classification of titres expresses that which is found on average after a single inoculation of inactivated whole virus antigen in the presence of Freund's complete adjuvant.

immune response to FMDV was not inefficient in exactly the same manner as it was against HCG (1), since inoculation of concentrations greater than 20 μg/mouse made little significant difference, but concentrations less than 20 μg had reduced immunostimulatory potential (Table 3.5). In contrast, both the route of inoculation (Table 3.6) and the immunisation schedule (Table 3.7) had significant influences on the generation of plasma cells in the immune spleen and specific antibodies in the antiserum. However, as with the immunisation schedule of Stähli *et al.* (1), this procedure will not necessarily be as effective with some antigens as with others. For example, the murine immune response against inactivated poliovirus or coxsackievirus (B3, B4 or B6) is more efficient than that against inactivated FMDV. The 'common' immunisation procedure of a priming followed by a boosting after four weeks is adequate for these viruses (K.C. McCullough & R.N. Butcher, unpublished data). Similar conclusions have been made when comparing live FMDV with inactivated virus. There is also a second consideration to be taken into account: the quality of the immune response. Although the most substantial immune response against inactivated FMDV was obtained with multiple boosts at 14 day intervals, the hybridomas generated from spleens thus stimulated produced antibodies with a high degree of cross-reactivity between FMDV isolates. The priming plus single boost type of immunisation, although less efficient at stimulating the immune response, pro-

Table 3.4. *Influence of immunisation schedule of foot-and-mouth disease virus on the generation of antigen-specific antibody-secreting cells in the spleen of Balb/c mice*

Method	Schedule[1]	PFC[3] per 10^6 splenocytes
I	20 μg iv splenectomy after 10 days	0.1–1
II	20 μg FCA[2] ip 20 μg iv after 4 weeks splenectomy after 3 days	3–17
III	20 μg FCA ip 20 μg FCA ip after 4 weeks 20 μg ip after 4 weeks splenectomy after 3 days	20–31
IV	20 μg FCA ip 20 μg FCA ip after 4 weeks 20 μg ip after 4 weeks 20 μg ip after 10 days 20 μg iv after 10 days splenectomy after 3 days	73–162
V	20 μg FCA ip 20 μg FCA ip after 8 weeks 20 μg ip after 12 weeks 20 μg iv after 12 weeks 20 μg ip after 16 weeks splenectomy after 3 days	84–212

Notes:
[1] iv, intravenous; ip, intraperitoneal.
[2] FCA, Freund's complete adjuvant at 50% (v/v) final concentration.
[3] Plaque-forming (antibody-secreting) cell as detected by the Jerne PFC assay.

duced hybridoma antibodies with a higher degree of specificity for a particular FMDV isolate.

Since efficient stimulation of the spleen was concomitant with efficient generation of specific Ab-secreting hybridomas derived from these spleens (Table 3.5), the above reports demonstrated that a combination of the optimised dose of antigen, the optimised route of inoculation and a multiple-boost hyperimmunisation programme should provide an efficient stimulation of mouse spleens. The reasoning behind the hyperimmunisation comes from the manner in which the immune response against a particular antigen expands and is amplified by each encounter with that antigen (see §1.4.9, Memory). If an antigen stimulates a spleen poorly, the few cells stimulated will produce only a small number of memory cells, slightly greater in number than the original antigen-

Table 3.5. *Effect of concentration of FMDV antigen on the stimulation of antibody-secreting plasma cells in the spleen of Balb/c mice, and the number of hybridomas subsequently produced*

Inoculations[1]			PFC[2] per 10^6 splenocytes	% hybridomas[3]
1st	2nd	thereafter		
1 μg	1 μg	—	1 (±1)	8
2.5 μg	2.5 μg	—	3 (±3)	9
5 μg	5 μg	—	4 (±3)	12
10 μg	10 μg	—	6 (±4)	19
20 μg	20 μg	—	13 (±5)	27
50 μg	50 μg	—	15 (±7)	25
100 μg	100 μg	—	14 (±5)	30
20 μg	20 μg	100 μg	16 (±7)	28
20 μg	20 μg	20μg[4]		
		1 μg		
		100 μg		
		100 μg		
		100 μg		
		100 μg	15 (±4)	29

Notes:

[1] The first, second and third (where applicable) inoculations were at 4 week intervals. All were intraperitoneal except the last (3 days before taking the spleens), which was intravenous. The first inoculation was emulsified in Freund's complete adjuvant (50% v/v).

[2] Plaque-forming cells using the Jerne plaque assay.

[3] The percentage of wells seeded giving antibody-producing hybridoma cultures which could be passaged.

[4] The fourth inoculation was 4 weeks after the third, the fifth was after a further 3 days and the rest at daily intervals. The last five inoculations were all intravenous, and the spleens were taken one day after the last inoculation.

reactive cells. As these memory lymphocytes are in turn stimulated by a second inoculation of antigen, an even greater population of memory cells will be generated, and this expansion will continue with each encounter of the memory cells with antigens. Hence the requirements of the multiple-boost immunisation programme (and hence the term hyperimmunisation).

As mentioned above, the problem with the hyperimmunisation procedure is that it can increase the proportion of low affinity and/or cross-reactive antibodies. In order to overcome this problem and produce dominant high affinity response from a hyperimmunisation, the immune system should be rested for a number of months between boosts. With hybridoma technology, individual workers must decide between the rapid

Table 3.6. *Influence of the route of inoculation of FMDV antigen on the production of antibody-secreting cells in the spleen, and antibody in the serum, of Balb/c mice*

Inoculations[1]			
1st	2nd	PFC/10^6 splenocytes[2]	Ab titre[3]
ip	ip	5 (±3)	32
ip	iv	14 (±4)	128
im	im	10 (±2)	64
im	iv	15 (±2)	128
sc	sc	8 (±4)	64
sc	iv	15 (±2)	256
ip/iv	iv	20 (±3)	512
im/iv	iv	15 (±4)	256
sc/iv	iv	26 (±4)	1024

Notes:

[1] All inoculations used 20 μg/mouse in Freund's complete adjuvant (50% v/v) either intraperitoneally (ip), intravenously (iv), intramuscularly (im), subcutaneously (sc) or combinations of these, followed one month later by 20 μg/mouse in the absence of adjuvant and either by the same route or iv.

[2] Plaque-forming cells from the Jerne plaque assay; values are means plus or minus standard deviation.

[3] Antibody (Ab) titre $\times 10^{-3}$, as measured by the amplified sandwich ELISA (see Chapter 4).

but least efficient priming plus single boosting procedure and the much longer (several months to one year) but most efficient hyperimmunisation procedure. The choice will depend on the time available, the type of immune response required, the efficiency of the substance under study as an antigen, and the ease with which that substance can be modified to make it more antigenic without destroying the antigenic determinants against which an immune response is desired.

Thus, different antigens, particularly those which are poorly immunogenic, will probably require different procedures to enhance their immunogenic potential. A general rule of thumb is that if the antigen is of low molecular mass, aggregation will increase its molecular mass, probably enhancing the presentation of that antigen to the immune system and thus enhancing the immune response. Furthermore, if the immune system can be stimulated, albeit poorly, several rounds of immunisation (hyperimmunisation) will expand the population of antigen-reactive lymphocytes, again enhancing the immune response. These are only general rules; and the immunogenicity of each antigen should

Table 3.7. *The influence of both route and schedule of immunisation with FMDV antigen on the generation of antibody-producing cells in the spleen of Balb/c mice*

Immunisation protocol[1]		
Time[2]	Route	PFC/10^6 splenocytes
d 0 d 0 + 4 wk	ip (FCA[3]) iv	12 (±4)
d 0 d 0 + 4 wk	ip (FCA) + iv iv	21 (±4)
d 0 d 0 + 4 wk	sc (FCA) + iv iv	25 (±3)
d 0 d 0 + 4 wk d 0 + 8 wk d 0 + 12 wk	ip (FCA) ip (FCA) ip iv	121 (±18)
d 0 d 0 + 4 wk d 0 + 8 wk d 0 + 12 wk	ip (FCA) + iv ip (FCA) + iv ip iv	180 (±21)
d 0 d 0 + 4 wk d 0 + 8 wk d 0 + 12 wk	sc (FCA) + iv sc sc iv	240 (±28)

Notes:

[1] Immunisations were with 20 μg/mouse of antigen, and the routes were intraperitoneal (ip), intravenous (iv), subcutaneous (sc), ip + iv, or sc + iv.

[2] The times of inoculations were at day 0 (d 0) and either 4, 8 or 12 weeks (wk) thereafter.

[3] FCA: Freund's complete adjuvant at 50% (v/v).

be assessed beforehand and an efficient immunisation programme determined prior to the removal of immune spleens for fusion with myeloma cells. The efficiency of the immune response can be monitored constantly by taking tail vein or cardiac test bleeds, and assaying for antigen-reactive antibodies. These assay procedures will be described in Chapter 4.

3.2. Source of myeloma cells

The influence of the genotype of the myeloma cells on the success of hybridoma generation was discussed in detail in §2.5.8. Generally speaking, the more closely related the myeloma cells and splenocytes, the greater the chance of success. However, syngeneic (myeloma cells and splenocytes from the same strain of animal, e.g. Balb/c mouse) combinations are not essential, since allogeneic mixes can give similar results. Furthermore, xenogeneic combinations using closely related animal species, e.g. rat myeloma cells with mouse splenocytes, can also be as successful. It is only when more distantly related animal species are used that difficulties are encountered. This is not to say that such xenogeneic fusions as between rabbit and mouse, human and mouse, and pig and mouse will not generate hybridomas. The initial culturing conditions have to be more strictly defined but heterohybridomas can be produced, albeit at an efficiency of less than 20% of that observed with homohybridomas (mouse myeloma cells + mouse splenocytes). It may be desirable to raise MAb using lymphocytes from humans, rabbits, pigs, etc. If the donor is suffering from an immediate-type hypersensitivity or an auto-immune disorder, only antibodies from that species of animal can help to understand the humoral responses involved in that type of reaction. Furthermore, the antibody repertoire generated against a particular pathogen may not be exactly the same in the mouse as in the human or the bovine. Antibody from the host for that pathogen is more desirable. Such antibodies will also allow a study of the antibody-dependent immune reactions (see §§ 1.4.8–1.6.4) against a pathogen in the natural host, and may also prove to have prophylactic potential.

The theory behind the lower success rate of generating heterohybridomas, and the more strictly defined culture conditions for them, are given in detail in §2.5.8. Section 2.4 also demonstrates the relative efficiency of different mouse–mouse, rat–rat and rat–mouse combinations on the generation of hybridomas, based on the work of Milstein and co-workers (5).

3.3. Source of PEG

The fusion agent in current use for generating hybridomas is polyethylene glycol (PEG). As its name suggests this chemical is a polymer of ethylene glycol. There are a number of preparations of this polymer available, with average M_r ranging between 2000 and 10 000. Fazekas de St Groth & Scheidegger (6) compared different PEG preparations with respect to hybridoma production; a summary of their results is shown in Table 3.8. There was considerable variation in the efficacy of PEG as an agent for generating hybridomas, with respect to commercial source, molecular mass and batch. This variation may reflect the efficiency with which the

Table 3.8. *The influence of different sources and relative molecular masses of polyethylene glycol, used in the fusion of Balb/c splenocytes and myeloma cells, on the efficiency of generating hybridoma cells*

PEG source and rel. molecular mass			% wells seeded, positive for hybridoma growth
BDH	200		1.4
BDH	1000		5.6
BDH	4000		16.7
Merck	200		4.2
Merck	1000		51.4
Merck	4000		94.4
Merck	20 000		38.9
Serva	200		0
Serva	1000		23.6
Serva	4000		55.5
Sigma	6000	Batch *1[1]	69.4
Sigma	6000	Batch *2[1]	95.8

Note:
[1] Two different lot numbers of the same product purchased from Sigma.

different PEG materials 'prime' cell membranes for fusion. It is also probable that some PEG sources are toxic or otherwise harmful to cells. Results from other laboratories have supported the above observations, and it is recommended that *before* the technology of hybridoma production is tackled, several sources and molecular masses of PEG should be tested for their efficiency at generating hybridomas. This procedure is now routine in most laboratories. The optimum batch of PEG tested is ordered in large quantities (usually kilogram amounts) such that it will last many years.

3.4. **Fusion ratio**

The ratio of splenocytes to myeloma cells in a fusion mixture (the fusion ratio) was mentioned in §2.6.2. Generally speaking, a ratio of 5 splenocytes to 1 myeloma cell has been used, but this can vary from 10 : 1 to 1 : 1. The higher proportion of splenocytes was initially used because the excess splenocytes were required as feeder cells. Supplementation of the recently fused cells with additional feeder cells – splenocytes, thymocytes, peritoneal exudate cells (PEC) or 3T3/A31 cells (see §3.7.5) – will allow the fusion ratio to be reduced. Ratios of 2 : 1 to 5 : 1 (splenocytes : myeloma cells) have been successfully used in the presence of feeder layers. Fig. 3.1 summarises this work, comparing the efficiency

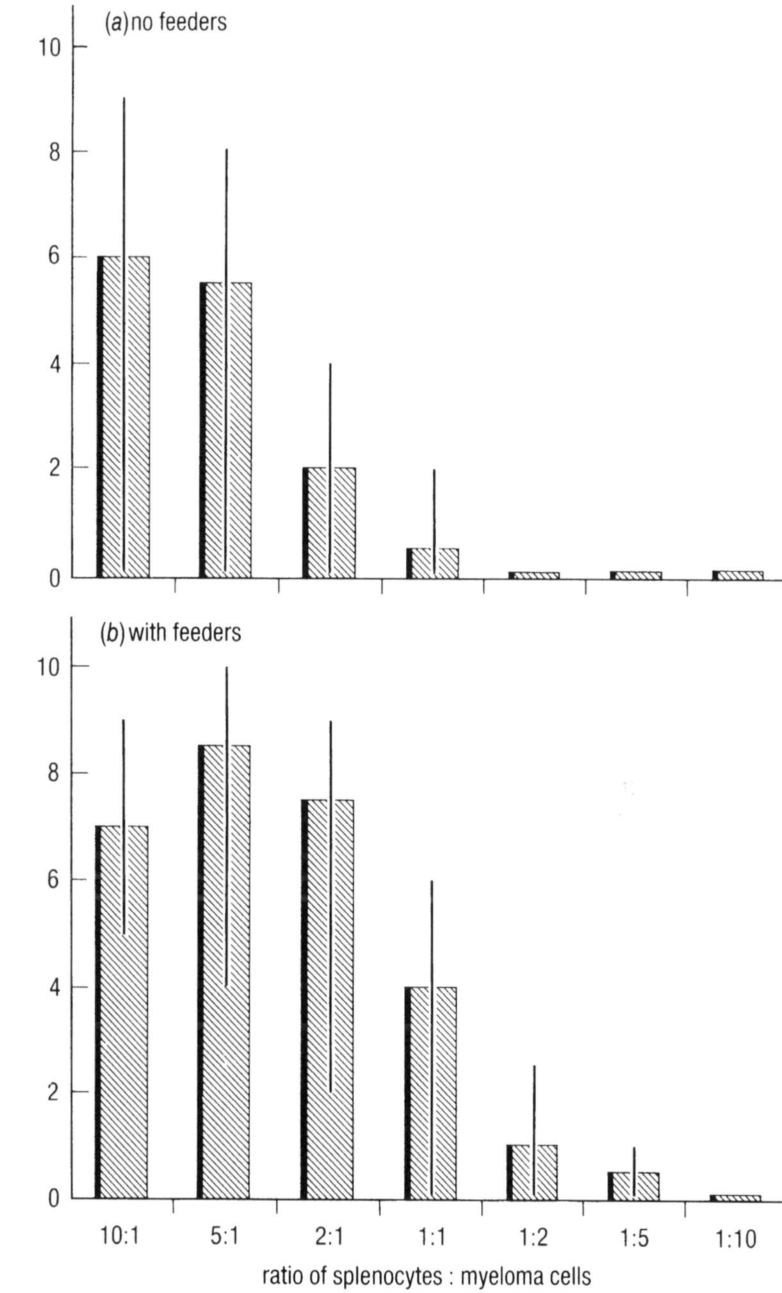

Fig. 3.1. The influence of the fusion ratio (ratio of splenocytes to myeloma cells in a fusion mixture) on the generation of hybridomas in the absence (*a*) or the presence (*b*) of macrophage or 3T3/A31 feeder cells (see Figs 3.13 and 3.14). The bars indicate the maximum and minimum values from different experiments.

of different fusion ratios at generating hybridomas in the presence or absence of PEC or 3T3/A31 feeder layers.

When feeder layers are used, the major controlling factor in a fusion is the number of myeloma cells. With five- to tenfold excess of splenocytes in the fusion mixture, as many as 8–10 hybridomas per 10^5 myeloma cells may be generated (7,8), although this figure can vary considerably and should only be regarded as a maximum (4). With some fusions, the majority of wells will not yield hybridomas, and the overall picture in such cases would be less than 1 hybridoma/10^5 myeloma cells. By optimising the technology for the generation of hybridomas secreting antibody against either foot-and-mouth disease virus (FMDV), vesicular stomatitis virus (VSV) or the measles virus/rinderpest virus (MV/RPV) group, 8–10 hybridomas per 10^5 myeloma cells in a fusion mixture could be generated using splenocytes from animals immunised with either VSV or MV–RPV, but only 3.5 hybridomas per 10^5 myeloma cells could be generated using splenocytes from animals immunised with FMDV (4).

This variation in the expected number of hybridomas obtained from a fusion is because the success of a fusion is dependent on the lymphoblastoid status of the splenocyte population. That is, the greater the stimulation of the secondary lymphoid organs by the immunising antigen, the larger the proportion of stimulated antigen-specific B lymphocytes (lymphoblasts) in the spleen, and hence the greater the likelihood of a myeloma cells fusing with one of these in a fusion mixture. This likelihood may be increased by using mitogens, because mitogen-stimulated splenocytes generated more antibody-secreting hybridomas than did unstimulated splenocytes (9). Thus, the success of generating antibody-secreting hybridomas is related to the ratio of viable myeloma cells to antigen-reactive lymphoblasts (and, hence, to the potency of the immunogen).

3.5. Source of media and media supplements

The early reports of hybridomas secreting antibodies of predefined specificity used RPMI 1640 or DMEM. Since then, the variety of media used has expanded, as have the supplements to these media (Table 3.9).

3.5.1. *Comparisons of different sources of the medium*

The first reports on comparisons of different sources of media come from Fazekas de St. Groth & Scheidegger (6) and McCullough *et al.* (4). They confirmed the usefulness of DMEM and RPMI 1640 for the culturing of hybridomas, although the two groups disagreed about the *relative* efficacy of these media. McCullough *et al.* (4) also noted certain advantages of Eagle's (Glasgow modification) medium, GMEM (Table 3.10). Cells grew more slowly in this, but eventually attained the cell

Table 3.9. *The potential supplements for media used in the culturing of hybridoma cells*

Class	Supplement
essential	serum (e.g. foetal calf serum) at 5–10% (v/v) or a serum substitute (see Tables 3.11–3.13); glutamine at 2 mM final concentration.
not essential but useful	sodium pyruvate at 10 mM final concentration; non-essential amino acids at a 1:100 dilution of commercially available '× 100 stock'; HEPES at 20 mM final concentration.
of variable efficacy	2-mercaptoethanol at 0.02 mM final concentration

Table 3.10. *The influence of different media on the growth of hybridoma cells*

Medium[1]	Maximum density of cells	Maximum viability	Mean generation time	Duration of stationary phase[2]	Duration of death phase[3]
RPMI 1640–FCS	2×10^6	>95%	20 h	12 h	30 h
RPMI 1640–HS	1×10^6	>95%	20 h	12 h	30 h
RPMI 1640–OS	0.5×10^6	50%	24 h	—[4]	—
DMEM–FCS	0.8×10^6	90%	36 h	10 h	20 h
DMEM–HS	0.7×10^6	90%	40 h	10 h	20 h
DMEM–OS	0.2×10^6	80%	72 h	—	—
GMEM–FCS	1×10^6	>95%	28 h	72 h	54 h
GMEM–HS	0.8×10^6	>95%	36 h	72 h	54 h
GMEM–OS	0.5×10^6	70%	60 h	—	—
Iscove's-FCS	2×10^6	>95%	18 h	16 h	30 h
Iscove's–HS	1×10^6	>95%	20 h	20 h	48 h
Iscove's–OS	0.6×10^6	70%	24 h	—	—

Notes:
1 FCS, 10% (v/v) foetal calf serum; HS, 10% (v/v) horse serum; OS, 10% (v/v) adult bovine serum.
2 Maintenance of cells at a single density and viability greater than 90%.
3 Time taken for cell viability to fall from 90% to less than 10%.
4 —: The cultures did not attain 90% viability.

densities, with high viability, found in DMEM and RPMI 1640 media. RPMI 1640 medium-fed cultures could be maintained at a high viability for longer (72 h) than DMEM-fed cultures (24 h). Eagle's medium-fed cultures maintained high viabilities (but with lower cell densities) for 96 h.

After attaining maximum cell densities, culture viability rapidly decreased to less than 10% in DMEM-fed cultures (30 h) and RPMI 1640-medium fed cultures (42 h). In contrast, 120 h after attaining maximum cell densities, Eagle's medium-fed cultures still had 40% viability. Hence, if it was desirable to maintain hybridoma cultures for longer periods, Eagle's medium would be most useful. Eagle's medium would also prove most useful if the hybridoma culture were to be used for continued secretion of antibody as opposed to viable cell production. Many hybridomas increase their antibody secretion rate after they attain the maximum cell density possible in a particular medium source (see §6.3).

Fazekas de St. Groth & Scheidegger (6) also tested Iscove's medium, a modification of DMEM or RPMI 1640 medium (10). Two sources of this are available commercially: incomplete Iscove's modification of DMEM (IDMEM) and complete IDMEM. Table 3.11 shows that IDMEM is DMEM supplemented with non-essential amino acids, sodium pyruvate and 2-mercaptoethanol. The incomplete form can then be supplied with serum, as in DMEM, Eagle's medium and RPMI 1640 medium. In contrast, complete IDMEM is a 'serum-free' medium in which the serum is replaced by transferrin, lipid, albumin and selenite. This 'serum-free' medium will be discussed in the following section (§3.5.2), relating to the observations by Fazekas de St. Groth & Scheidegger (6) that their hybridomas grew most efficiently in IDMEM.

There has been little consideration of the influence of different media on the secretion of antibody by hybridomas. Antibody secretion by some, but not all, hybridomas can be influenced by the medium in which they were cultured. When this antibody secretion is dependent on the composition of the culture medium, the optimum conditions are often a rapid growth of the cells (MGT = 14–20 h) with high viability, and rapid decrease in this viability after the exponential (growth) phase. The media which fulfil these requirements are RPMI 1640, IDMEM and Iscove's modification of RPMI 1640. There were, of course, exceptions to this rule, in which Eagle's medium can be the most appropriate.

Hence, four media appear useful for culturing hybridomas routinely, namely DMEM, RPMI 1640, Iscove's modification of DMEM or RPMI 1640, and Eagle's (Glasgow modification) medium. Some hybridomas will show little variation in which medium they prefer. If, however, it is desired to maintain hybridomas in culture over longer periods of time, i.e. a slower growth rate, but still with high cell viability (over 90%), Eagle's (Glasgow modification) medium is useful. When the antibody, rather than the cells, is required, either Eagle's medium, RPMI 1640 medium or the Iscove's modified medium should be used, depending on the hybridoma. McCoy's medium and Ham's F16 medium have also been used. Hybridomas therefore vary considerably in their media requirements. In our experience, Eagle's medium has proved to be the most

Table 3.11. *Composition of Iscove's medium (complete and incomplete)*

Iscove's modification of DMEM (IDMEM)
Values are quantities in milligrams per litre

Constituent	IDMEM complete	IDMEM incomplete	DMEM
L-alanine	25	25	—
L-arginine, HCl	84	84	84
L-asparagine, H_20	28.4	28.4	—
L-aspartic acid	30	30	—
L-cystine, Na_2	82.8	82.8	56.78
L-glutamic acid	75	75	—
L-glutamine	584	584	584
Glycine	30	30	30
L-histidine, HCl.H_20	42	42	42
L-isoleucine	105	105	104.8
L-leucine	105	105	104.8
L-lysine, HCl	146	146	146.2
L-methionine	30	30	30
L-phenylalanine	66	66	66
L-proline	40	40	—
L-serine	42	42	42
L-threonine	95	95	95.2
L-tryptophan	16	16	16
L-tyrosine Na_2	104.2	104.2	89.5
L-valine	94	94	93.6
biotin	0.013	0.013	—
D-calcium pantothenate	4	4	4
choline chloride	4	4	4
folic acid	4	4	4
i-inositol	7.2	7.2	7
nicotinamide	4	4	4
pyridoxal, HCl	4	4	4
riboflavin	0.4	0.4	0.4
thiamin, HCl	4	4	4
vitamin B_{12}	0.013	0.013	—
$CaCl_2.2H_20$	218.6	218.6	264.9
$Fe(NO_3)_3.9H_20$	—	—	0.1
KCl	330	330	400
KNO_3	0.076	0.076	—
$MgSO_4.7H_20$	200	200	200
NaCl	4505	4505	6400
$NaHCO_3$	2520	2520	3700
$NaH_2PO_4.2H_20$	141.3	141.3	141.3
D-glucose	4500	4500	4500
HEPES	5962	5962	5962
sodium pyruvate	110	110	110
sodium selenite	0.0713	0.0173	—
bovine serum albumin	400	—	—
pure human transferrin	1	—	—
soybean lecithin	100	—	—

universally applicable both to different hybridomas and to different culture requirements (growth of cells, production of antibody, long-term culture, large-scale culture). Of course, the different supplements used with media can have a significant influence on the growth of, and antibody secretion by, hybridomas.

3.5.2. *Medium supplements*

(i) Serum
The medium supplement which has received most attention is serum. Dulbecco (11) identified a number of functions of serum as required for the growth and replication of transformed cell lines. He suggested that one role was in the initiation of DNA synthesis after appropriate environmental stimuli (that is, counteracting the phenomenon of 'contact inhibition'; the real situation is probably a balance between these two factors). A second role was to prevent irreversible changes in cells which would lead to cell death, and a third role was concerned with mitosis. He suggested that the functions of DNA synthesis initiation, counteracting 'contact inhibition' and the influence over mitosis were separable functions effected by different factors in serum. It is conceivable that all three functions are related (or have the same overall effector mechanism) although different serum factors could be involved in similar functions.

Most reports on hybridoma production use medium supplemented with 10–20% (v/v) foetal bovine serum (foetal calf serum, FCS), horse serum or combinations of these. FCS and horse sera have similar effects on the growth of hybridoma cells, but medium supplemented with adult bovine (ox) serum is the least efficient at supporting these cells (Fig. 3.2). The FCS and horse sera also give relatively low levels of batch variation, in contrast to the ox serum. This latter serum was collected from a local abattoir, and of ten batches obtained over 18 months, only one could be considered suitable as a source of serum supplement for the media of hybridoma cultures. In contrast, batches of the other sera gave a maximum variation in hybridoma growth of only 10% (Fig. 3.3).

Newborn calf serum (taken within the first five days after birth) gave a lower growth rate of hybridoma cells than FCS, but otherwise maintained a culture of high viability during the exponential growth phase of the cells (Fig. 3.4). Donor calf serum (taken from animals more than one week old) was similar to the FCS with respect to the growth and viability of hybridoma cells in media supplemented with them. Donor calf serum batches show similar variability to foetal calf serum batches for the maintenance of hybridoma cell growth.

The influence of the relative amount of foetal calf serum supplement on the growth of, and antibody production by, hybridomas secreting antibody against foot-and-mouth disease virus has been studied as shown

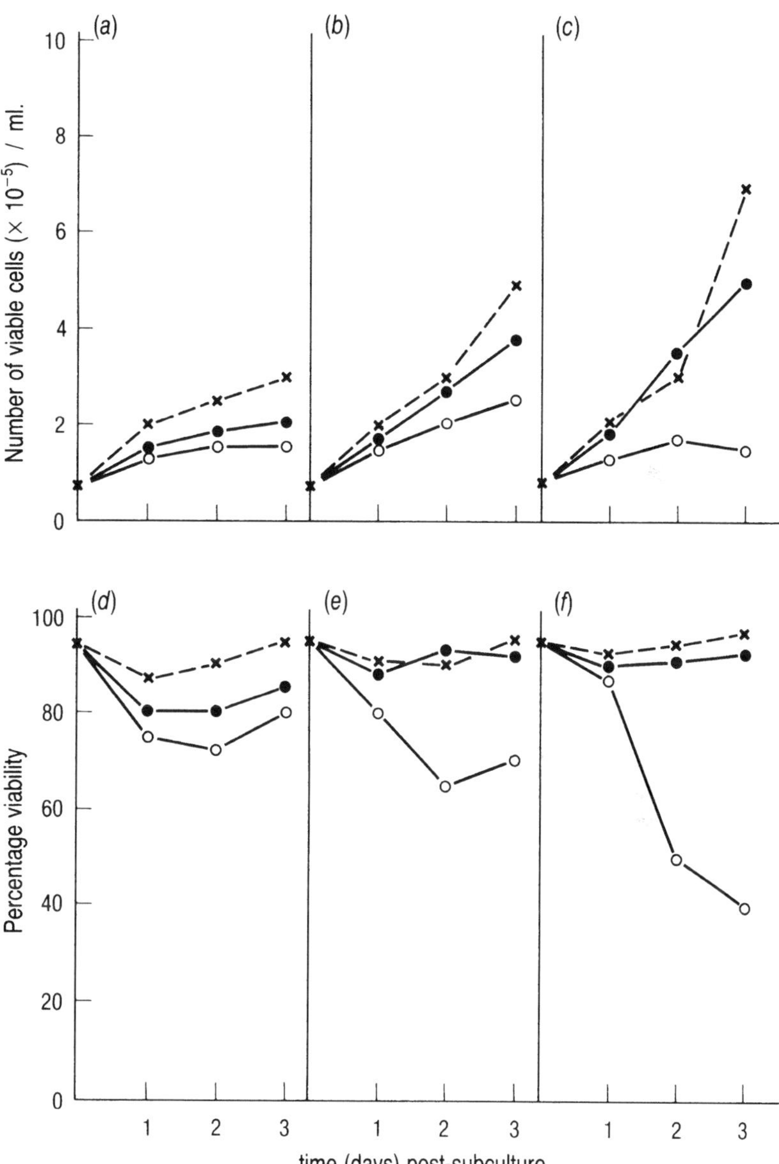

Fig. 3.2. The influence of different compositions of media and different sources of serum supplement on the generation of anti-foot-and-mouth disease antibody-secreting hybridomas (see McCullough *et al.* (21)). (*a*), (*d*), DMEM; (*b*), (*e*), GMEM (BHK-21 medium; Glasgow modification of Eagle's); (*c*), (*f*), RPMI 1640. (*a*)–(*c*), number of viable cells/ml; (*d*)–(*f*), percentage viability. x, foetal calf serum; •, horse serum; ○, adult bovine serum from an abattoir.

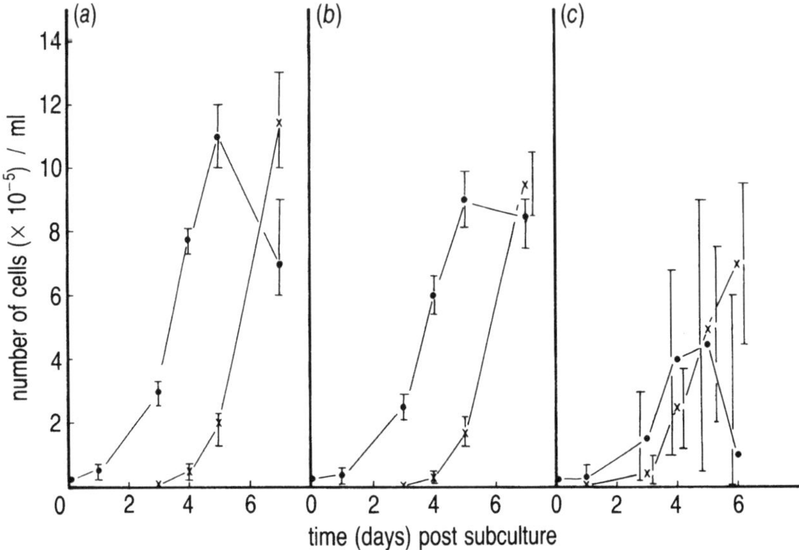

Fig. 3.3. The growth of hybridoma cultures in RPMI 1640 medium supplemented with foetal calf serum (*a*), horse serum (*b*) or abattoir-derived adult bovine serum (*c*). •, Number of viable cells; x, number of dead cells. The bars represent the variations obtained with different batches (6–10) of each type of serum.

in Fig. 3.5. Between 2% and 10% (v/v) supplement of foetal calf serum maintained the cell viability at over 90% during the exponential phase of the growth cycle. The mean generation time (the time for the number of cells to double) increased with decreasing levels of serum supplements. Antibody production did not, however, increase concomitantly. Taken as antibody produced per cell, the maximum productivity occurred just after subculture of the cells, but an increase in this relative secretion could also occur when the cells approached a stationary phase. No single level of serum supplement could be considered ideal for increasing antibody productivity by the hybridomas tested. An interesting observation was that the ideal percentage of serum supplement for maintaining the highest viability in an *established* hybridoma culture was 5% v/v.

(ii) L-glutamine

L-glutamine is an essential amino acid for hybridoma growth, without which attempted hybridoma cell culture is unsuccessful. It has a short half life, and when hybridoma cells are subcultured in RPMI 1640 medium DMEM or the Iscove's media, L-glutamine must be added. Hybridomas may be cultured in Eagle's medium (Glasgow modification) without the addition of L-glutamine, but the additional presence of this amino acid provides more consistent growth rates between different hybridomas, more rapid growth and as efficient recovery of hybridomas

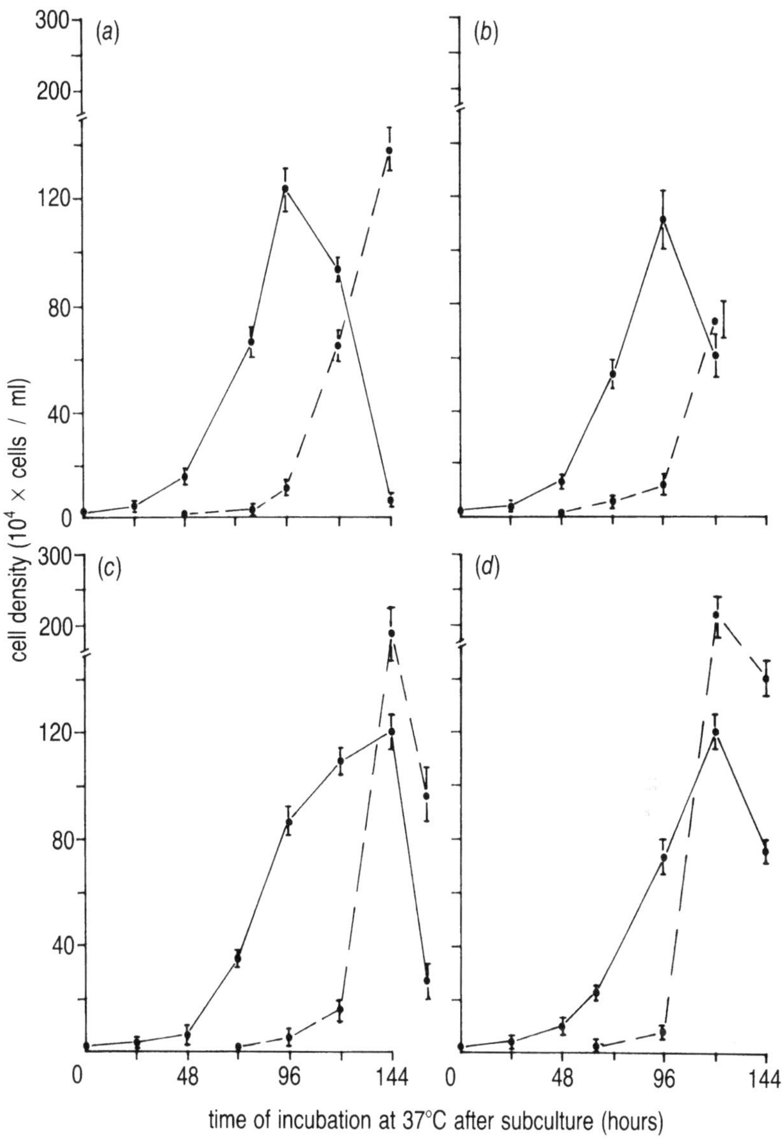

Fig. 3.4. The growth of hybridoma cells in RPMI 1640 medium supplemented with either foetal calf serum (*a*), donor calf serum (*b*), newborn calf serum (*c*), or abattoir-derived newborn calf serum (*d*). Solid lines, viable cells; broken lines, dead cells (see McCullough *et al.* (21)).

from a fusion as can be obtained with RPMI 1640 medium or DMEM supplemented with L-glutamine.

The influence of medium supplement depletion on the growth of antibody secretion by hybridomas has been studied (Fig. 3.6). Hyb-

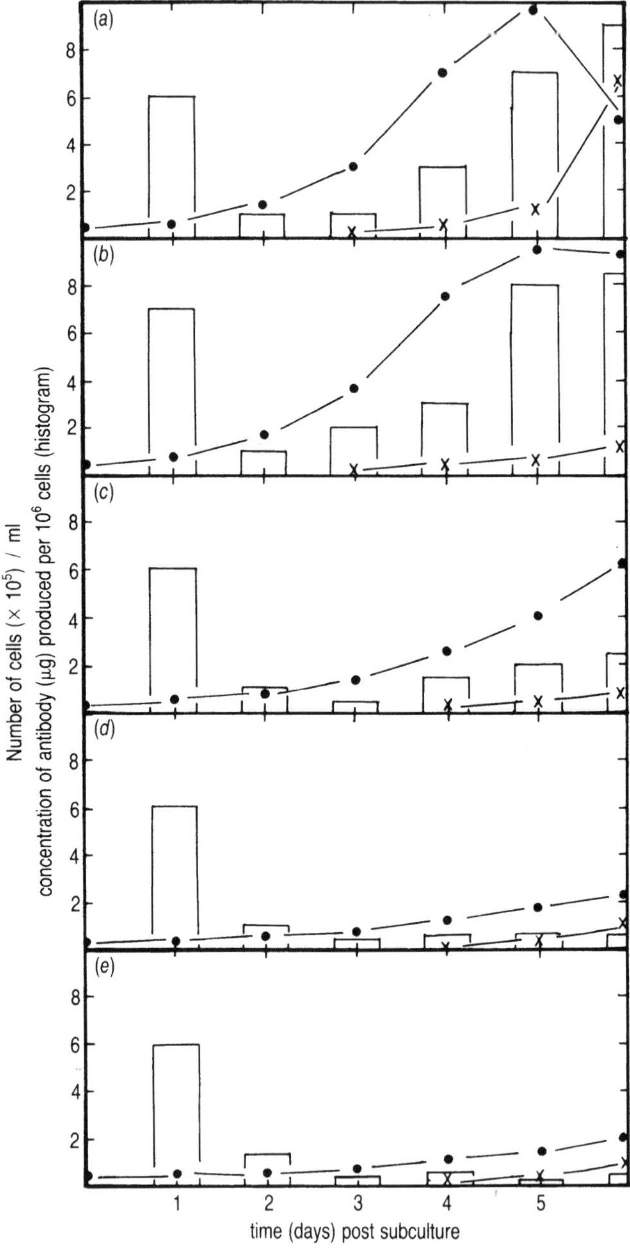

Fig. 3.5. Influence of different concentrations of foetal calf serum (FCB) supplement to RPMI 1640 medium on the growth of anti-foot-and-mouth disease virus antibody-secreting hybridoma cells, and the production of antibody: (*a*), 10% (v/v) FCS; (*b*), 5% (v/v) FCS; (*c*), 2% (v/v) FCS; (*d*), 1% (v/v) FCS; (*e*), 0.5% (v/v) FCS. Histogram, antibody produced from 10^6 cells; •, number of viable cells; x, number of dead cells.

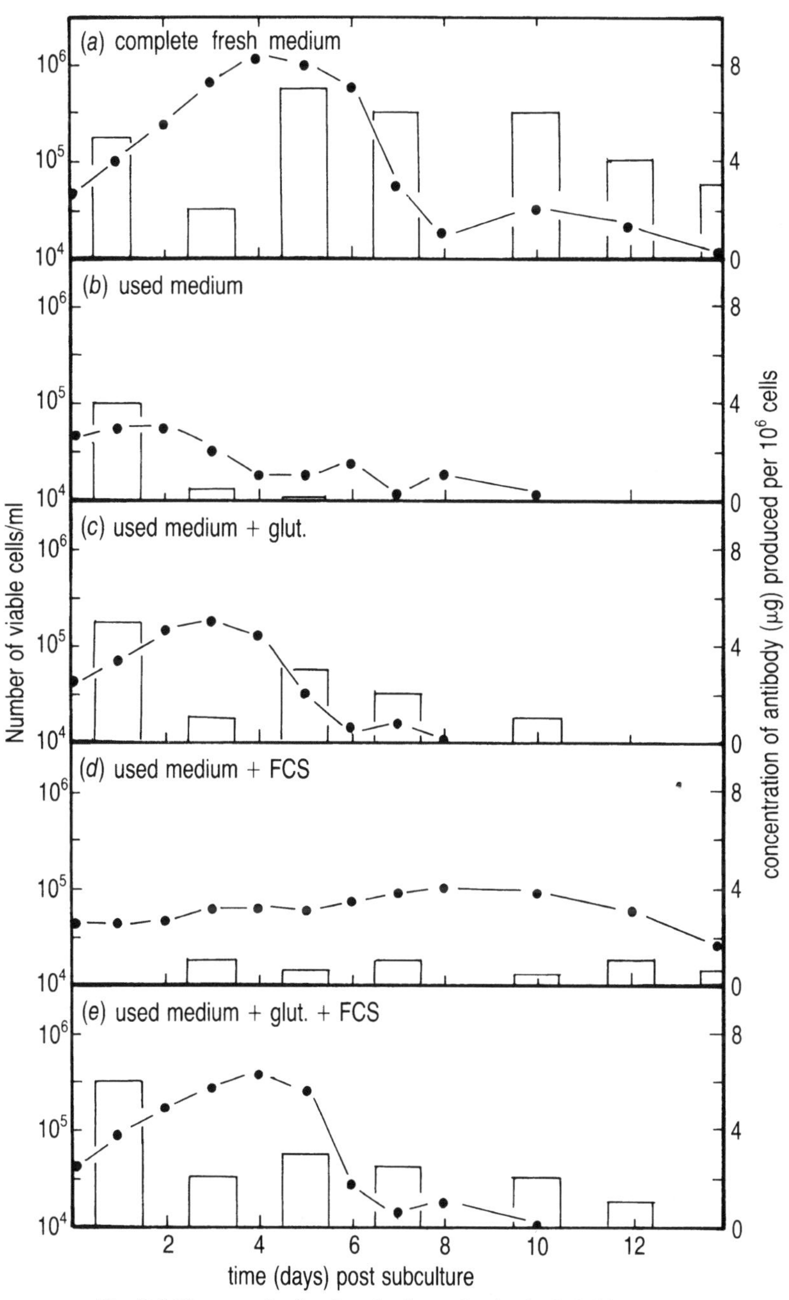

Fig. 3.6. The growth of and antibody production by hybridoma cells in complete fresh medium (*a*), or in myeloma cell medium 72 h old ('used medium') without supplementation (*b*), with added 2 mM glutamine (*c*), with added 10% (v/v) FCS (*d*), or with both glutamine and FCS (*e*). Histogram, antibody produced from 10^6 cells; •, number of viable cells/ml.

Table 3.12. *Supplements which, when added to DMEM or RPMI 1640 medium, will give Iscove's modification of DMEM or RPMI 1640 ('serum-replaced media')*

Supplement	Concentration[1]
L-alanine	25 mg/l
L-asparagine	25 mg/l
L-aspartic acid	30 mg/l
L-cystine	22 mg/l
L-glutamic acid	75 mg/l
L-proline	40 mg/l
sodium pyruvate	110 mg/l
vitamin B_{12}	0.013 mg/l
biotin	0.013 mg/l
sodium selenite	0.0173 mg/l
water	200 ml/l (to obtain the correct osmolarity of 280 mOsm for the medium)[2]
α-thioglycerol	7.5×10^{-5} M
HEPES (pH 7.3)	25 mM
sodium bicarbonate	30 mM
human transferrin[3]	1 mg/l (1×10^{-8} M)
bovine serum albumin (delipidated)[4]	275 mg/l
bovine serum albumin (in association with soybean lipid)	125 mg/l
soybean lipid[5]	100 mg/l

Notes:

1 Concentrations are given per litre of DMEM or RPMI 1640 medium.

2 In place of adding extra water to obtain the correct osmolarity of the medium, a special formulation of medium can be used in which NaCl is reduced to 4505 mg/ml, KCl to 330 mg/ml and $CaCl_2$ to 165 mg/l. Osmolal: molecular mass of osmotically active compounds per litre (e.g. 1M NaCl = 2 Osm NaCl); measured on an osmometer as a depression in freezing point, which is related to the molecular mass of osmotically active compounds per litre.

3 Stock solution of transferrin was prepared as follows: 90 mg/ml in the medium containing the additional amino acids and co-factors, and of the correct osmolarity; $\frac{1}{3}$ saturated with Fe^{3+} by adding 7.4×10^{-9} mol Fe^{3+} (as $FeCl_3$ dissolved in 0.1 mM HCl) per milligram transferrin; sterilised through a 0.2 μm filter; stored at 4 °C.

4 Bovine serum albumin (BSA) was delipidated as follows: 5 g BSA was dissolved in 100 ml deionised water; pH adjusted to 3.0 with concentrated HCl; 1 mg Dextran T40 was added per millilitre, as was 10 mg/ml activated charcoal; the mixture was incubated at 56 °C for 30 min with gentle agitation; the charcoal was removed by centrifugation and filitration; pH adjusted to 6.5 with 2 M NaOH; the solution was deionised with 1.5 ml Amberlite MB-1 resin per gram of BSA overnight at 4 °C (*no* agitation); concentrated four times over an Amicon Diaflo UM-10 membrane; filter sterilised; stored at 4 °C.

ridoma cells were passaged in 'used (conditioned) medium' – medium in which the hybridomas had been cultured through their exponential phase (usually 72 h at 37 °C) – with either no additional supplement, or replenished with 10% v/v foetal calf serum, 2 mM L-glutamine or both. When both the serum and glutamine were depleted, the hybridoma cells failed to grow or produce much antibody and rapidly died. In the absence of replenished glutamine, the cells either 'stuck' (remained in a lag phase without increase in cell number or decrease in viability) for up to ten days, or slowly increased in cell number for a short period and then slowly died. In the absence of replenished foetal calf serum, the cells grew moderately well (not as well as in fresh complete medium), but after 48–96 h the culture rapidly died. Even when both serum and glutamine were replaced, the cultures did not grow as well as those in fresh medium. No culture produced antibody as efficiently as those in fresh medium.

(iii) Serum-replaced media

There are two sources of medium supplement which can be used to increase the efficiency with which hybridoma cells may be subcultured, secrete antibody, or both. These two methods have in common the use of 'serum-free' media; it is not that the media are free of serum but that the serum is replaced by a number of chemicals, many of which are found in serum. The important omission is immunoglobulin; this makes purification of hybridoma antibody from such 'serum-free' media relatively straightforward. When hybridoma cells are cultured in conventional tissue culture media as above, the secreted MAb is contaminated with the immunoglobulin molecules of the serum supplement. Hence, purification of the MAb requires the use of anti-mouse immunoglobulin affinity columns. Iscove & Melchers (10) reported a serum-replaced medium for the culture of lymphocytes (the compounds which were used to supplement conventional media such as RPMI 1640 and DMEM and thus replace serum are shown in Table 3.12). This medium was subsequently used by Fazekas de St. Groth & Scheidegger (6) for the culture of hybridoma cells, and found to be optimum, among those tested, for hybridoma cell growth. No studies have yet been reported on the antibody-secretion by hybridomas cultured in such media.

Notes to Table 3.12. *(cont.)*

[5] Soybean lipid–cholesterol suspension was prepared as follows: 200 mg soybean lipid plus 50 mg cholesterol were completely dispersed in 50 ml acid medium (DMEM or RPMI 1640 WITHOUT sodium bicarbonate but containing 1% delipidated BSA and the pH adjusted to 5.1) by ultrasonication at maximum amplitude for 1 h at 0 °C using a 2 cm diameter titanium probe; sterilised by passage through 1.2 and 0.45 μm filters; stored at 4 °C.

Table 3.13. *Composition of the insulin-based 'serum-replaced' medium of Chang* et al. *(12)*

Constituent	Quantity
DMEM or RPMI 1640	1 l (as commercially available)
$NaHCO_3$ (if not already added to the commercially available medium)	2.75 g/l
L-glutamine	0.6 g/l
non-essential amino acids (×100 stock; commercially available from Gibco Ltd and Flow Labs Ltd)	1% (v/v)
insulin (Sigma)[1]	5 mg/l
transferrin (Sigma)[2]	5 mg/l

Notes:
[1] The insulin is added from a stock solution of 2 mg/ml prepared in distilled water adjusted to pH 2.5 by the addition of 1 M HCl.
[2] The transferrin is added from a stock solution of 2 mg/ml prepared in PBS.

The second type of serum-substituted medium was designed for the selection of antibody-secreting hybridomas. The composition of this medium was DMEM base supplemented with 2 mM L-glutamine, transferrin and insulin (Table 3.13). Chang *et al.* (12) produced evidence that this medium would select in favour of antibody-secreting cells, but confirmatory evidence has not been forthcoming. Suggestions have been made that the hybridomas must be cultured in this insulin–transferrin-containing medium from the moment of fusion for the ability to select antibody-secreting hybridomas to be effective.

(iv) Other medium supplements (Table 3.9)

Non-essential amino acids are sometimes used as a supplement to defined media such as the Iscove's media. As their name suggests, they are not always essential, but they do contribute to protein synthesis and can act as additional reservoirs of NH_4^+ for use in amino acid biosynthesis. Likewise, sodium pyruvate is not an obligate requirement for all media, but the advantage is that it can enter directly into the Krebs cycle (Fig. 3.7) as pyruvic acid. This cycle has two major functions. It provides a considerable portion of the biochemical energy requirements of the cell,

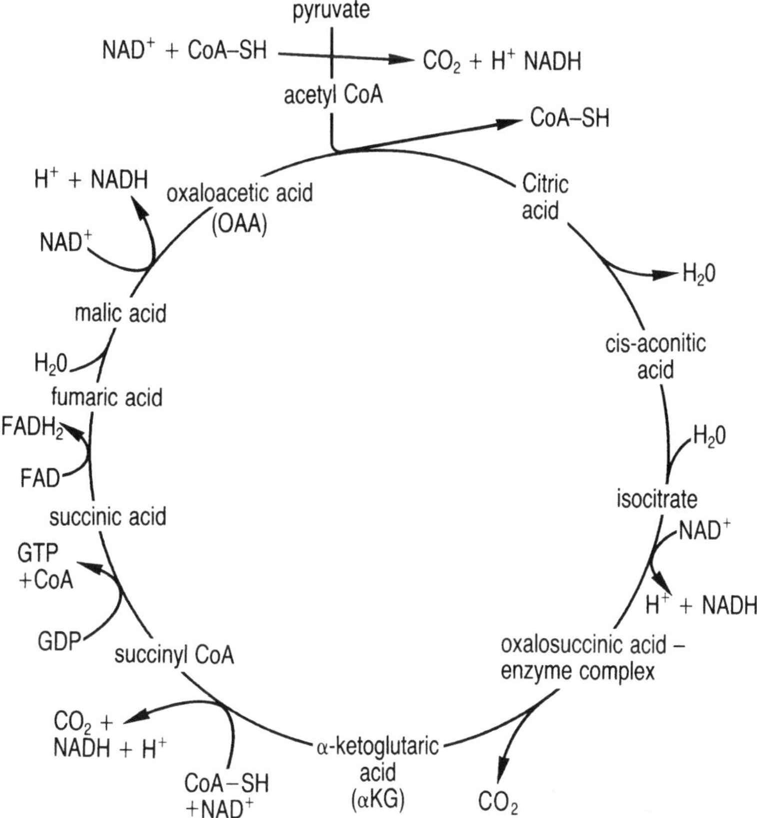

Fig. 3.7. The Krebs or TCA cycle: the major energy-producing biochemical pathway of the mammalian cell.

and is the starting material for the biosynthesis of many amino acids (Fig. 3.8). Since antibody is a protein, the presence of sodium pyruvate, in addition to the glutamine (as a source of NH_4^+, obligatory in the synthesis of amino acids from the Krebs cycle) normally added to hybridoma culture medium, is beneficial to the protein synthesis by hybridoma cells. The non-essential amino acids may further enrich the medium in this context.

The final medium supplement which requires mentioning is 2-mercaptoethanol (2-MCE). This is a higly toxic and degradative substance, but when used at 5×10^{-5} M is an obligatory supplement for the successful *in vitro* culture of lymphocytes (13, 14), as indeed are non-essential amino acids and sodium pyruvate. Thus, it should follow that 2-MCE would be a beneficial supplement for hybridoma cells, since they are derived from B lymphocytes (see Chapter 2). Mercaptoethanol has indeed been used in the culture of hybridomas (6). These authors did

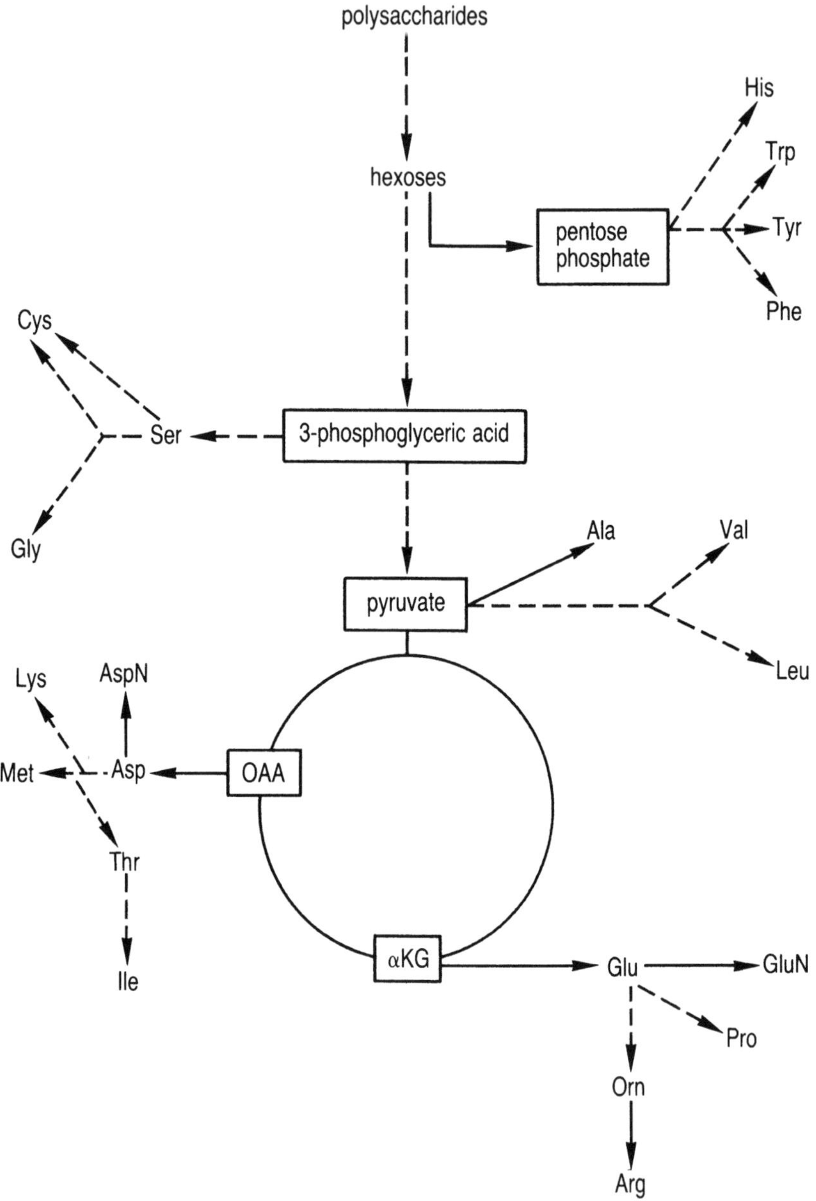

Fig. 3.8. How the Krebs cycle contributes to the synthesis of amino acids.

not determine whether or not the presence of the 2-MCE was obligatory. In contrast, McCullough *et al.* (4) found that 2-MCE had no influence on either the growth or the cloning (see §4.2) of hybridoma cells. Hence, the efficacy of 2-MCE as a growth supplement for hybridoma cells may vary for different cells lines, or, alternatively, its presence may be unnecessary. The relevance of 2-MCE to hybridoma growth requires the elucidation of its function as a growth supplement.

3.6. Physical factors

The previous section has dealt with the chemical aspects of culturing hybridoma cells, but these procedures would be ineffective if the physical conditions of the culture were unsuitable. The primary physical condition which can be altered readily is the means by which the cells are held in homogeneous suspension culture. Of other factors, d_{O_2}, d_{CO_2}, shear factors such as bubble size and distribution, pH (hybridomas, like lymphocytes in culture, prefer a pH just on the acidic side of neutral, about pH 6.8) and temperature are probably the most influential. These physical factors will be dealt with in more detail with respect to culturing conditions and scale-up to commercial production of hybridomas and their antibodies in Chapter 5.

3.7. Growth factors

Cells, whether in a culture flask or within a biological mass, are continually modifying the composition of their environment. Probably the most important of such contributions to *in vitro* cultures is that of growth factors. As mentioned previously, a cell creates a diffusion gradient of growth promotability around itself as proposed by Dulbecco & Elkington (15). Fig. 3.9. summarises the conclusions of their work. Dulbecco (11) had suggested that a number of 'medium factors', of which serum was a major one, contributed to the growth rate of cells in culture. Subsequently, Dulbecco & Elkington (15) showed that cells did not experience inhibition of growth on contact, but rather that it was due to a depletion of growth factors from the medium. In addition, the state of the cells was important, since isolated cells have better access to medium components than do crowded cells (16). Nevertheless, the cells cannot be too dispersed, because Dulbecco & Elkington (15) also demonstrated a 'distance-dependent helper effect between cells'. Thus, a balance has to be achieved between the ready accessibility of medium components and the effectiveness of the 'helper' relationship. Furthermore, Stoker identified the 'diffusion boundary layer', based on the earlier experiments of Rubin & Rein (17). The layer is formed by the cumulative effects of removal of molecules from the medium by cells adjacent to the layer and replenishment of these molecules by diffusion from other parts of the media. It is likely that production of growth factors by the cell would similarly be influenced by the diffusion boundary layer: highest concentrations close to the cells. This diffusion boundary layer and its

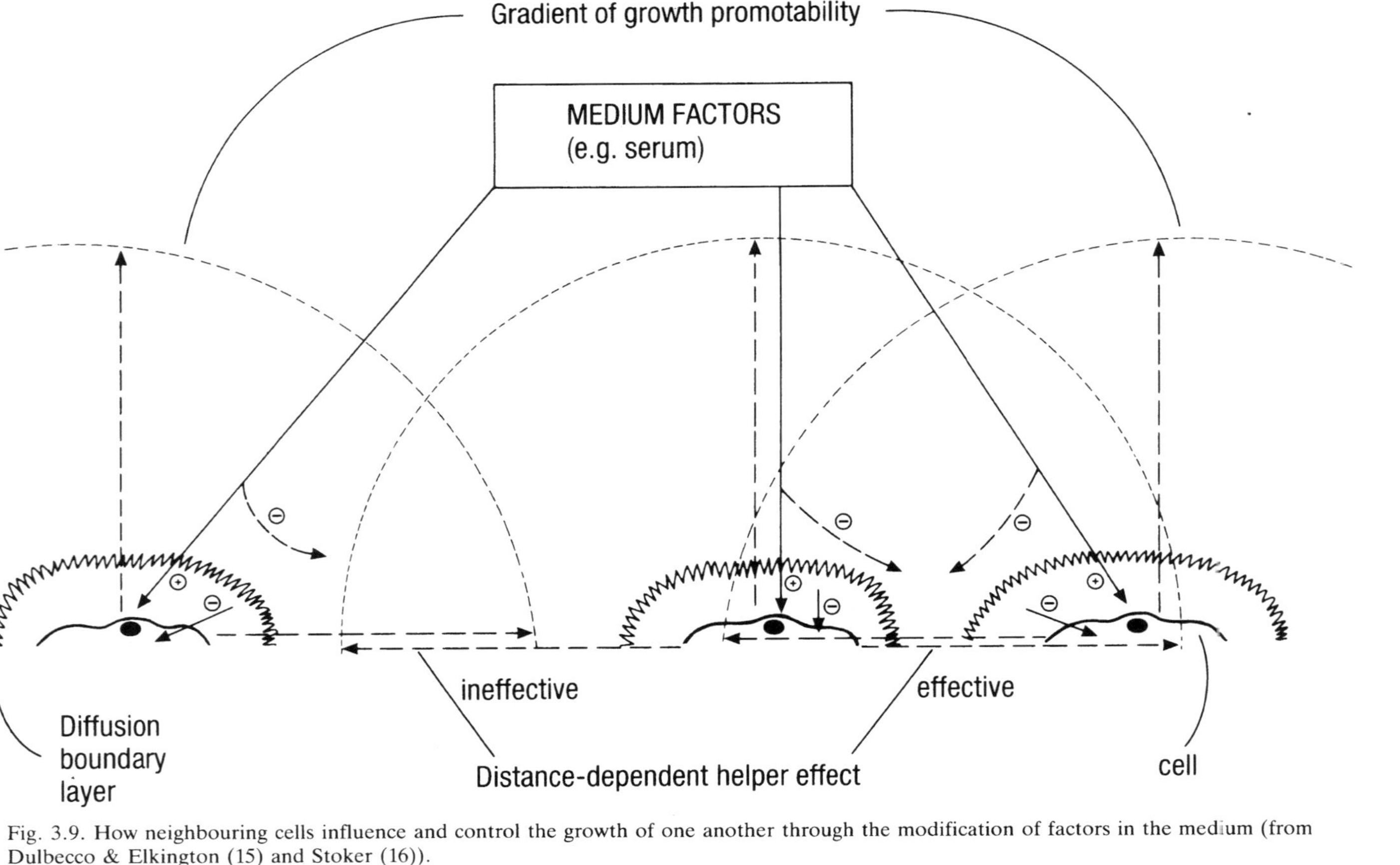

Fig. 3.9. How neighbouring cells influence and control the growth of one another through the modification of factors in the medium (from Dulbecco & Elkington (15) and Stoker (16)).

manipulation will be considered again in Chapter 5 with respect to the optimal physical conditions required for the culture of hybridoma cells.

These cellular 'growth factors' are still poorly defined, although some 'growth factor populations' have now been prepared commercially, mainly from endothelial tissue such as umbilical cord and nerve fibre cultures. It has been argued, however, that a more relevant population of 'growth factors' are those produced by lymphocytes and hybridomas.

After fusion, every millilitre of fusion mixture – that is, an original density of 10^5 myeloma cells and 10^6 splenocytes – will generally yield between 3 and 10 hybridoma clones (4, 7, 8). As can be seen from the models of Dulbecco & Elkington (15) and Stoker (16), these cells would be at too low a density to survive owing to a lack of essential cellular growth factors. However, the tenfold excess of splenocytes in the fusion mixture can provide many of the essential growth promoting substances. The T_h lymphocytes and macrophages are particularly capable of this 'feeder cell' function (see Chapter 1).

3.7.1. *Feeder cells as sources of growth factors*

The application of feeder cells in hybridoma technology will be dealt within §§3.7.2–3.7.5, 3.8.2 and 4.2. How these cells function as feeders, and the capacity to replace the cells with exogenous factors, will be discussed here.

The T_h cells have a selective role to play in that they produce the BCGF, BCMF and IL-2 substances described in Chapter 1, which directly or indirectly aid the growth and differentiation of B cells. They can similarly promote and sustain the replication of other T lymphocytes and mononuclear phagocytes, and they are essential for the majority of lymphocyte (B and T) responses *in vivo* and *in vitro*.

In contrast to lymphocytes, hybridomas do not require the strictly defined environmental conditions of the stimulated B or T lymphocyte. They are not antigen-driven and as such do not require antigen-specific T_h cells or antigen-presenting accessory cells (macrophages, dendritic cells, etc.). They are not 'MHC restricted'. Thus, no Ia recognition (class II MHC antigen recognition) is essential between hybridoma and feeder cell (in contrast to the B or T lymphocyte and its accessory cell). Any T lymphocyte which is producing growth factors should be capable of serving as a feeder cell for hybridomas, and the growth factors do not have to be so strictly defined for hybridomas as they are for B lymphocytes. An impure cocktail of growth factors will suffice.

Macrophages and monocytes are good examples of feeder cells for the provision of essential growth-promoting substances to hybridomas. These cells divide very slowly in culture, but continually synthesise cellular material, among which are growth factors. They can be relatively stable in culture: they can survive up to 2–3 months without cultivation in a specially defined medium. When used at relatively low concentrations, their metabolic rate is not sufficient to deplete the culture medium of essential nutrients, or produce toxic levels of metabolic waste, before the hybridoma cells have grown and established themselves.

The macrophages can be obtained from the splenocyte population used in the fusion. With many fusions this will be adequate. There are, however, situations in which additional feeder cells should be supplied. This is the case when a poor immunogen was used for stimulating the spleens, where a lower proportion of the splenocyte population will be B lymphocytes–lymphoblasts than when a more potent immunogen was used. Hence the frequency of viable hybridomas arising from such a fusion will be lower, and a higher level of growth factor supplement will required. A further complication arises due to the variability in immunoresponsiveness of different mice. It cannot always be assumed that a particular immunogen will always stimulate the spleens sufficiently to obviate a need for additional growth factor supplementation to a fusion mixture. Thus, it is prudent to adopt a routine of providing additional feeder cells to a fusion mixture.

3.7.2. *Splenocyte feeder layers*

A common method of providing additional cells to a fusion mixture is to supplement the mixture with a further tenfold excess of splenocytes. That is, the routine outlined in Fig.3.10. This is a very simple method, but the variation in effectiveness is high. The splenocytes will provide both macrophages–monocytes and lymphocytes as potential feeder cells. Their effectiveness will depend upon their state of activation and degree of differentiation. Different spleens will vary in both the proportions of different leukocyte subpopulations, and the proportions of cells at the correct stage to function as feeders for hybridomas. It is therefore desirable to have a more defined population of cells to act as feeders; that is, one in which the state of activation is more easily determined, and the homogeneity of cell type is more certain. Splenocyte feeders should not be ignored totally, because they can be very effective.

3.7.3. *Peritoneal exudate cell (PEC) feeder layers*

A more definable source of feeder cells is the washings of the peritoneal cavity of mice: the peritoneal exudate cells (PEC). These are a mixture of plastic-adherent macrophages and monocytes (mononuclear phagocytes), non-adherent lymphocytes, and dendritic cells. After two to three days in culture, the adherent cells, which are mainly mononuclear phagocytes, take on a fibroblastic appearance. Such cells can also be seen after culturing splenocytes, and again are the adherent monocytes. Some

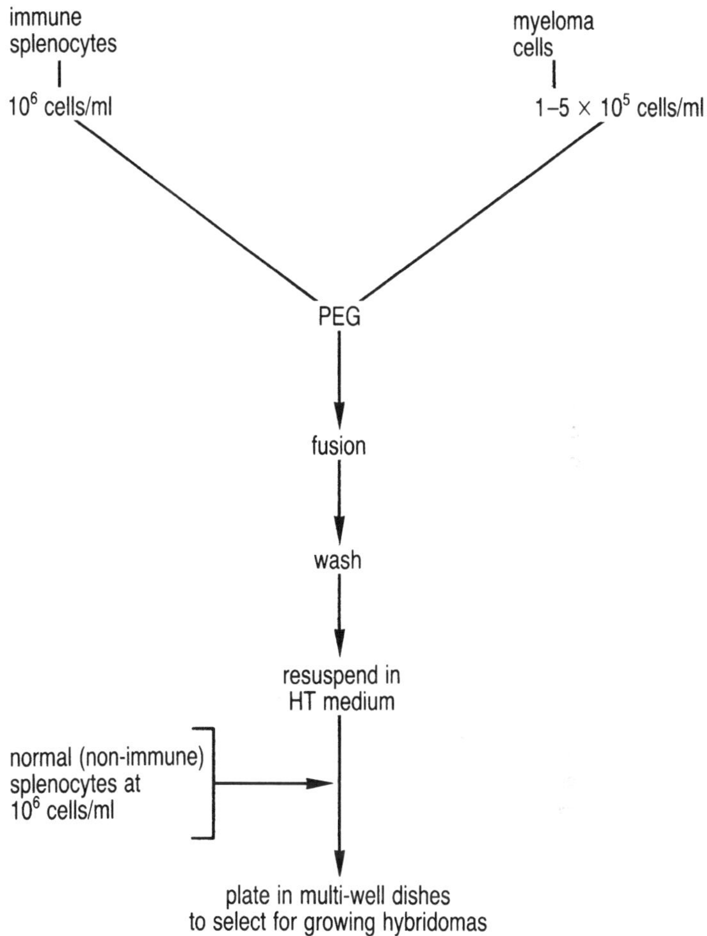

Fig. 3.10. Flow diagram to show when normal splenocytes should be added to a fusion mixture of antigen-stimulated splenocytes and myeloma cells, as a source of feeder cells. The normal splenocytes are usually used at a concentration up to ten times that of the cells in the fusion mixture.

workers favour the selection of adherent populations by culturing at 37 °C for 2 h and then washing off the non-adherent cells. Other workers may irradiate these feeder cells to prevent cell division. This is obligatory when using feeder cells such as splenocytes or lymphocytes to clone, for example, cytotoxic T lymphocytes (single T cells are placed on dense 'monolayers' of feeder cells at 10^6–10^7 cells/ml). For hybridoma culture and cloning, densities of PEC feeder cells in the range of 2 × 10^4 cells/ml are ideal (4). Under these conditions, a DNA replication-inhibitory procedure, such as irradiation, is unnecessary. Likewise, when PEC are

Table 3.14. *Methods for enhancing the quantity of monocytes in the peritoneal cavity of Balb/c mice*

Method[1]	Useful for generating feeder cells or phagocytes
no enhancement[2]	feeder cells
E. coli lipopolysaccharide	feeder cells and primed phagocytes
PPD	activated phagocytes
mineral oil (e.g. 0.5 ml pristane)	activated phagocytes
thioglycollate broth	activated phagocytes (and feeder cells; variable)

Notes:
[1] All inoculations are intraperitoneal.
[2] No enhancement: the resident, 'resting' monocytes of the peritoneal cavity are used.

used, the removal of non-adherent cells is unnecessary, since they also may produce growth-promoting substances without creating a toxic environment for the hybridoma cells.

The resident population of macrophages in the peritoneal cavity can be boosted by various treatments resulting in an influx of secondary mononuclear cells. Such treatments are certainly desirable for increasing the numbers of phagocytic cells in the peritoneal cavity. Comparison of stimulated and unstimulated PEC as feeder cells has not been reported. Table 3.14 lists the various procedures and their influence on the concentration of monocytes in the PEC.

Removal of the PEC is normally effected by vigorous washing of the peritoneal cavity, but great care must be taken not to rupture blood vessels (in which case contaminating erythrocytes must be removed) or the viscera (in which case bacteria or yeast could contaminate the PEC and render them useless as feeders). Such washings are best achieved by using a pipette with a hole in the side rather than at the end, as shown in Fig. 3.11. The procedure for washing peritoneal cavities is illustrated as a flow diagram in Fig.3.12.

3.7.4. *Endothelial cell feeder layers*

There are other sources of feeder cells (Table 3.15), most of which are a macrophage–monocyte population mixed with lymphocytes. Two exceptions are the endothelial and fibroblast cultures. Endothelial cells derived

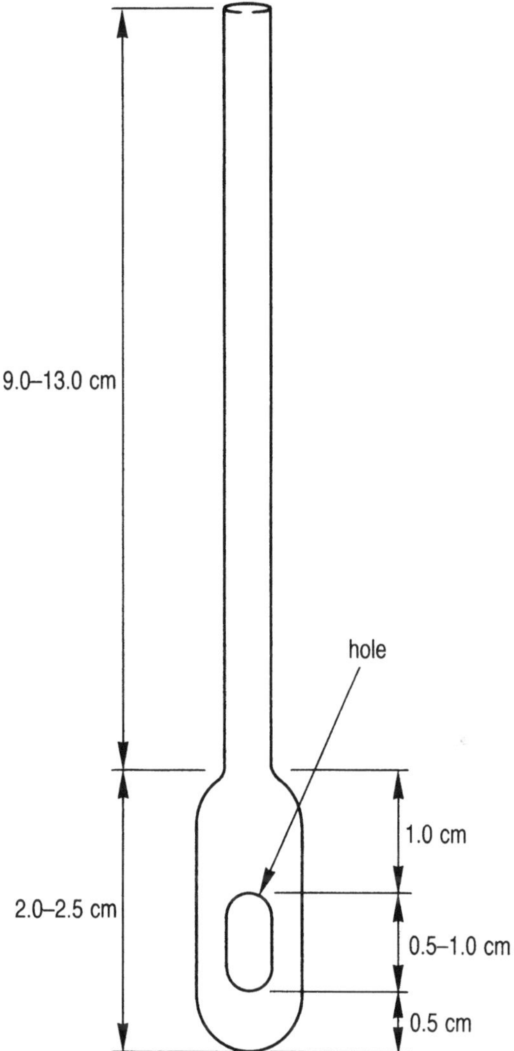

Fig. 3.11. A modified Pasteur pipette used for washing out the peritoneal cavity of mice and rats to obtain peritoneal exudate cells.

from the umbilical cord or nerve tissue have been reported to be a reliable source of growth factors which will sustain the growth of hybridoma cells (18). These and other authors (19) have reported that only the 'factor' (probably a heterogeneous mixture of many factors) is required, and thus medium from such endothelial cells (ECGS) will provide all the requirements made of feeder cells; ECGS were reported to be superior to freshly isolated macrophages at supporting hybridoma

kill mouse
(cervical dislocation)

|

Place mouse on its back

|

Wash peritoneal area thoroughly
with 70% (v/v) methanol in water

|

Make an incision through the skin in the peritoneal area,
running the length of the abdomen
(do not cut through the peritoneum)

|

Suspend mouse by means of two sterilised clips,
one attached to the edge of each flap of skin

|

Make an incision of 1–2 cm long in the peritoneum,
in the centre of the abdominal area and
running the length of the animal

|

Using the special pipette (see fig. 3.11) place 0.5 ml cold,
serum-free RPMI 1640 medium into the abdominal cavity, on each
side of the viscera.

|

Place 1.0 to 1.5 ml cold, serum-free RPMI 1640 medium into the
special pipette, and use this to wash one side of the abdominal
cavity, using the face of the pipette end opposite the hole to rub
against the walls of the abdomen and under the diaphragm.

|

Place the collected fluid into a sterile plastic
container in an ice-bath.

|

Repeat the procedure a total of three to four times
for each side of the abdominal cavity.

Fig. 3.12. The routine for washing out the peritoneal cavity of mice to obtain peritoneal exudate cells. The media should be serum-free, and both the medium and cells should be kept at 2–4 °C until ready for culturing (an ice bath is useful for maintaining media between 2 and 4 °C).

growth. However, McCullough *et al.* (4) reported that PEC feeder cells are optimally used after 5–10 days culture at 37 °C. Extending these observations, Butcher *et al.* (20) showed that ECGS was inferior to seven day old PEC cultures as feeders. Attempts to replace the feeding potential of PEC by using PEC conditioned media (from seven day old cultures of PEC), splenocyte-conditioned media, or ‘Con A activated splenocyte soups’ (media from splenocytes stimulated three to five days previously with the T lymphocyte mitogen concanavalin A, and reputed to be a source of IL-2) also failed to duplicate the efficacy of PEC as feeder cells.

Table 3.15. *Different sources of feeder layers which have been used in the generation of hybridoma cells*

peritoneal exudate cells
splenocytes
thymocytes
lymph node cells
umbilical cord epithelial cells (human)
spinal cord (embryonic) cells (different animals)
Balb/c embryo fibroblast cells: 3T3/B
3T3/A31
activated lymphocytes (72 h activation by LPS, 72 h activation by ConA, 48 h activation by PHA[1])

Note:
[1] LPS, 1 μg/ml bacterial lipopolysaccharide; ConA, 5 μg/ml concanavalin A; PHA, 10 μg/ml phytohaemagglutinin.

3.7.5. *Fibroblastic (3T3/B and 3T3/A31) cell feeder layers*

The other non-monocyte source of feeder cells used in hybridoma technology has proven to be the most reliable of all feeders. These are the embryonic Balb/c mouse fibroblast cells, 3T3/B and 3T3/A31. In contrast to PEC, these cells grow very rapidly; although their optimum seeding concentration as feeders is 2×10^4 cells/ml, their cell division must be inhibited without impairing their feeding potential. To achieve this, DNA replication is blocked by either irradiation or treatment with mitomycin C. Fig. 3.13 outlines both procedures. As with macrophages, the treated 3T3/B or 3T3/A31 cells are cultured at 37°C before use as feeder cells, in this instance for 3–5 days (Fig. 3.14). The advantages of these cells over macrophages are firstly, that they are a tissue culture cell line and therefore more readily available and less expensive to prepare (one mouse will yield approximately 10^6 macrophages; one 75 cm^2 flask of 3T3/B or 3T3/A31 cells will yield 1×10^7 cells); and secondly, that they are more consistent as feeder cells. Although PEC can be just as effective as 3T3/A31 cells as feeders, they are more variable (standard deviation of mean number of hybridoma colonies developing with macrophage feeders was ± 60% (20)). Thus, it is preferable to use 3T3/B or 3T3/A31 cells routinely as feeder cells both for the original fusion mixtures and for cloning hybridomas (see §4.2). The 3T3/A31 subline is the most efficient in this respect.

Once we have established a fusion mixture, containing hybridomas, and optimised the culture medium and environmental factors (chemical, physical and biological), the final parameter required is an efficient protocol for culturing the hybridomas and adapting them to growth *in*

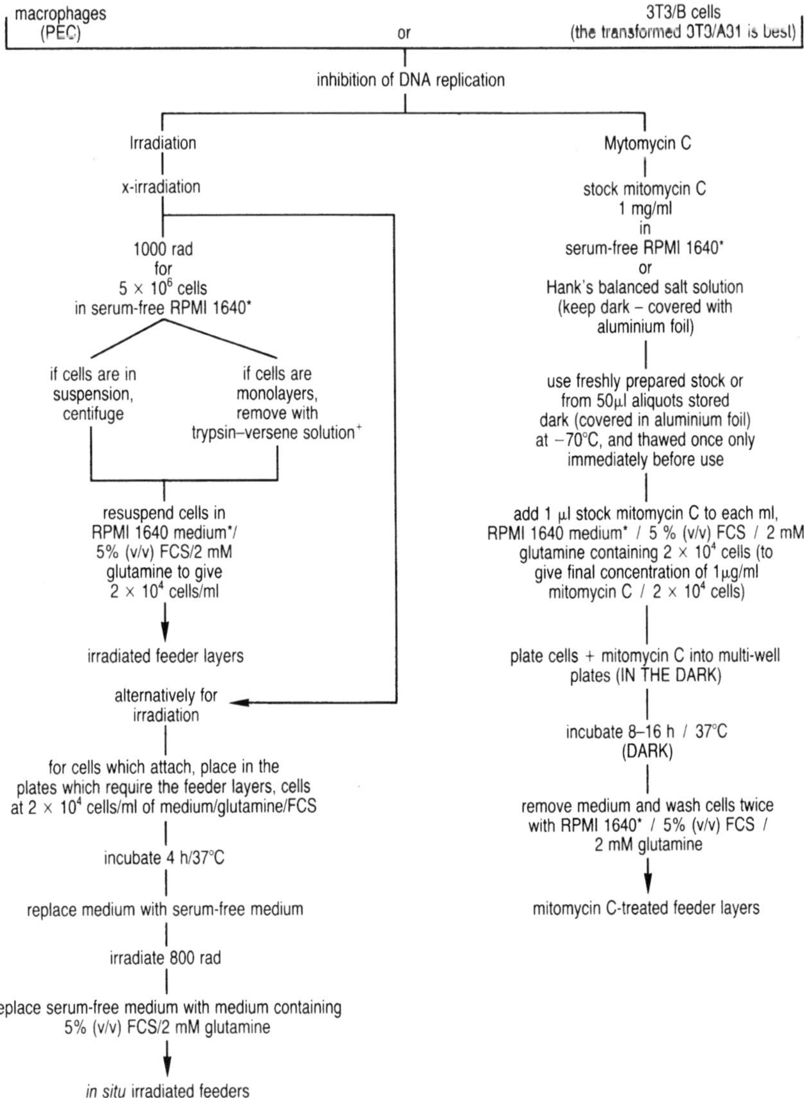

* GMEM (Glasgow modification of Eagle's medium) can be used in place of RPMI 1640 medium

+ Wash cell monolayer twice with pre-warmed (37°C) trypsin–versene solution (0.05% w/v trypsin '1–250'; 0.02% w/v EDTA; 0.1% w/v glucose; 0.04% KCl; 0.8% w/v NaCl; 0.058% w/v $NaHCO_3$), add 5 ml of the trypsin–versene solution / 75 cm^2 flask of cells, leave about 30 s at room temperature, then remove all but a small amount of trypsin–versene. Rock the bottle gently to spread the remaining trypsin–versene over the surface, then tap the side of the bottle forcefully. The cells should then detach from the surface. Resuspend the cells immediately in 10 ml medium/FCS and count the number of cells.

Fig. 3.13. The procedures for the irradiation and the mitomycin C treatment of 3T3/A31 cells prior to their use as feeder cells.

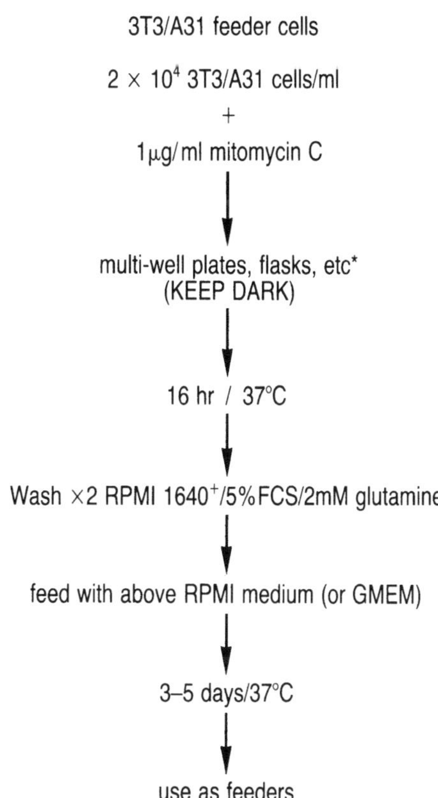

Fig. 3.14. The procedure for using 3T3/A31 cells or peritoneal exudate cells as feeder layers for hybridoma cultures. *Seeding or feeding volumes for plates and flasks are: for 96 well (w) plates, 0.1 ml/well; for 24 w plates, 1 ml/well; for 12 w plates, 1.5 ml/well; for 6 w plates, 2 ml/well; for 25 cm^2 flasks, 5 ml; for 75 cm^2 flasks, 20 ml. +DMEM or GMEM could also be used.

vitro. The next section will therefore deal with these procedures, presenting a stepwise description of the manipulations involved. Various alternatives will also be described.

3.8. Culturing protocols

This aspect of hybridoma technology is critical, since improper culturing of the cells will result in total failure of the technology. However, not all hybridoma cultures will behave identically, even from within the same fusion; the cells in some wells may grow faster than others and some may be weaned off feeder cells before others.

3.8.1. *Initial growth of hybridomas after fusion*

The multi-well dishes known as 24 well (6 × 4) plates have been shown to be the most efficient at supporting the growth of antibody-secreting hybridoma cells which could subsequently be passaged (Fig. 3.15)(21).

The growth of these hybridomas after the fusion relies on two environmental phenomena: the supply of nutrients from the medium, and the production of 'growth factor' gradients by feeder cells. In order to achieve the maximum benefits from both phenomena during this initial growth of hybridomas after fusion, a particular feeding schedule has been devised. Initially, the plates are left, in the main, undisturbed for the first seven days post fusion; then half of the medium in which the cells are growing is removed and replaced with fresh medium. This is critical

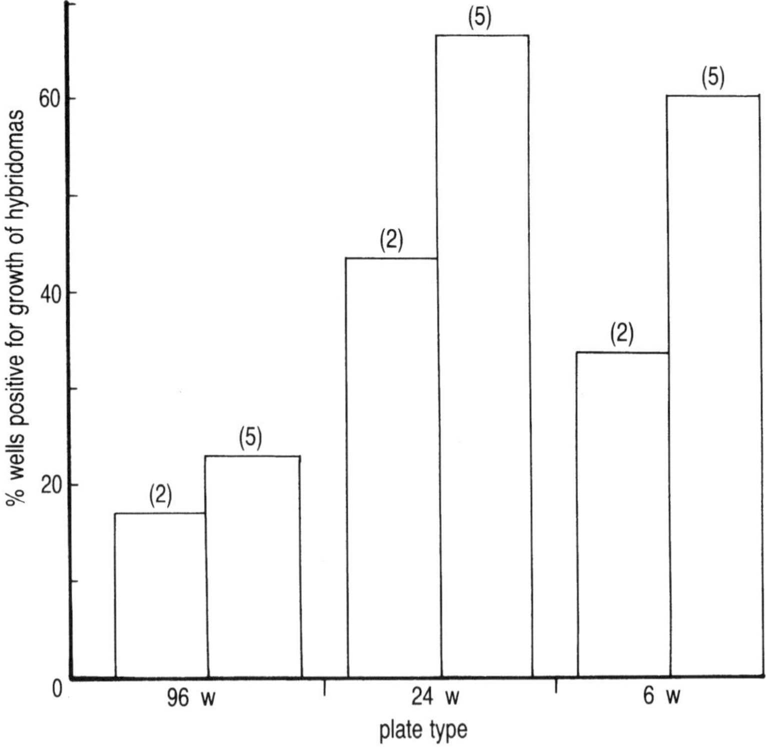

Fig. 3.15. The relative growth of hybridoma cultures in plates of 96 wells (96 w; 12 × 8), 24 wells (24 w; 6 × 4), or 6 wells (6 w; 3 × 2). The fusion mixture was plated in HAT medium incubated at 37 °C for 7 days and then fed with HAT medium by replacing half of the old medium. Further feedings were every two days thereafter. The numbers (2 and 5) in parentheses above the histograms indicate the percentages of wells containing viable hybridomas 2 and 5 weeks after fusion, respectively.

to the success of hybridoma recovery after fusion because the undisturbed incubation probably permits growth factor gradients to be established. Such gradients could then assist or sustain the division of the surviving hybridoma cells. This and other regimes for the first feeding schedule have been compared (6, 21), and the findings (summarised in Fig. 3.16) have proved this 'seven day rest' before feeding to be the most effective.

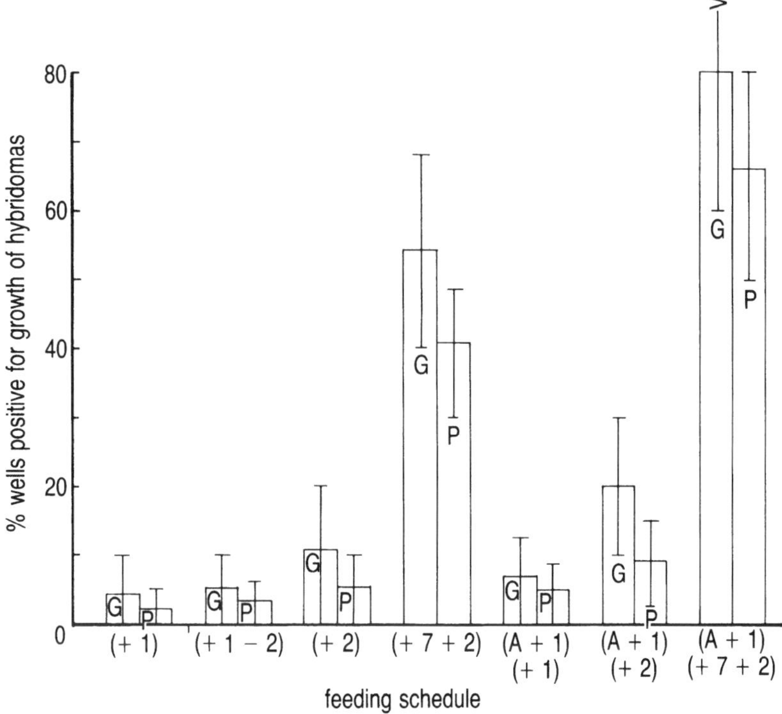

Fig. 3.16. The relative efficacy of different feeding schedules for hybridoma cultures after fusion on the generation of viable hybridoma cells which could be subcultured. (+1), cultures fed every day by replacing half of the old medium with new HAT medium; (+1−2), as for +1 except that after 7 days, the feedings were every second day; (+2), feedings were every two days; (+7+2), the first feeding was 7 days after fusion, and then every two days thereafter; (A+1)(+1), aminopterin was not added until one day after the fusion, and then the cultures were fed every day with HAT medium as for +1; (A+1)(+2), aminopterin was added after one day and the cultures were then fed every 2 days with HAT medium; (A+1)(+7+2), aminopterin was added after one day, the cultures were left at 37°C for another 7 days and then fed with HAT medium by replacing half of the old medium every two days. G, wells with growing hybridomas; P, wells from which the hybridomas could be subcultured successfully. The bars indicate the variation in efficiency which can be obtained when a fusion has been successful (unsuccessful fusions usually give less than 10% of the wells with growing hybridomas, and then only with the feeding schedule (A+1)(+7+2)).

It should be necessary to view the hybridomas during this seven day period only once, and that is 24 h after fusion. The culture should be carefully checked for fungal or yeast contamination. If found, the wells must be emptied, washed and the medium replaced with an equal volume of saturated copper sulphate solution. During this observation, the plates should be kept out of the incubator for the minimum period possible, since a small increase in pH into the alkaline range will be detrimental to the hybridomas. These manipulations 24 h after fusion are made more feasible because this is the optimum time for the addition of aminopterin. Thus, the hybridomas should experience little impairment to their growth since the myeloma cells, which have been capable of a limited degree of growth during this time, will have 'conditioned' the medium with growth factors, to supplement those produced by the feeder layers. The benefits of the myeloma cell products will soon cease after their death through addition of aminopterin; hence the cultures and their surviving growth factor gradients should be undisturbed for seven days.

On the seventh day, the medium will require replenishing owing to a build-up of toxic metabolites and a loss of activity of glutamine and other serum factors. The cultures can also be screened microscopically for hybridoma cells at this time, but again adhering to the principle at all times of keeping the cultures out of the incubator for the minimum period possible. With many fusions, especially those in which potent immunogens were used, cells will be easily seen, and over the next few days they will grow rapidly. Some fusions, however, do not yield many hybridomas. In such cases, the cells should be disturbed as little as possible until the hybridomas are seen to be growing; in other words, time should not be spent looking for hybridomas. When the cells are ready for subculture, their presence will be detected very easily.

The general rule is that at the seventh day post fusion, half of the medium in each well of the multi-well dish should be carefully removed without disturbing the cells. This is replaced by an equal volume of fresh HAT medium (ensure the pH is 7.0 ± 0.2). When hybridoma cells are easily seen, the wells will probably need feeding every two days, but if only a few cells are present, feeding every 3–5 days may be more appropriate. The times of feeding are governed by the rate of growth of hybridoma cells. The faster they grow, the more often they will require feeding (the same 50% replacement described above).

3.8.2. *Subcultures of hybridomas*

When the hybridoma cells have grown substantially (that is, they cover 60–80% of the available growing surface: '60–80% confluence') they may be subcultured. Fig. 3.17 demonstrates how this is best achieved. No time scale is given since this will vary considerably for different

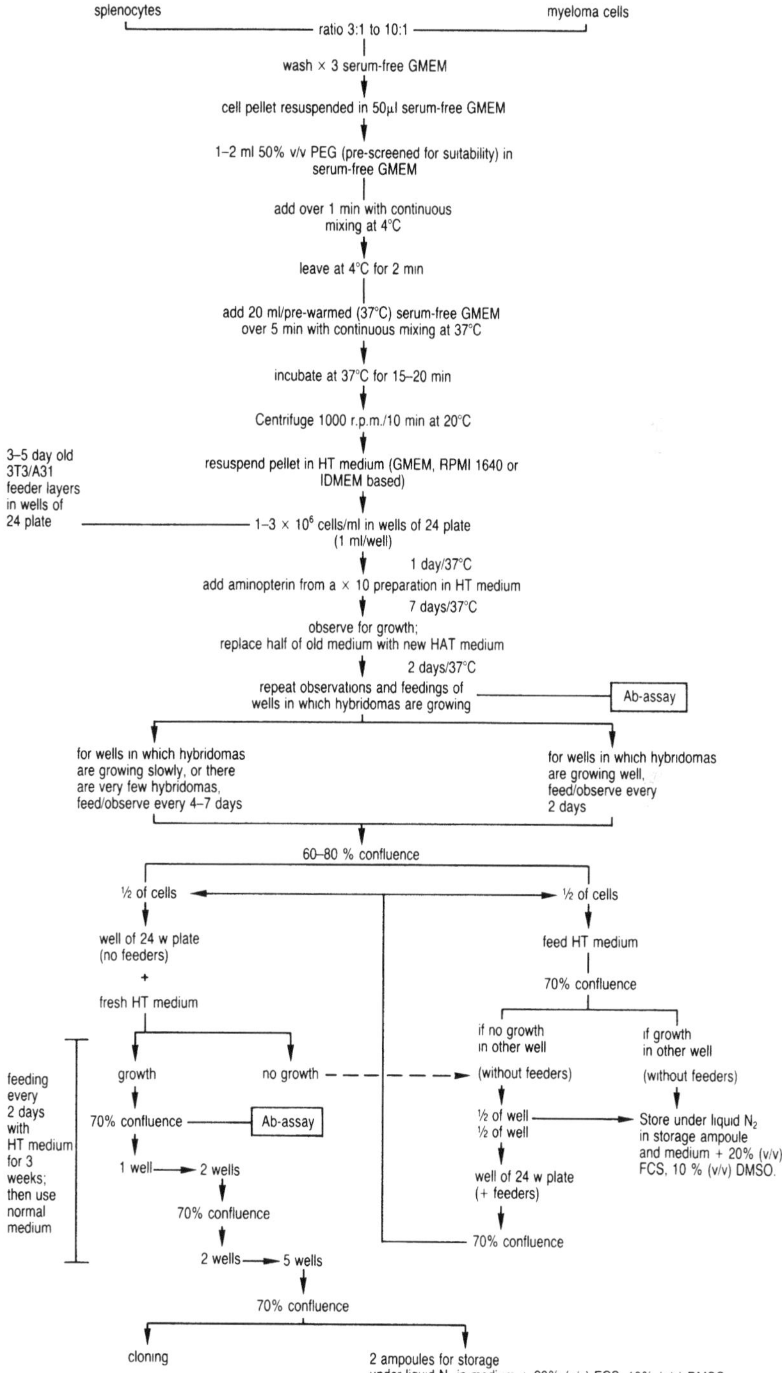

Fig. 3.17. The optimum routine for generating and culturing hybridoma cells.

cultures. In a single fusion, some wells containing hybridomas will require subculturing 10–14 days after fusion, whereas others may not be ready until after 4–5 weeks. The secret of successful subculture is knowing how to handle the particular hybridoma being subcultured. The first step is to determine how efficiently the cells are growing. This will become obvious during the first 14 days after fusion. Secondly, the adaptability of the hybridoma cells to *in vitro* culture must be ascertained. The cells are subcultured into fresh wells, or wells with new feeders to ensure that any detrimental effect of passage is minimised. The next subculture of the cells on new feeders, when at 60–80% of confluence, should be attempted without feeder cells ('weaning off the feeders'). If either weaning fails, the subculture must be repeated with feeders. This is possible because a *maximum* of half of the cells is removed from a well during subculture. Thus, if the transferred cells do not grow, the remaining cells normally do, because they are in a more conditioned environment. When these cells have regrown to between 60 and 80% of confluence, they can again be subcultured. The attempted weaning should be repeated in this fashion until the hybridoma cells can grow without feeder cells. The time taken to achieve this also varies considerably with different hybridomas, as does their growth rate in the absence of feeder cells.

This weaning of hybridoma cells from their dependence on feeder cells is desirable if successful storage and cloning is to be achieved. The less dependent the hybridomas are on feeder layers, the more beneficial will be the effects of adding feeder cells to the hybridomas when breaking them out from storage or when cloning. Thus, hybridoma cells are ideally stored or cloned when they grow independently of feeder cells. Fig. 3.17 shows the points at which these manipulations may successfully be achieved.

The split levels shown at each passage in Fig. 3.17 are the optimum dilution of the hybridoma cells which will permit growth of the subcultured cells. However, the number of subcultures before cloning should be kept to a minimum to prevent overgrowth of the non-producing hybridoma cells (see §§2.3.1 and 2.6.3). The ideal time post fusion for cloning (and for storing), if all cultures behaved identically, would be after two to four weeks to allow the hybridomas to stabilise (see §§2.3.1 and 2.6.3) but to keep the overgrowth of the culture by the non-producing antibody cells to a minimum. This, of course, is not always possible because of the variation between cultures in the time required to wean the cells off feeder layers and stabilise their growth *in vitro*. Consequently, a compromise must be reached, such that the hybridomas are stored and/or cloned as soon as they have adapted to *in vitro* growth in the absence of feeder cells. Should the stable uncloned hybridomas be passaged further, cell density measurements can now be made more readily, because the cells can be grown in flasks as opposed to multi-well plates.

The density range within which the cells should be cultured is 2×10^4 to 4×10^5 cells/ml. However, it is best not to give these uncloned hybridomas more than three to four subcultures, and as such it may not be possible to passage the cells into flasks. It is preferable to clone as soon after fusion as is feasible, and it is likely that this may be done when the cells are still in multi-well dishes.

3.8.3. *Removal of aminopterin*

The final consideration for culturing hybridomas after fusion is when to change to HT medium. Hybridomas should be cultured in HAT medium for at least one, and preferably two subcultures. This should remove most hybridomas which revert to a myeloma cell phenotype due to chromosomal losses (§§2.3.1 and 2.5.9). The cells then have to be given enough medium changes with HT medium to ensure that no toxic levels of aminopterin remain either extracellularly or intracellularly (see §2.3.2). An ideal number is seven (consisting of feedings, subcultures and storage followed by 'break-out').

3.8.4. *Screening for antibody production, and cloning of cells*

Attempts to detect antibody too early will produce inconclusive results, owing to the presence of splenocyte antibody and the fact that chromosomal chain losses may still be occurring (see §§2.6.3 and 2.5.9). Fig. 3.17 shows suitable time points (= Ab-assay) at which cultures may be tested for antibody. The first point is chosen to prevent time and effort being wasted in passaging non-producing cultures. The second assay confirms that the initial observations were not due to extraneous antibody or from hybridomas which subsequently lost the capacity to secrete antibody. Procedures for assaying hybridoma cultures for the presence of antibody will be described in Chapter 4.

Having successfully generated, subcultured, tested and stored hybridoma cells, the final procedure is to clone the cells. From this activity, the object of the exercise – to produce monoclonal antibody – is achieved. This procedure, and that of determining antibody secretion by the hybridomas, will be dealt with in §§4.2–4.4.

3.9. **Summary**

Manipulation of every facet of hybridoma technology, from the immunisation of the animals to the composition of the culture medium, can influence the success rate of generating antigen-specific antibody-secreting hybridoma cells.

The immunisation protocol must be designed to stimulate a large number of B cell lymphoblasts in the secondary lymphoid organ of choice (normally the spleen) on the day of the fusion (three days after the final inoculation of the animals). Not all antigens are equally immunogenic, and various mechanisms have been used to increase this immunogenicity, ranging from simple treatments of the antigen (such as aggregation) to multi-step immunisation protocols (hyperimmunisation).

The conditions for fusing the lymphoblasts with myeloma cells require selection of the optimum from several batches and molecular weight ranges of PEG. Subsequent culturing requires certain media supplements (in particular foetal calf serum, and 2 mM glutamine, or replacement of serum by the transferrin–lipid–albumin–selenite composition of IDMEM), and the correct pH (6.8–7.2, with the CO_2 concentration in the atmosphere set at 7% v/v).

Growth factors are one of the most important culturing aspects of hybridoma technology, in particular shortly after fusion, owing to the very low concentration of hybridomas (often only 3–10 cells/ml). The most effective method of supplying these factors is through the use of feeder cell layers. The ideal feeder cells appear to be mitomycin C-treated or irradiated 3T3/A31 cells at 2×10^4 cells/ml.

Finally, the optimum culturing protocol is where the fused cells are placed into wells of 24 well plates, aminopterin is added after 24 h, and the fusions are left untouched for seven days after addition of the aminopterin (this permits the establishment of growth factor diffusion gradients and hence hybridoma cell colony growth). Half of the medium in each well is then replaced every 2–3 days until the cells cover about 70% of the available growing surface, at which point they are subcultured and slowly weaned off the feeder cells as shown in Fig. 3.17. Once adapted to growth without feeder layers, the hybridomas are maintained at between 2×10^4 and 4×10^5 cells/ml.

Having now established hybridoma cultures *in vitro*, the antibody-secreting cells of choice must be selected. This requires screening of the cultures for the production of antigen-specific antibody, and the subsequent cloning of the cells. It is on these two topics that Chapter 4 will concentrate.

4 Selection of monoclonal antibody-secreting hybridoma cell lines

The production of monoclonal antibodies can be divided into a number of phases. (i) Immune splenocytes are fused with myeloma cells, and the resultant hybridomas are selected and adapted to growth in tissue culture. (ii) The hybridoma media (culture supernatants) are tested for the presence of antibody. (iii) Positive cultures are 'weaned off' feeder cells and, when fully adapted to growth *in vitro*, are cloned. (iv) Growing colonies of hybridoma cells are tested for secretion of antibody specific for the appropriate antigen, and positive cultures expanded (by growth and passage) and recloned. (v) Of these 're-clones', those secreting the highest relative quantities of antibody (relative to the cell concentration) are selected for expansion and eventual storage. Chapters 2 and 3 dealt in detail with the preparation and passage of hybridoma cultures, and the conditions required for successful hybridoma production. This chapter will describe the methods for detecting antibody in hybridoma cultures, and the procedures of isolating monoclonal hybridomas (cloning).

The antibody-detecting assays will be described in approximate order of frequency of use in reports of hybridoma technology, and only the major assays will be discussed in detail. Other procedures will be mentioned, but the assays described in detail are those which should prove most applicable to hybridoma technology.

The three most commonly reported methods of cloning hybridoma cells will be described; the theoretical and practical advantages and disadvantages will be discussed. These procedures are cloning established hybridomas by limit dilution, isolation of colonies from the 'masterplate' (plate used for seeding the fusion mixture) – micromanipulation – and isolation of colonies in semi-solid ('sloppy') agar. A more recent adaptation, that of cloning hybridoma cells immediately after fusion, will also be described.

To complete the technological requirements of hybridoma generation, monoclonality must be confirmed, and to this end the various applicable procedures will be described. Finally, the culturing protocol for monoclonal hybridoma cells will be shown, with the aid of a comprehensive flow diagram, to encompass the various alternative routines which must be considered.

4.1. Screening of polyclonal hybridomas

The various assay systems for detecting antibody in hybridoma culture supernatants can be broadly classified into those for general screening and those for a more defined characterisation (Table 4.1). In the former class are the immunoassay and immunodiffusion–immunoelectrophoresis procedures. These can be subdivided into those for detecting the secreted hybridoma cell products – enzyme-linked immunosorbent assay (ELISA); radioimmunoassay (RIA); passive haemagglutination (PAH); Ouchterlony double immunodiffusion (DID); single radial immunodiffusion (SRID); radial haemolytic assay (RHA) – and those for the detection of the antibody-secreting hybridoma cell: haemadsorption (HAd); direct and indirect antiglobulin rosetting reactions (DARR, IARR); Jerne plaque assay for antibody-secreting cells (PFCA); replica plate assay (RPA).

The second class of assays which will be described are those which can be used for determining the functional activity of the MAb: haemagglutination inhibition (HAI), neuraminidase inhibition (NI) and haemolysin inhibition (HLI) for detecting reactivity against the glycoprotein antigens of certain viruses; virus neutralisation assays, which detect antibody with the capacity to inhibit virus infection of susceptible host cells; opsonisation assays, which are used to detect MAb reactivity against bacterial antigens, although most antigens can be opsonised; immunofluorescence for detecting antigens in infected mammalian cells (infected by intracellular parasites such as viruses, chlamydia, mycobacteria and certain protozoa), antigens on the surface of bacteria and other unicellular and multicellular parasites, and antigenic determinants on mammalian cells such as leukocytes; and cytolytic assays, which will also identify antigens on bacteria, parasites and mammalian cells with the aid of the antibody-dependent complement-mediated cytolytic processes (as with the opsonisation assays, these procedures detect an antibody-dependent function which can be directly related to *in vivo* immune defence mechanisms).

4.1.1. *Enzyme-linked immunosorbent assay (ELISA)*

The ELISA can be divided into the sandwich ELISA, indirect ELISA, amplified ELISA, indirect sandwich ELISA, double sandwich ELISA and liquid phase ELISA. Variations, in the form of additional steps, in the three major ELISA formats (sandwich, indirect and liquid phase) may be used. From these come the amplified ELISA and tests such as the indirect and double sandwich ELISA. Fig. 4.1 is a schematic of the steps involved in each ELISA (only one example is given for the amplified, indirect sandwich and double sandwich ELISA in order to

Table 4.1. *The major assays applied to the detection of monoclonal antibodies*

Assay type	Assay
general screening	enzyme-linked immunosorbent assay
	radioimmunoassay
	passive haemagglutination
	Ouchterlony double immunodiffusion
	single radial immunodiffusion
	radial haemolysis
	haemadsorption
	direct rosetting
	indirect rosetting
	Jerne plaque assay
	replica plate assay
	immunoelectrophoresis
defined characterisation	haemagglutination inhibition
	neuraminidase inhibition
	haemolysin inhibition
	virus infectivity neutralisation
	opsonisation
	immunofluorescence
	cytolytic assays

demonstrate how ELISA procedures can be adapted and amplified). As can be seen, the common feature is an immobilisation of the immunoreactions to a solid phase. This was originally developed in polystyrene tubes (1) and later adapted to microtitre (96-well) plates (2), which is now the accepted procedure. There are now a number of commercially available ELISA plates; comparison of their characteristics and performances in ELISA have been reported by McCullough & Parkinson (3,4). The basic requirements for ELISA are listed in Table 4.2. There are alternative buffering systems in that either lactalbumin yeast hydrolysate (LYH), bovine serum albumin V (BSA) or, with certain ELISA plates, ovalbumin (OA) can be used to supplement the PBS–Tween 20 diluting buffer (3,4). The source of LYH, BSA or OA should be chosen carefully since different sources or even different batches from the same supplier can produce aspecific binding of conjugates or unconjugated enzyme which has not been removed after a conjugation procedure.

The central theme to ELISA – immobilising the reaction on the solid phase – can be achieved by one of the following (Fig. 4.2).

(i) Antigen or immunoglobulin (purified immunoglobulin or IgG must be used, since serum proteins other than immunoglobulin,

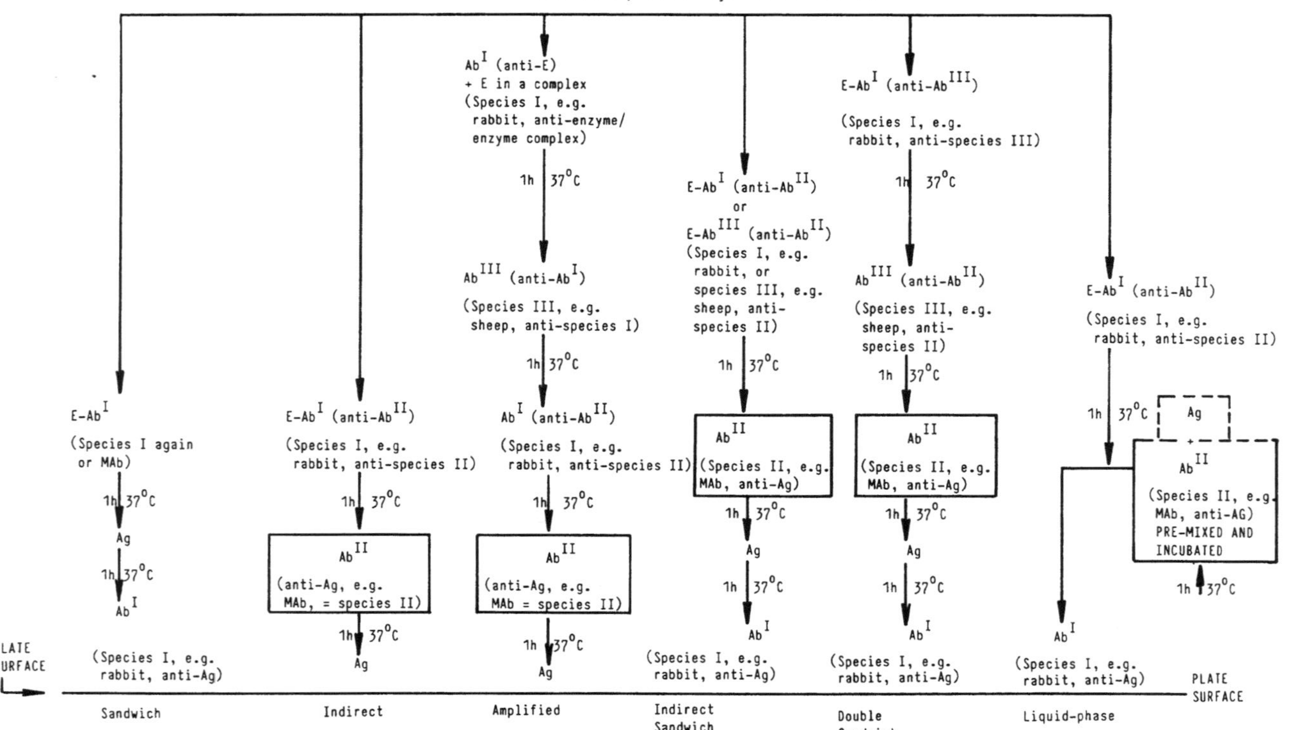

Fig. 4.1. The various incubation steps involved in the sandwich, indirect, amplified, indirect sandwich, double sandwich and liquid-phase ELISA. Ab, antibody (of species I, II or III); Ag, antigen; E-Ab, enzyme-conjugated antibody.

Table 4.2. *ELISA requirements*

Plates:

Nunc Immunoplate I
Dynatech M129B immunoassay plate
Falcon immunoassay plate

Coating buffer:

8 ml 0.2 M Na_2CO_3 anhydrous
17 ml 0.2 M $NaHCO_3$
75 ml distilled H_2O
pH 9.6

Diluting buffer (blocking buffer) PBS/T20/albumin:

PBS: 8 g NaCl
0.2 g KH_2PO_4
2.9 g $Na_2HPO_4.12H_2O$
0.2 g KCl
made up to 1 litre with H_2O
pH 7.4
0.05% (v/v) Tween 20
1% (w/v) lactalbumin yeast hydrolysate
(or bovine serum albumin fraction V
or ovalbumin)

Conjugates:

anti-species (usually mouse) immunoglobulins
labelled with (a) horseradish peroxidase (HRPO)
(b) alkaline phosphatase type VII (AP)
(c) β-galactosidase (gal)
(d) biotin (Bio)
(e) glucose oxidase (GO)

Substrates:

(a) for HRPO: *o*-phenylenediamine (OPD) – H_2O_2
or tetramethylbenzidine (TMB) – H_2O_2
(b) for AP : *p*-nitrophenylphosphate
(c) for gal : *o*-nitrophenyl-ß-galactoside (ONPG)
(d) for Bio : Streptavidin–HRPO conjugate followed by the substrate for HRPO (a).
(e) for GO : ß-D-glucose–nitro-blue tetrazolium

in particular albumin, can compete for the binding of the IgG to the plastic) is diluted in coating buffer (Table 4.2) tc a final concentration of 10 μg/ml (4), applied to the wells of the ELISA plate at 50 μl/well for 2–3 h at 37 °C or room temperature, or overnight at 4 °C.

(ii) Repeat of (i) but using PBS (Table 4.2) as opposed to coating buffer. With several antigens, the binding is reversible to a degree, and incubation should not exceed 2 h. Although coating buffer is preferable, PBS is sometimes required owing to the labile nature of certain antigens at the pH (9.6) of coating buffer.

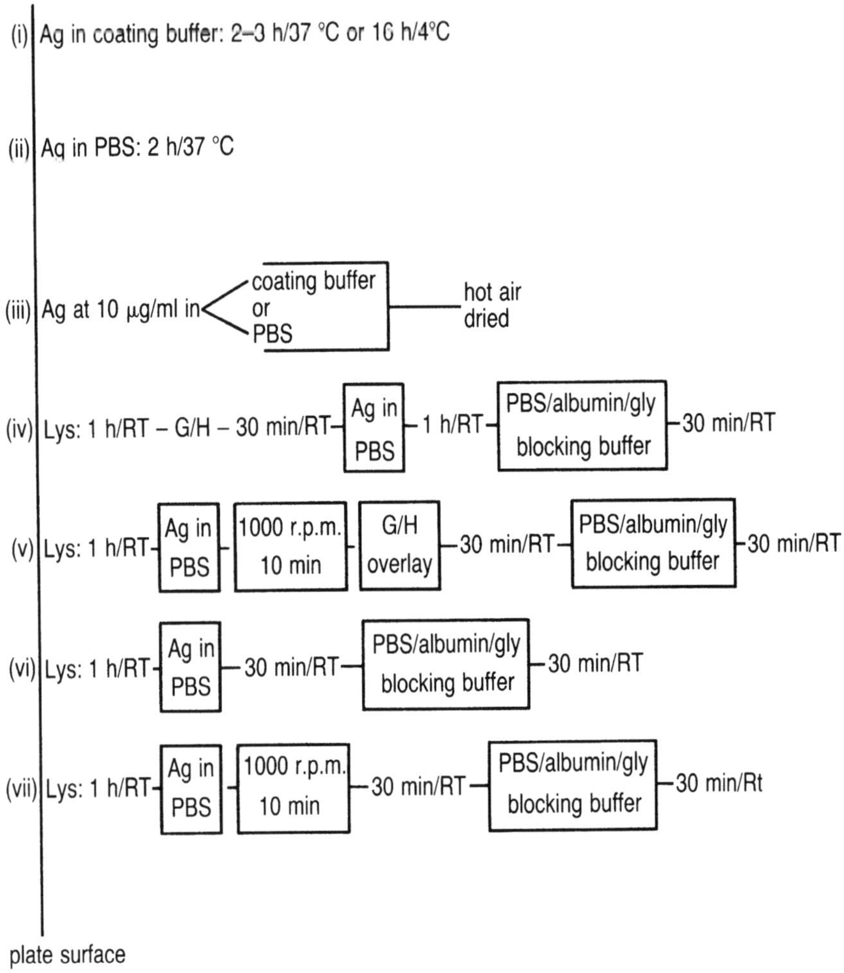

(i) Ag in coating buffer: 2–3 h/37 °C or 16 h/4°C

(ii) Ag in PBS: 2 h/37 °C

(iii) Ag at 10 μg/ml in coating buffer or PBS — hot air dried

(iv) Lys: 1 h/RT – G/H – 30 min/RT – Ag in PBS – 1 h/RT – PBS/albumin/gly blocking buffer – 30 min/RT

(v) Lys: 1 h/RT – Ag in PBS – 1000 r.p.m. 10 min – G/H overlay – 30 min/RT – PBS/albumin/gly blocking buffer – 30 min/RT

(vi) Lys: 1 h/RT – Ag in PBS – 30 min/RT – PBS/albumin/gly blocking buffer – 30 min/RT

(vii) Lys: 1 h/RT – Ag in PBS – 1000 r.p.m. 10 min – 30 min/RT – PBS/albumin/gly blocking buffer – 30 min/Rt

plate surface

Fig. 4.2. Various methods used for the adsorption of antigen to the surface of ELISA plates. Ag, antigen; Lys, poly-L-lysine; G/H, glutaraldehyde; RT, room temperature; gly, glycine.

(iii) Antigen is diluted in PBS or coating buffer and dried on to the ELISA plate using a source of hot air such as a hair drier. This is not recommended for IgG or antigens which are extremely labile to heat. It is, however, more suitable than (i) or (ii) for binding whole cells, such as bacteria, protozoa and mammalian cells such as lymphocytes. When using coating buffer, only fixed cells can be used, since the pH (9.6) would disrupt live cells.

(iv) Poly-L-lysine (M_r 70 000–400 000) is diluted in carbonate–bicarbonate coating buffer to give 10 mg/ml. 50 μl are added to each well of an ELISA plate, and incubated for 2 h at 37 °C. The plates are washed three times with PBS (Table 4.2) and 50 μl/well of 0.25%–0.0125% (v/v) glutaraldehyde solution (the lower concentrations are favoured owing to the denaturing activity of glutaraldehyde on certain antigens) added for 30 min at room temperature. The plates are again washed, and the cellular antigen (or other antigen which is difficult to bind to the ELISA plate by using procedures (i) or (ii)) added at a pre-determined concentration. The plates are incubated for 1 h at 37 °C. Alternatively, the cells may be added before the glutaraldehyde, pelleted onto the poly-L-lysine – 1000 r.p.m./10 min at 4 °C – and the cells then overlayed with glutaraldehyde and incubated at room temperature for 15 min before washing. The remainder of the ELISA is similar to that when other binding procedures are used. This procedure has been used primarily for binding whole cells to an ELISA plate.

(v) An alternative procedure to that described in (iv) has been reported by Epstein & Lunney (5) in which the concentration of glutaraldehyde was reduced tenfold and the poly-L-lysine step was found to be unnecessary. That is, whole cells in PBS were pelleted on to ELISA plates (1000 r.p.m./10 min at 4 °C), and glutaraldehyde then added to give a final concentration of 0.0125% (v/v). The plates were incubated for 15 min at room temperature, and washed as in (iv). The remainder of the ELISA was again similar to when other binding procedures were used.

In Fig. 4.1, each joining line represents an incubation step. Excepting the coating procedure (binding antigen or immunoglobulin to the ELISA plate), all reagents are diluted in PBS/T20/albumin (Table 4.2) and incubation steps are 1–2 h at 37 °C or overnight at 4 °C. After each incubation step, plates are washed by flooding with PBS wash solution (Table 4.2), flicking off the PBS, and repeating three more times. Excess wash solution is removed by vigorously shaking the plates or forcefully blotting them on paper towelling.

Reaction is detected by an appropriate antibody conjugated with either alkaline phosphatase or horseradish peroxidase (HRPO) (Tables 4.3 and 4.4. show these conjugation procedures, and many conjugated antibodies are commercially available). Antibody conjugated with biotin (Table 4.5) can also be used, but requires incubation (1–2 h at 37 °C) followed by washing and then incubation with HRPO-conjugated streptavidin (1 h at 37 °C). Bound enzyme-conjugated antibody is detected by adding the appropriate substrate and stopping the reaction after a pre-determined time (Table 4.6). Degraded substrate is measured spectrophotometrically (Table 4.6). In the indirect ELISA, the enzyme-conjugated anti-mouse Ig can be replaced by enzyme-conjugated protein

Table 4.3. *Method for conjugating antibody with alkaline phosphatase (AP)*

1. Take 0.3 ml of the AP suspension (Sigma type VII) and centrifuge at 1000 r.p.m. for 10 min at 4 °C to remove the enzyme from the ammonium sulphate solution.
2. Dissolve the pellet in 0.1 ml of immunoglobulin solution (5 mg/ml) in PBS.
3. Dialyse against PBS overnight at 4 °C.
4. Add 10 μl glutaraldehyde (25% solution, Sigma grade II, diluted to give a 2% solution) for 2 h at 20 °C with continuous mixing.
5. Dilute to 1 ml with PBS.
6. Dialyse extensively against PBS for 48 h at 4 °C (frequent changes of dialysate).
7. Dilute to 10 ml with 0.05 M Tris–HCl (pH 8) containing 0.001 M magnesium carbonate and 10 mM sodium azide.

Table 4.4. *Methods for conjugating antibody with horseradish peroxidase (HRPO)*

(a)

1. Dissolve HRPO (Sigma type VI, 8 mg) in 1.0 ml freshly prepared 0.3 M sodium bicarbonate, pH 8.1.
2. Add 100 μl of 1.0% (v/v) dinitrofluorobenzene (CAUTION) in absolute ethanol.
3. Mix gently for 60 min at 20 °C.
4. Add 1.0 ml of 0.08 M sodium periodate in distilled water.
5. Mix gently for 30 min at 20 °C.
6. Add 1.0 ml of 0.16 M ethylene glycol (ethanediol) in distilled water.
7. Mix gently for 60 min at 20 °C.
8. Dialyse (3 changes of 1 l) against 0.01 M sodium carbonate, pH 9.5, at 4 °C.
9. Add the activated HRPO solution to the immunoglobulin solution at the ratio of 1.33 mg HRPO to 5 mg of immunoglobulin.
10. Leave the mixture at 20 °C for *at least* 3 h.
11. Add 5 μl of a 200 mg/ml solution of sodium borohydride per milligram of HRPO used.
12. Leave at 4 °C for *at least* 3 h.
13. Dialyse against PBS, pH 7.4.
14. Store in small aliquots at −20 °C.

(b)

1. Dissolve 4 mg HRPO in distilled water.
2. Add 200 μl 0.1 M sodium periodate.
3. Mix and leave for 30 min at 20 °C.
4. Dialyse against 1 mM sodium acetate, pH 4.4 (1 l), for 16 h at 4 °C.
5. Add 100 μl 0.2 M sodium carbonate, pH 9.5. Immediately add 8 mg immunoglobulin in 1 ml 10 mM sodium carbonate, pH 9.5.
6. Check that pH is greater than 9.0.
7. Incubate for 2 hours at 20 °C.
8. Add 100 μl of a 4 mg/ml solution of sodium borohydride.
9. Incubate for 2 h at 4 °C.
10. Dialyse against PBS, pH 7.4, for 16 h at 4 °C.
11. Add glycerol to 50% (final volume) and store at −20 °C, or store in aliquots (no glycerol) at −70 °C.

Table 4.4. *(cont.)*

(c) 1. Dissolve 5 mg HRPO in 0.5 ml 0.1 M sodium bicarbonate, pH 8.1.
2. Add 0.5 ml 16 mM sodium periodate. (Use a small tube in order to have a small air gap.)
3. Close tube and leave in the *dark* for 2 h at 20 °C.
4. Dissolve 15 mg immunoglobulin in 1.5 ml 0.1 M sodium carbonate, pH 9.2, and add to the HRPO solution.
5. Add 0.167 g Sephadex G25 per millilitre immunoglobulin–HRPO solution.
6. Place in a plugged Pasteur pipette.
7. Incubate *at least* 3 h at 20 °C in the *dark*.
8. Open the bottom of the Pasteur pipette and collect the eluate by eluting with 0.1 M sodium carbonate, pH 9.2.
9. Add $\frac{1}{20}$ of the volume of sodium borohydride solution (5 mg/ml in 0.1 M NaOH).
10. Incubate for 30 min at 20 °C.
11. Add $\frac{3}{20}$ of the volume of the sodium borohydride solution and leave for 60 min at 20 °C.
12. Dialyse against PBS, pH 7.4.
13. Store as in method (b) (step 11).

Table 4.5. *The use of biotinylated antibody*

1. Dialyse antibody (1 mg/ml) against 0.1 M sodium bicarbonate.
2. Dissolve Biotin *N*-hydroxysuccinimide ester in dimethyl sulphoxide to give 1 mg/ml.
3. Add 125 µl of the biotin solution to every millilitre of antibody solution.
4. Incubate for 4 h at room temperature.
5. Dialyse extensively against PBS, pH 7.4.
6. Divide into aliquots and store at 4 °C in the presence of 10 mM sodium azide.
7. When used in an assay, the presence of biotinylated antibody in the reaction is identified by adding a pre-determined dilution of streptavidin conjugated with either alkaline phosphatase or horseradish peroxidase for 1 h at 37 °C, followed (after washing) by the appropriate substrate; both of these streptavidin conjugates are commercially available.
8. The sensitivity of this type of assay is due to high avidity of binding between biotin and avidin (streptavidin in this case).

A. This binds to many mammalian species of immunoglobulin, although with variable efficiency. It cannot, however, be used when immunoglobulins other than the MAb are present, since it will also bind to these.

The detection of antibody bound to an antigen (or anti-immunoglobulin, in certain forms of sandwich ELISA) can be enhanced by using the amplified ELISA (6). The amplification relies mainly on the bridging antibody and peroxidase–anti-peroxidase (PAP) complexes (Fig. 4.1). The latter are produced by incubating, for example, rabbit anti-horseradish peroxidase with the enzyme to form large complexes. If the anti-

Table 4.6. *The different substrates commonly used with the enzyme conjugates employed in ELISA*

Enzyme	Substrate	Incubation time	Wavelength for reading
horseradish peroxidase	(a) 0.4 mg/ml *o*-phenylene-diamine (OPD) plus 0.04% (v/v) stock (30%) H_2O_2 freshly added to a buffer of 0.05 M citric acid, 0.1 M NaH_2PO_4, pH 5.0 (stopping solution: 1M H_2SO_4)	5–15 min, room temperature	492 nm
	(b) Amersham ABTS substrate: (2.2′-azino-di (3-ethyl-benzthiazoline sulphonate) (stopping solution: 0.01% NaN_3)	as required	410 nm
ß-galactosidase	(a) 1.5×10^{-5} M 4-methyl umbelliferyl-ß-D-galactoside in 0.05 M Tris–HCl, pH 7.4, containing 1 mM $MgCl_2$ (100 μl) + 50 μl 0.05 M Tris–HCl, pH 7.4, containing 0.15 M NaCl, 1 mM $MgCl_2$, 5 mM $CaCl_2$, 0.2% (w/v) albumin (stopping solution: 0.1 M glycine–NaOH, pH 10.3)	1h. 37 °C	excitation 360 nm; emission 450 nm
	(b) 33 mM *o*-nitrophenyl-ß-D-galactoside in 10 mM sodium phosphate buffer, pH 7.0, containing 0.3 M NaCl and 1 mM $MgCl_2$ (stopping solution: 3 mM NaOH)	30 min, room temperature	420 nm
	(c) Amersham ONPG substrate: *o*-nitrophenyl-ß-D galactopyranoside (stopping solution: Na_2CO_3)	as required	410 nm
alkaline phosphatase	(a) 1 mg/ml Sigma phosphatase substrate (*p*-nitrophenyl phosphate) in 0.5 M carbonate –bicarbonate buffer, pH 9.6, with 0.5 mM $MgCl_2$ (stopping solution: 3 M NaOH)	1h, 35 °C	405 nm
	(b) Sigma 104 phosphatase substrate tablets (*p*-nitrophenyl phosphate, disodium) dissolved in diethanolamine buffer (97 ml diethanolamine, 200 mg NaN_3, 100 mg $MgCl_2.6H_20$ per litre,	30–60 min, 37 °C	405 nm

Table 4.6. *(cont.)*

Enzyme	Substrate	Incubation time	Wavelength for reading
	pH 9.8) (stopping solution: 3 M NaOH)		
glucose oxidase	1 mg/ml ß-D-glucose plus 7.5 mg/ml 3-(4,5-dimethyl-thiazol-2-yl)-2,5-diphenyl tetrazolium (MTT), or nitro-blue tetrazolium (NBT), plus phenazine methosulphate (PMS) in PBS, pH 7.5 (stopping solution: 1 M HCl)	1h, 37 °C	570 nm

mouse immunoglobulin (anti-Ab^{II}) is also rabbit, a sheep anti-rabbit Ig is used as a bridging antibody, but a dilution must be chosen such that it reacts with both rabbit antibody species and not just one. This amplification procedure increases the ratio of enzyme molecules bound per MAb molecule. For example, if one rabbit anti-mouse antibody molecule was bound by each MAb in an indirect ELISA, then only the number of enzyme molecules which could be conjugated to a single antibody would be immobilised. In contrast, one or more sheep anti-rabbit antibodies could bind, and these in turn would immobilise at least one PAP complex for every sheep antibody bound. Hence, the *minimum* number of enzyme molecules bound per MAb in the amplified ELISA would be the number associated with one PAP complex; many more than could be conjugated to an antibody molecule.

The liquid phase ELISA (7) is used to determine MAb reactivity against antigen in what is probably its 'natural' conformation, and is related to the liquid phase RIA (see §4.1.2), but obviates the need for dangerous radiochemicals and expensive scintillation or gamma counters. MAb and antigen are diluted in PBS–T20–albumin, mixed and incubated for 1 h at 37 °C. The mixtures are then transferred to plates pre-sensitised with an IgG specific for the antigen. If MAb has reacted with the antigen, it will also be trapped, and can be detected by using enzyme-conjugated anti-mouse immunoglobulin.

In summary, the basic ELISA procedures can be divided into three types: the indirect, the sandwich or trapping, and the liquid phase ELISA.

(i) Indirect ELISA

1. Antigen is diluted in 0.05 M Na_2CO_3–$NaHCO_3$ coating buffer, pH 9.6, to give 10 µg/ml and added to the wells of an ELISA

plate (Nunc Immunoplate I, Dynatech M129B or Falcon 3912) at 50 μl/well.

2. The plates are incubated at 37 °C for 2–3 h or overnight at 4 °C.
3. The plates are washed by flooding with PBS containing 0.05 % (v/v) Tween 20 (PBS/T20), and then shaking vigorously to remove the PBS. This is repeated a total of four times. After the final wash, excess PBS is removed by tapping the plates forcefully (wells downward) onto paper towelling.
4. Hybridoma supernatants are diluted in PBS–T20 supplemented with 1% bovine serum albumin, lactalbumin yeast hydrolysate or ovalbumin (PBS/T20/albumin) and added to the wells of the now sensitised ELISA plate at 50 μl/well. As a positive control, dilution of a mouse antiserum known to react with the antigen to give, in ELISA, an A_{492} of 1.0 is added to at least three wells of each plate. The negative control is myeloma cell supernatant medium.
5. The plates are incubated at 37 °C for 2–3 h or overnight at 4 °C.
6. The plates are washed as in 3.
7. HRPO-conjugated rabbit-anti-mouse immunoglobulins (e.g. DAKOPATTS preparation at a 1 : 1000 dilution) diluted in PBS/T20/albumin is added to each well (50 μl/well).
8. The plates are incubated at 37 °C for 1 h or overnight at 4 °C.
9. The plates are washed as in 3.
10. The OPD–H_2O_2 substrate (Tables 4.2 and 4.6) is added (50 μl/well). The development of colour is monitored, and the reaction stopped with 50 μl/well of 1M H_2SO_4 when enough colour has developed in the positive control but before substantial colour development has taken place in the negative controls. With practice it will be possible to estimate a colour development in the positive controls of 0.2. In most tests, the time of incubation with the OPD–H_2O_2 substrate will vary from 5 to 15 minutes at room temperature. (ABTS- or TMB-substrates can also be used.)
11. The colour development in the plates is read with a spectrophotometer set for A_{492}, or with an automatic ELISA reader using the filter setting of 492 nm (410 nm for ABTS).

(ii) Trapping ELISA

1. A polyclonal IgG preparation prepared against the antigen of choice (usually rabbit or chicken IgG is best) is diluted in coating buffer to give 10 μg/ml, and 50 μl are added to each well of an ELISA plate.
2. The plates are incubated for 2–3 h at 37 °C, or overnight at 4 °C, and then washed as in step 3 of the indirect ELISA.
3. Antigen is diluted in PBS/T20/albumin to give 1 μg/ml, and 50 μl added to each well of the ELISA plate.

4. The plates are incubated for 1–2 h at 37 °C or overnight at 4 °C, and then washed as in step 3 of the indirect ELISA.
5. Hybridoma supernatants, positive control and negative control are prepared and added to the ELISA plates as in step 4 of the indirect ELISA. The remainder of the ELISA is as in steps 5–11 for the indirect ELISA. Care should be taken that the HRPO conjugate does not react with the trapping antibody of step 1 in the trapping ELISA.

(iii) Liquid phase ELISA

1. ELISA plates are sensitised with a trapping antibody as in step 1 of the trapping ELISA.
2. In another microtitre (96 w) plate, but of low protein binding capacity (e.g. Nunc bacteriological microtitre plates, number 26217), hybridoma supernatants and the positive and negative controls are diluted in PBS/T20/albumin to give 25 μl/well. To these wells are added 25 μl/well of antigen diluted to give 2 μg/ml in PBS/T20/albumin.
3. This reaction mixture from step 2 is incubated for 1–2 h at 37 °C.
4. The sensitised ELISA plates from step 1 are washed as in step 3 of the indirect ELISA.
5. The reaction mixture from step 2, after incubation (step 3), is transferred to the sensitised ELISA plate.
6. The plates are incubated at 37 °C for 1–2 h or overnight at 4 °C.
7. The plates are washed as in step 3 of the indirect ELISA.
8. HRPO-conjugated anti-mouse immunoglobulin (which does not react with trapping antibody of step 1) is added as described in step 7 of the indirect ELISA, and the remainder of the procedure is as for steps 8–11 of the indirect ELISA.

There are a few important technical points which need mentioning, in particular the determination of the correct concentration of antigen, trapping antibody and positive control antibody which should be used. The above procedures use 1–10 μg/ml of antigen, depending on the ELISA, but this cannot always be determined easily with different antigens. Instead, a checkerboard titration is used.

The principle of the checkerboard titration is described by McCullough *et al.* (7). A 96 w microtitre plate is used. When the solid-phase substance is to be titrated, 100 μl of the first dilution (usually 10 : 1) in coating buffer is placed in each well of the first column, marked '1' on the plate and containing 8 wells, 'A'–'H'. The remaining 88 wells (11 columns marked '2'–'12') receive 50 μl per well of coating buffer alone. Using a multichannel pipette (Titertek, Flow Laboratories Ltd) with eight pipette tips fitted, 50 μl are transferred from each well of the first column to each well of the second column. This second dilution is mixed by pipetting the volumes in each well up and down using the multichannel pipette, and 50 μl are transferred to each well of the third column. The dilution procedure is continued across the plate, and the plates then incubated. After washing, the second substance is applied. If this also has to be a dilution series, it follows the same principle as the first, with two exceptions. Firstly, the diluent is PBS/T20/albumin. Secondly, the dilution series is made down the plate. The first dilution is applied to each well of the first row, marked 'A' on the plate and containing 12 wells, '1'–'12'. The first transfer is from row 'A' (12 wells) to row 'B', and subsequent transfers continue down the plate through the 8 rows ('A'–'H'). After incubation and washing, the subsequent steps use single concentrations.

For this checkerboard titration, any two of the substances used in the ELISA can be titrated; it need not necessarily be the first two in the order of the scheme: steps 1, and 3, or 2 and 3, etc. can be titrated. In addition, the first titration can use rows instead of columns and the second titration can then use columns. By this means, reactants can be titrated against one another to obtain the optimum conditions for the assay. Only the positive control can be titrated against single concentrations of the other reactants, since it is the other reactants which require estimation of optimal proportions.

4.1.2. *Radioimmunoassay (RIA)*

Solid phase RIA procedures are identical to the ELISA, with the exception that the enzyme-conjugated antibody is replaced by ^{125}I-labelled antibody (Table 4.7). The amplified ELISA does not have an RIA counterpart. The RIA equivalent of the liquid phase ELISA was one of the original RIAs to be described. This used radioactively labelled antigen which was reacted with antibody for 1 h at 37 °C, in suspension, and both complexes and unreacted antibody precipitated using pansorbin (whole, inactivated *Staphylococcus aureus* strain Cowan as a source of protein A) or rabbit anti-mouse immunoglobulin. Detection of radioactive counts in the immunoprecipitate reflected antibody reactivity against the antigen. As an alternative to precipitation, the pansorbin or rabbit anti-mouse immunoglobulin could be immobilised on a solid phase, much as in the liquid phase ELISA. Fig. 4.3 outlines the procedures for these three variations on the liquid phase–solid phase RIA.

4.1.3. *Passive haemagglutination (PHA)*

The PHA techniques can be considered similar to ELISA with the enzyme-conjugated antibody replaced with sensitised red blood cells (rbc). There is no immobilisation of the reaction to a solid phase (but

Table 4.7. *Iodination of hybridoma antibodies*

1. Place 50 μl of the antibody preparation (preferably purified immunoglobulin at 1 mg/ml in PBS) into a V-bottomed tube.
2. Add 1 mCi carrier-free ^{125}I in 10 μl PBS.
3. Add 30 μl *FRESHLY* prepared Chloramine-T solution (0.30 mg/ml in 0.5 M phosphate buffer, pH 7.2).
4. Immediately mix well.
5. Mix for 15 s.
6. Add 100 μl saturated L-tyrosine solution in PBS.
7. Mix well.
8. Transfer the contents of the tube on to a pre-prepared column (in a disposable 1 ml syringe fitted with an 18 gauge (1.20 mm) needle) of Amberlite IRA 400.
9. Wash the iodinated protein (detected with a hand monitor) through with PBS containing 1% BSA (the free iodine is retained in the column).

see pp.205–207, MRSPAH), and the positive reaction is detected through aggregation of the sensitised rbc: haemagglutination. The technique is referred to as passive haemagglutination since the agglutinating component on the rbc is artificially added (the sensitisation procedure; see below), in contrast to the haemagglutination effected by certain viruses reacting with natural receptors on certain species of rbc. Before considering the various adaptations of the technique, the sensitisation procedures for preparing the rbc will be described. It is these procedures which are central to the success of the passive haemagglutination assays.

(i) Sensitisation of rbc (8–16)

Rbc from several species of animal have been successfully used for sensitisation. However, some cells are less suitable than others, due mainly to non-specific agglutinins in assay material, instability during or after sensitisation, or incompatibility for sensitisation with particular antigens or species of antibody. The human type O rbc, donkey rbc and sheep rbc have been the most widely applied, and as such are probably the most suitable for these purposes. Owing to their ready availability, it is recommended that sheep rbc should be used for sensitisation.

An antigen-specific assay can be designed by sensitising the rbc with the antigen against which it is hoped the MAb will react. Conversely, a more general assay for mouse immunoglobulin in hybridoma culture supernatants would use rbc sensitised with rabbit IgG anti-mouse immunoglobulin. The result with a 'positive' hybridoma supernatant will be the same. At the correct concentration of MAb, rbc and antigen on the surface of the rbc, the MAb will react with antigen on adjacent rbc (Fig. 4.4). As several MAb enter this reaction, a lattice-work is built

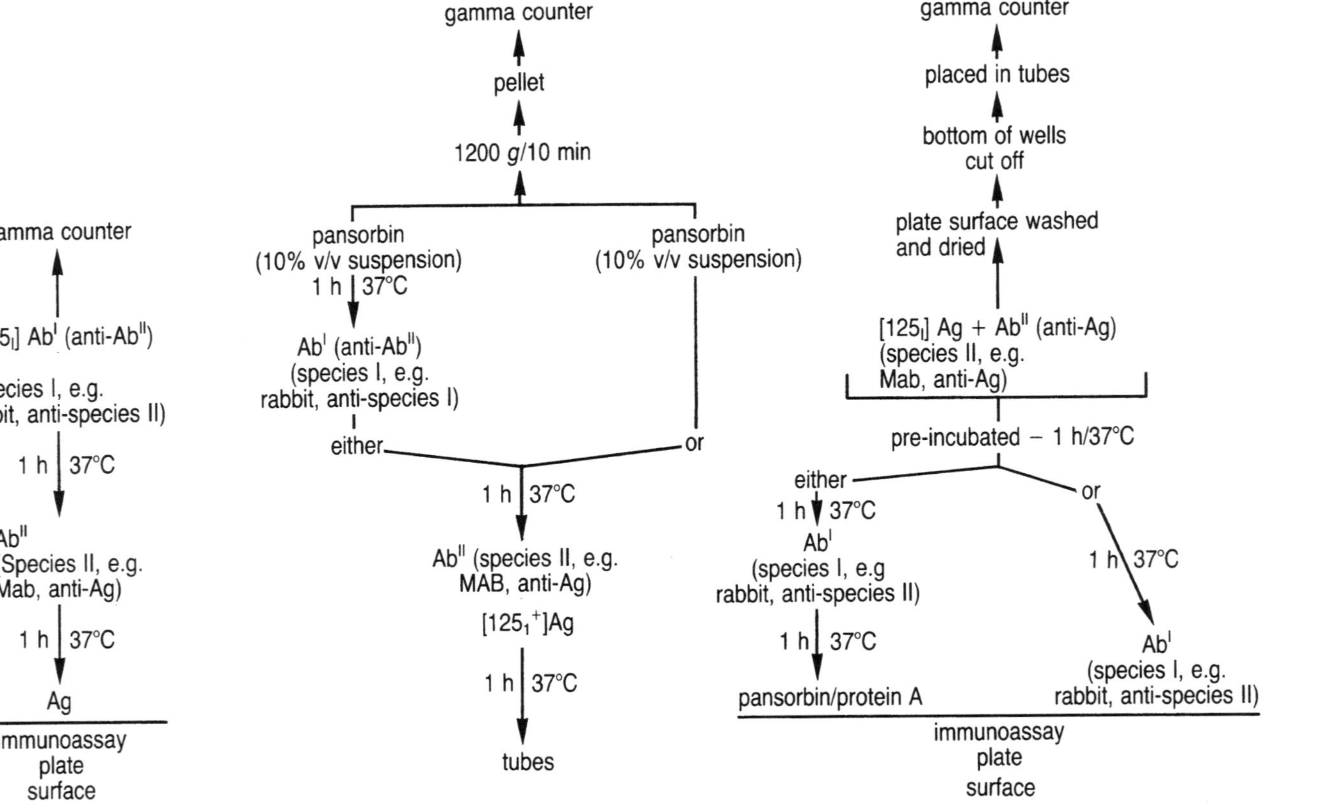

Fig. 4.3. The various incubation steps involved in the solid-phase indirect, liquid-phase (direct and indirect), and capture liquid-phase RIA. Ag, antigen; Ab, antibody; ^{125}I-Ab, iodinated antibody; ^{125}I-Ag, iodinated antigen.

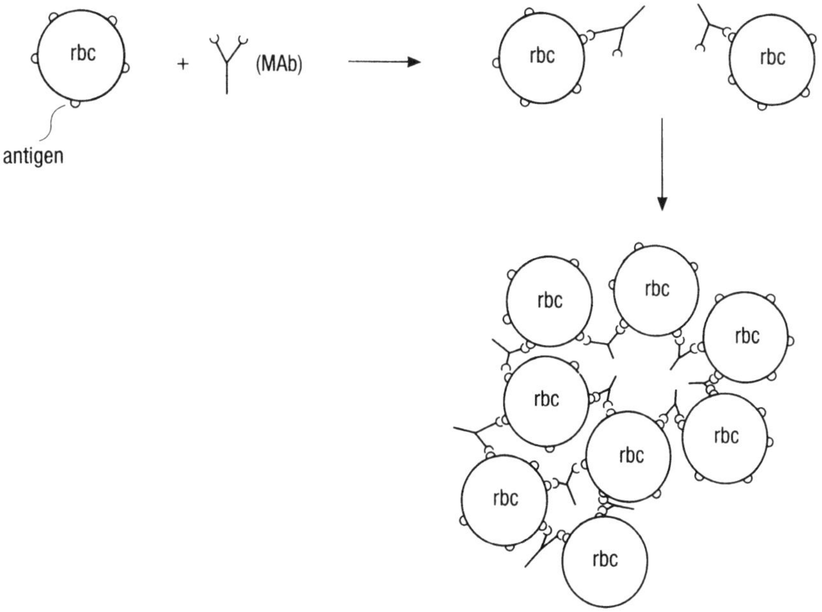

Fig. 4.4. Passive haemagglutination reaction where antigen-specific MAb reacts with antigen on the surface of antigen-sensitised erythrocytes (rbc), forming complexes and then visible lattices.

up, resulting in agglutination. This agglutination becomes visible to the eye after at least 10^6 rbc have entered into the lattice-work. If the rbc are sensitised with anti-mouse immunoglobulin, a similar reaction occurs, except that the sensitising antibody on the rbc binds to sites on the MAb. Thus, the concentration of anti-mouse immunoglobulin on the rbc is not as critical as the concentration of antigen. If the latter is too high, MAb may react with two antigen molecules on the same rbc and thus fail to agglutinate. Furthermore, if the MAb is monovalent (see §2.4), only the reaction using anti-mouse immunoglobulin-sensitised rbc will succeed; the monovalent MAb can only ever bind to one antigen molecule, hence only one rbc, and hence no agglutination, whereas more than one anti-mouse immunoglobulin on rbc can still react with one monovalent MAb and result in lattice formation. The major procedures for sensitising rbc are tanning, chromic chloride sensitisation, sensitisation in piperazine buffer, and the use of other cross-linking agents. Rbc can be 'derivatised' with certain haptens, but this is not applicable as a general sensitisation procedure. Tables 4.8–4.11 outline the steps and buffers of these procedures. The method which is currently in favour is the chromic chloride method, first reported by Jandl & Simmons (17) and elaborated into the reverse passive haemagglutination assays by Coombs and co-workers (8–12).

Table 4.8. *Sensitisation of rbc by tanning*

1. Wash rbc 3 times with 40 volumes of PBS (Table 4.11) and centrifuge at 300 *g* for 10 min.
2. Adjust rbc to 4% v/v in PBS.
3. Make tannic acid solution of 2.5 mg per 50 ml PBS; add equal volume to the 4% rbc.
4. Incubate at 37 °C for 15 min.
5. Centrifuge *very gently* (to prevent auto-agglutination) at 100 *g* for 20 min.
6. Divide into two aliquots, one for antigen or antibody coating and the other for control cells, and wash each with 1 volume PBS (N.B. 100 *g* for 20 min).
7. Resuspend the aliquot for sensitisation in PBS to give 4% (v/v) and add an equal volume of antigen or antibody. (The optimum concentration of the antigen or antibody can vary greatly for the particular protein, and must be pre-determined; examples are 10 μg/ml to 25 mg/ml for albumins; 100 μg/ml to 10 mg/ml for IgG; 10 μg/ml to 1 mg/ml for certain virus antigens; 2 μg/ml to 2 mg/ml for enzymes, hormones and plasma proteins; 10 μg/ml to 1 mg/ml for cellular antigens; 75 μg/ml for helminth antigens.)
8. Incubate at 37 °C for 30 min.
9. Wash gently as in 5., and resuspend cells in borate–succinate buffer (Table 4.11) to 2% v/v.
10. Resuspend control cells likewise in borate–succinate buffer.
11. Add $\frac{1}{10}$ volume 40% (v/v) formalin (aqueous) dropwise with constant stirring over 20–30 min.
12. Leave overnight at 4 °C.
13. Add a further $\frac{1}{10}$ volume of 40% (v/v) formalin.
14. Leave 24 h and pour off supernatant.
15. Resuspend cells in borate–succinate buffer, and again leave 24 h to settle.
16. Repeat 14 and 15.
17. Adjust cell suspension to 1% (v/v) and add formalin to a final concentration of 0.2% (v/v) as a preservative.

Source: From Hudson & Hay (13).

(ii) Comments on erythrocyte sensitisation

(i) Some erythrocytes, notably ovine and bovine, can produce unwanted agglutinations; trypsin-treatment of the erythrocytes prior to sensitisation (Coombs *et al.* (10)) may therefore be advisable.

(ii) If antisera are used in any of the tests, they may contain anti-erythrocyte activity, and this should be removed by incubating the heat-inactivated (56 °C for 30 min) sera with an equal volume of packed rbc for 1 h at 37 °C, pelleting the rbc and using the 'adsorbed' supernatant.

Table 4.9. *Sensitisation of erythrocytes with chromic chloride**

1. Wash rbc five times in saline (0.85% (w/v) aqueous NaCl), centrifuging at 400 *g* for 10 min at each step.
2. Immediately before use, prepare a solution of $CrCl_3.6H_2O$ in saline at 6.6 mg/ml, and dilute 1 : 100 in saline.
3. Mix 100 μl packed rbc with 100 μl protein (again the optimum concentration should be pre-determined, but rabbit IgG anti-mouse immunoglobulin may be used at 1–5 mg/ml).
4. Add 1 ml of the 1 : 100 $CrCl_3.6H_2O$ solution.
5. Rotate for 1 h at 30 °C (or room temperature).
6. Add 6 volumes PBS (phosphate inhibits the reaction) and centrifuge at 400 *g* for 10 min.
7. Wash twice with PBS.
8. Resuspend in PBS to 20% (v/v) for storage.

Source: From Coombs and co-workers (8–12).

Note:
* *Sensitisation of rbc with chromic chloride in piperazine buffer is done in the same way, except that the protein and 1 : 100* $CrCl_3.6H_2O$ *are prepared in piperazine buffer (Table 4.11) and after reaction the cells are washed in 0.9% (w/v) aqueous NaCl.*

Table 4.10. *Sensitisation of rbc using other cross-linking agents*

(a) bis-diazotised benzidine (BDB) (14)

1. Dissolve 0.23 g benzidine in 45 ml cold 0.2 M HCl in an ice–salt bath (0 °C).
2. Add 0.175 g $NaNO_2$ dissolved in 5 ml cold distilled water.
3. Leave 30 min with stirring.
4. Divide the BDB into aliquots of 1 ml in chilled tubes and freeze quickly in a solid CO_2 – acetone bath.
5. Store at −70 °C.
6. Wash rbc three times in PBS.
7. Resuspend to 50% (v/v).
8. To 1 volume 50% rbc add:
   8 volumes PBS
   2 volumes antigen or antibody
   20 volumes phosphate buffer (Table 4.11).

(Control cells receive 2 volumes 0.5% (v/v) gelatin in phosphate buffer in place of the antigen or antibody).

9. Thaw 1 ml BDB.
10. Add to 14 ml phosphate buffer.
11. Mix and add immediately 5 volumes (where 1 vol. = 1 vol. in step 8) to the rbc–antigen (or antibody) mixture and 5 volumes to the control cell mixture.
12. Mix well and leave 10–12 min at room temperature.
13. Centrifuge at 500 *g* for 5 min at 4 °C.
14. Resuspend cells in 30 volumes 0.1% (v/v) gelatin solution, in phosphate buffer, and centrifuge as in 13.

Table 4.10. *(cont.)*

15. Repeat 14, three times.
16. Resuspend in 30 volumes 0.1% (v/v in phosphate buffer) gelatin solution and store at 4 °C.

(b) 1,3-difluoro-4,6-dinitrobenzene (DFDNB) (15)
1. Dissolve 2 g DFDNB in 100 ml acetone and store at 4 °C.
2. To 1 volume 10% (v/v) rbc add 2 volumes EDTA buffer, pH 8.4 (Table 4.11) and 1 volume of the DFDNB diluted 1 : 10 in EDTA buffer.
3. Incubate for 30 min at room temperature.
4. Centrifuge the cells (400 *g* for 10 min).
5. Resuspend in 2 volumes EDTA buffer, pH 8.4.
6. Add pre-determined concentration of antigen or IgG in 1 volume EDTA buffer.
7. Incubate for 1 h at 37 °C.
8. Wash three times with EDTA buffer, pH 7.5, containing 0.1% (w/v) gelatin.
9. Resuspend in 40 volumes EDTA buffer, pH 7.5.

(c) 1-ethyl-3-(3-dimethylaminopropyl)-carbodiimide–HCl (ECDI) (16).
1. Wash rbc four times in cold 0.85% (w/v) saline.
2. Wash rbc once in cold mannitol solution (Table 4.11) (any clumping of the rbc may be ignored since the cells dissociate after the conjugation).
3. Resuspend to 10% (v/v) in cold mannitol solution.
4. Add 10 volumes 10% (v/v) rbc to 1 volume antigen or antibody in mannitol solution, pH 7–8 (10 μg/ml to 20 mg/ml).
5. Mix well and rotate for 10 min at 4 °C.
6. Add 1 volume of 100 mg/ml of ECDI in mannitol solution (freshly prepared).
7. Rotate for 30 min at 4 °C.
8. Wash twice in a balanced salt solution or tissue culture medium containing 0.1% (w/v) gelatin.
9. Resuspend to 6–10% (v/v) in balanced salt solution (Table 4.11).

(iii) With BDB, the optimal BDB : protein ratio for coupling must be determined beforehand. In addition, the protein and gelatin must be added to the rbc before BDB since the cells are more stable in the presence of gelatin.

(iv) When conjugating with ECDI in mannitol solution, should the clumping not re-dissolve after suspension of the rbc in balanced salt solution, 1 drop of 0.1 M NaOH per millilitre of 10% rbc should help. In addition, performing all steps at 4 °C reduces the clumping.

(v) Erythrocytes can be preserved for longer periods if they are fixed with formalin (18) or glutaraldehyde (19).

(vi) Some antigens naturally agglutinate certain species of erythrocyte, and as such can be used to sensitise erythrocytes directly. Examples are the lipopolysaccharides of Gram-negative bacteria onto several species of fresh or formalinised erythrocytes; toxoplasma antigen onto pyruvic aldehyde fixed erythrocytes; extracts of tubercle bacillus onto fresh erythrocytes; influenza virus or haemagglutinin protein onto chicken erythrocytes; parainfluenza virus or haemagglutinin protein onto chicken cells; measles virus – haemagglutinin onto rhesus monkey cells; certain subtypes of foot-and-mouth disease virus onto guinea pig erythrocytes.

Table 4.11. *Buffers for sensitisation of erythrocytes*

1. PBS (for tanning) 0.2 M, pH 7.2
   12.2 g KH_2PO_4 (0.02 M)
   40.4 g Na_2HPO_4 (0.06 M)
   36 g NaCl (0.12 M)
   5 l distilled water
2. Borate–succinate buffer 0.15 M, pH 7.5
   Solution A: 19 g sodium tetraborate $Na_2B_4O_7.10H_2O$ (0.05 M)
   1 l distilled water
   Solution B: 5.9 g succinic acid (0.05 M)
   1 l distilled water
   Add B to 1 l A until pH is 7.5
   Add NaCl to 0.14 M, and 1% (v/v) (final concentration) heat-inactivated (56 °C for 30 min) horse serum.
3. Saline 0.14 M (0.85% w/v)
   8.5 g in 1 l distilled water. (Prepare for storage as ×10 stock: 85g/l.)
4. PBS 0.1 M (= ×10 stock; dilute to 0.01 M for use), pH 7.2 (for $CrCl_3.6H_2O$ and other cross-linking agents)
   20.5 g $NaH_2PO_4.H_2O$
   179.9 g $Na_2HPO_4.7H_2O$
   4 l distilled H_2O
   Adjust to pH 7.2–7.4.
   Add 701.3 g NaCl.
   Make up to 8 l with distilled H_2O
   Dilute 1 : 10 for use.
5. Piperazine buffer (0.27 M, pH 7)
   Prepare a piperazine solution in water to give 1 M
   (86.14 g plus 1 l distilled H_2O)
   Take 27 ml of this solution.
   Add 1 M HCl to obtain the desired pH.
   Make up to 100 ml with distilled H_2O.
6. Phosphate buffer 0.15 M, pH 7.2–7.4
   Solution A: 20.7 g $NaH_2PO_4.H_2O$ (0.15 M)
   1 l distilled water
   Solution B: 40.2 g $Na_2HPO_4.7H_2O$ (0.15 M)
   1 l distilled water
   270 ml A + 930 ml B
   Adjust to pH 7.2–7.4 by adding solution A or solution B.

Table 4.11. *(cont.)*

7. EDTA buffer, pH 7.5 *or* 8.4
   21.7 g EDTA (disodium salt)
   500 ml distilled water
   Adjust to pH 7.5 *or* 8.4 with 2M NaOH.
   Make up to 1 l with distilled water.
   Add equal volume 0.85% (w/v) NaCl.
8. Mannitol solution: 0.35 M mannitol–0.01 M NaCl
   63.7 g mannitol
   0.58g NaCl
   Make up to 1 l with distilled H_2O
   (buffering does not appear to be essential).
9. Balanced salt solution
   Solution A: 10.0 g dextrose
   0.6 g KH_2PO_4
   3.58 g $Na_2HPO_4.7H_2O$
   0.5% phenol red solution
   Make up to 1 l with distilled H_2O.
   Solution B: 1.86 g $CaCl_2.2H_2O$
   4.0 g KCl
   80.0 g NaCl
   1.04 g $MgCl_2$ (anhydrous)
   2.0 g $MgSO_4.7H_2O$
   Make up to 1 l with distilled H_2O.
   Mix 1 vol. solution A with 1 vol solution B.
   Make up to 10 vols with distilled H_2O.
   The pH should be 7.2–7.4; conductivity should be 14–16 mS.

(iii) Reverse PHA

The reverse passive haemagglutination is simply as follows.

1. Serial dilutions of antigen in PBS are made in 25 μl volumes in the wells of 96 w microtitre plates.
2. Add 30 μl/well of a 1% (v/v) suspension of antigen-specific antibody-coupled erythrocytes in PBS.
3. Incubate at room temperature or 4 °C until observable buttons of red blood cells (no agglutination) form in the negative controls (no antigen).

The techniques elaborated by Coombs and co-workers (8–12) are termed the MRPAH (mixed reverse passive antiglobulin haemagglutination) and MRSPAH (mixed reverse solid phase passive antiglobulin haemadsorption) systems. These are shown in Figs 4.5 and 4.6. With MRPAH, the antigen must be large enough to be centrifuged, e.g. bacteria, protozoa, yeast, mammalian cells, tumour cells or mammalian cells infected by virus and expressing virus antigen on their surface. The procedure is as follows.

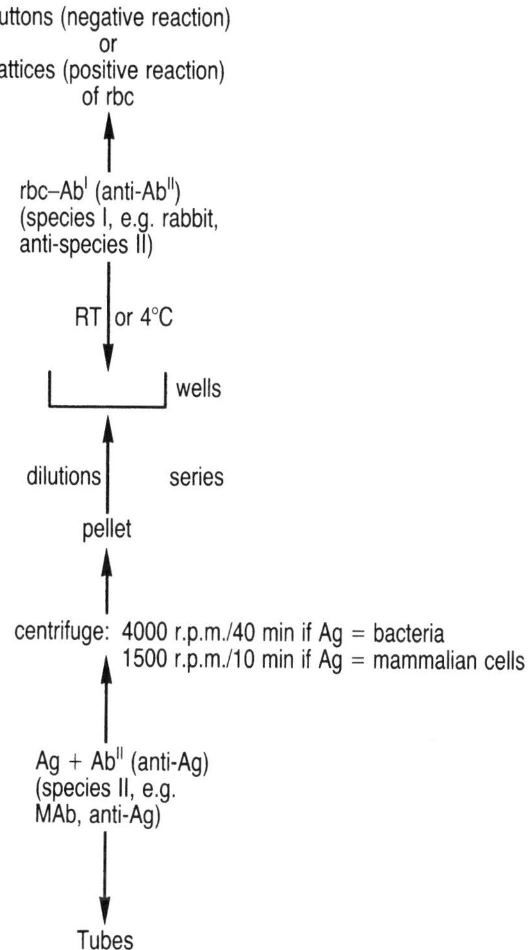

Fig. 4.5. The passive haemagglutination reaction termed MRPAH. Ag, antigen; Ab, antibody; RT, room temperature; rbc-Ab, erythrocytes sensitised with antibody.

1. Mixtures of, for example, bacteria and serial dilutions in PBS of anti-bacterial antibody, test antiserum (heat inactivated), negative antiserum (heat inactivated) or PBS are incubated for 30 min at 37 °C with agitation.
2. The bacterial preparations are centrifuged at 2000 *g* for 40 min (with mammalian cells, the speed is reduced to 300 *g* for 10 minutes), and washed six times using PBS and centrifugation.
3. Serial twofold dilutions of the washed preparations are prepared in 25 μl volumes of PBS in the wells of 96 w microtitre plates.

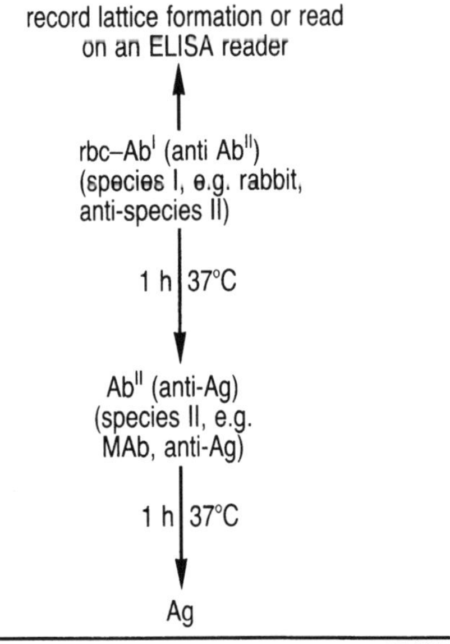

Fig. 4.6. The passive haemagglutination reaction termed MRSPAH. (Abbreviations as for Figs 4.1 and 4.5.)

4. 25 μl/well of anti-globulin (specific for the species of antibody used in step 1) sensitised erythrocytes (1% v/v) are added.
5. The plates are incubated at room temperature or 4 °C until buttons of red cells form in the negative controls (no antigen).

The MRSPAH uses antigen bound to a solid phase, such as the surface of an ELISA plate, instead of being used in suspension.

1. Adsorb antigen to the surface of an ELISA plate and wash as described for ELISA.
2. Titrate antigen-specific antiserum or test samples, again as described for ELISA.
3. Wash the plates as for ELISA and add 25 μl/well of a 1% (v/v) suspension of anti-globulin-sensitised erythrocytes; incubate as in step 5 of MRPAH.

Considerable time has been devoted to this topic of passive haemagglutination because, like ELISA, it is a rapid test, and the sensitisation procedures are identical to those used with tests for detecting antibody-secreting cells. These tests – HAd, DARR, IARR, PFC – are more sensitive than ELISA–RIA or PAH since they can detect a single positive cell after 1 h incubation. The ELISA–RIA and PAH have the advantage when the cell density is low, since 10^3 cells/ml are ideally required for the microscopy techniques used with HAd, DARR and IARR. (Only the PFC assay does not suffer this restriction.) Fewer than 10^3 cells/ml makes enumeration of cell numbers (rosetted with rbc and non-rosetted) difficult and inaccurate. In addition, ELISA–RIA and PAH do not require any manipulation of the hybridoma cells in order to detect the antibody. The tests for detecting the antibody-secreting cells as opposed to detecting the antibody will be described in §§4.1.8–4.1.12.

Both the ELISA–RIA–PAH group of tests and the HAd–DARR–PFC group can detect low levels of antibody or antibody-producing cells. If the concentrations of antibody are high, as in established monoclonal hybridomas, assays based on immunoprecipitation reactions may be employed. They may also be applicable for the general detection of murine antibody since this relies on the precipitating qualities of the anti-mouse IgG (for example, rabbit IgG is a very potent immunoprecipitator). However, the specific reaction of the MAb with antigen may be incapable of producing precipitates, especially if the MAb is of low affinity for the antigen or is monovalent. Certain small antigens such as haptens and low molecular mass 'soluble' proteins may also be incapable of forming precipitates with antibody. Nevertheless, the immunoprecipitation tests have been used, in particular for the differentiation of MAb isotype. They can be broadly classified into double immunodiffusion (DID), single radial immunodiffusion (SRID) and radial haemolysis (RH). The information obtained from immunoprecipitation can be increased by incorporating an electrophoresis step into the procedure. These immunoelectrophoresis methods will be dealt with separately in §4.1.7.

4.1.4 *Ouchterlony DID*

The DID assays have stemmed from the work by Ouchterlony (20). The majority of DID tests today use an agarose gel poured on to plastic Petri dishes, glass plates or microscope slides. Once set, holes are cut in the agar in a symmetrical pattern using a commercially available template and cutting apparatus. The most common arrangement of holes (wells) is as shown in Fig. 4.7. Antigen is placed in the central well, and samples of hybridoma supernatant or appropriate positive and negative controls are applied to the outer wells. For a more general detection of mouse antibody, the central well may contain rabbit anti-mouse immunoglobulin (or anti-mouse immunoglobulin isotype for isotypic determination of the MAb). Alternatively, a MAb sample may be applied to the central well and different antigen preparations to the outer wells to determine the relative specificity (degree of cross-reactivity) of the MAb.

The plates are incubated in a humid atmosphere at a constant temperature, during which time both MAb and antigen (or anti-mouse

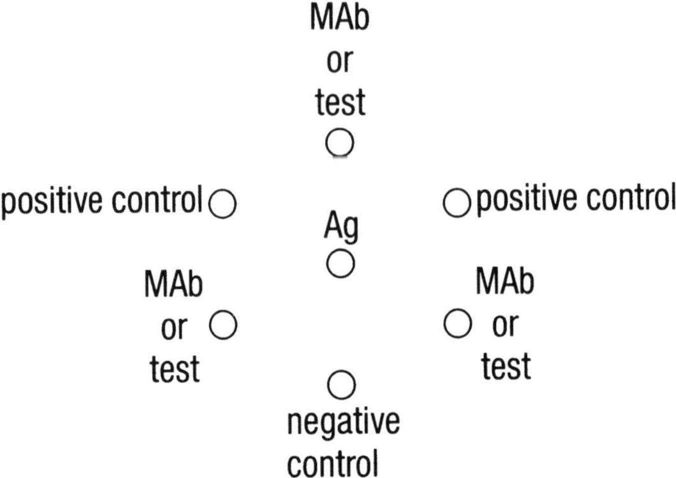

Fig. 4.7. Arrangements of 'wells' (hole template) for the DID test.

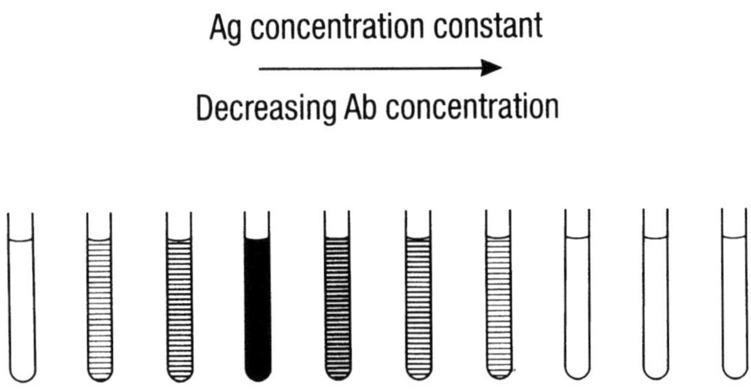

Fig. 4.8. Production of antigen–antibody aggregates at conditions of optimal proportions (of antigen and antibody) in the tube flocculation test.

immunoglobulin) will diffuse into the agarose. The arrangement of wells means that at least part of the sample in each outside well diffuses towards the sample in the central well and vice versa. If the two samples can react with one another, complexes of antibody with antigen (or anti-mouse immunoglobulin) will form. In order to produce precipitable complexes, both components have to be at a minimum concentration in the complex and at the correct ratio. If one of the reagents is too concentrated, a prozone phenomenon is experienced. This can be demonstrated in the tube flocculation test, in which a constant concentration of antigen is mixed with concentrations of antibody in a liquid medium (Fig. 4.8).

At too low a concentration of antibody, aggregates with antigen cannot form. As the antibody concentration increases, the complexing of the antibody with antigen begins to form lattice-works or aggregates containing several molecules of antibody and antigen. When these aggregates are large enough they become visible to the naked eye and form a flocculation or precipitate. As the antibody concentration increases, the size of the aggregates also increases, but at too high a concentration, more antibody molecules bind per antigen molecule and thus inhibit the cross-linking of antigen by antibody necessary to form a lattice-work. Thus, the precipitate does not form at too high a concentration of antibody: the prozone phenomenon. The same observation would be made if the antibody concentration were constant and the antigen concentration varied.

In a gel system (agarose) the flocculation of the liquid system can be seen as a line of precipitation at optimal proportions of antibody and antigen. Should the concentration of one or both reagents be too low, no visible precipitation will form. The detecting system (antigen or anti-mouse immunoglobulin) should therefore be carefully titrated beforehand, and, when using to test hybridoma supernatants, more than one dilution should be used. In addition, only those hybridomas which are well established, and should therefore be producing relatively high concentrations of MAb, can be used. The immunoprecipitation assays are not the most ideal test for screening hybridomas early after fusion or cloning (see above).

(i) DID procedure

1. Weigh agarose to give 2% w/v in barbitone buffer (dissolve 12 g sodium barbital (5.5.diethylbarbituric acid, Na salt) in 800 ml distilled water; dissolve 4.4 g barbital (5.5.diethylbarbituric acid) in 150 ml distilled water at 95 °C; mix the two solutions and adjust pH to 8.2 with concentrated NaOH; add 0.15 g merthiolate–thimerosal as a preservative and make up to 1 l).
2. Heat agarose in boiling water bath until melted, and hold at 56 °C.
3. Pour agar on to 3 cm Petri dishes (2 ml each), 4 cm × 4 cm glass plates (5 ml each) or microscope slides (0.5 ml each). Before addition of the agar, the glass plates or microscope slides are passed over a bunsen flame to heat slightly (prevents the agarose from solidifying too quickly) and placed on a level stand. Aliquots of agarose held at 56 °C are dispensed on to the Petri dish, glass plate or slide using a pipette which has been pre-treated by passing through the bunsen flame (again to prevent the agar solidifying prematurely). The pipette is placed in the centre of the Petri dish, glass plate or slide and agarose slowly released while moving the pipette in a spiral away from the centre so as to quickly cover the Petri dish, glass plate or slide

with a constant thickness of agarose. Care should be taken at the edges that the agarose does not flow over.

4. Allow to set.
5. Punch the pattern of holes using the appropriate template.
6. Suck out the agarose plugs using commercial apparatus (Miles).
7. Fill the wells with the appropriate antigen, MAb or anti-mouse immunoglobulin until the meniscus just disappears.
8. Place the Petri dish, plate or slide in a humid box at 37 °C for 3 h or overnight at 4 °C.

Under the appropriate ratios of antibody and antigen (or anti-mouse immunoglobulin) lines of precipitation will develop. Visualisation of these may be enhanced by staining with Coomassie blue R.

(ii) Staining of precipitin bands

1. Remove non-precipitated proteins by washing *carefully* with 0.1 M NaCl (2 × 30 min), followed by deionised water (2 × 30 min). Keep plates horizontal, otherwise the gels may slip off. (If Petri dishes are used, it is best to remove the gels by using water displacement, and put onto glass plates.)
2. Fill the wells with water, place a layer of wet filter paper on top of the gel (avoid trapping air bubbles), and a 2–3 cm layer of paper towelling on top of this.
3. Place a glass plate on top and apply a pressure of 10 g/cm^2 for 10–15 min.
4. Remove all layers.
5. Dry the gel under a stream of hot air (using a fan heater or hair drier) or use a commercially available gel drying apparatus.
6. Place the gel in the following staining solution for 10 min:
   450 ml ethanol (96%) + 100 ml acetic acid;
   add to this 5 g Coomassie blue (brilliant) R-250;
   leave overnight at room temperature;
   filter and make up to 1 l with deionised water.
7. Transfer the gel to the following destaining solution for 10 min:
   450 ml ethanol (96%) + 100 ml acetic acid + 450 ml deionised H_2O (can be regenerated by filtering through activated charcoal).
8. Repeat the staining/destaining twice.
9. Dry the gel as in step 5.

(iii) Patterns of antigen–antibody reactions

If a number of MAb are used in the outer wells against an anti-mouse immunoglobulin or a single antigen in the central well, their relationship to one another can be observed by DID as shown in Fig. 4.9. Alternatively, the relationship between different antigen samples can also be

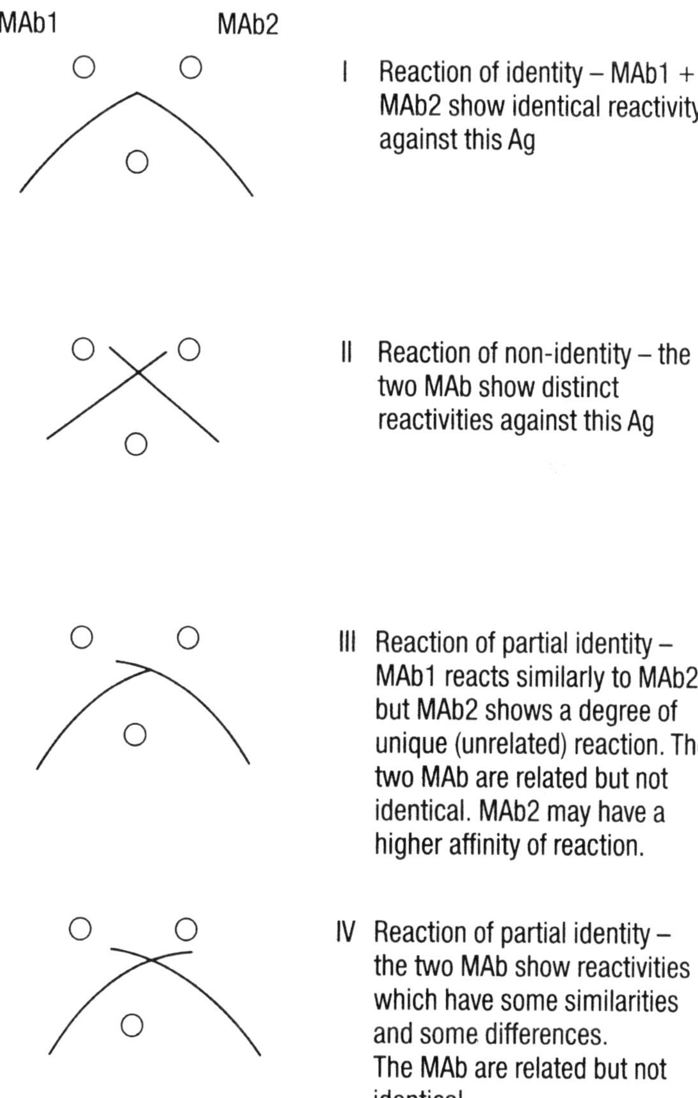

MAb1
MAb2
I Reaction of identity – MAb1 + MAb2 show identical reactivity against this Ag
II Reaction of non-identity – the two MAb show distinct reactivities against this Ag
III Reaction of partial identity – MAb1 reacts similarly to MAb2 but MAb2 shows a degree of unique (unrelated) reaction. The two MAb are related but not identical. MAb2 may have a higher affinity of reaction.
IV Reaction of partial identity – the two MAb show reactivities which have some similarities and some differences. The MAb are related but not identical.

Fig. 4.9. The different patterns of antigen–antibody precipitation lines in DID.

determined if these are in the outer wells and a single MAb in the central well.

4.1.5. *Single radial immunodiffusion (SRID)*

This technique is similar to the DID except that only one of the reagents is placed in a well while the other reagent is incorporated into the

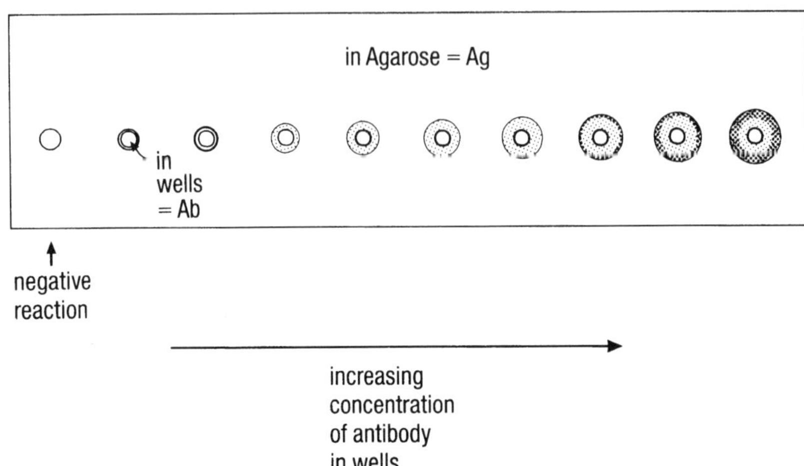

Fig. 4.10. The development of rings of antigen–antibody precipitation, as a function of antibody concentration in the 'wells', in the SRID test.

agarose. Thus, as the first reagent diffuses into the gel, it reacts with the second reagent. As the diffusion proceeds, an area of optimal proportions is reached, and a visible precipitate is formed (a precipitation ring) (Fig. 4.10). If the concentration of the reagent in the agarose is too low, no visible precipitate can form. If the concentration of the reagent in the wells is too low it either will not form a precipitate in the agarose, or forms a precipitate at the edge of the well which is very difficult to see. In this latter situation, the reagent in the well will be impaired from diffusing into the agarose owing to the proportionally much higher concentration of agarose-associated reagent. Thus, careful titration of reagents must again be made. Since the agarose-associated reagent is the more easily manipulated, test samples (hybridoma supernatants) are applied to the wells and either antigen or, preferably, rabbit IgG anti-mouse immuno-globulin is incorporated into the agarose. Nevertheless, the restrictions imposed on the applicability of DID to testing hybridoma supernatants apply equally in the SRID.

(i) SRID procedure

1. Prepare the agarose as for DID; see §4.1.4(i).
2. Hold the agarose at 56 °C and add a predetermined concentration of antigen or rabbit anti-mouse immunoglobulin. (This concentration is critical since the diameter of the precipitin ring is inversely proportional to antibody or MAb concentration.) It is advisable that several aliquots of agarose containing different concentrations of antigen or rabbit anti-mouse immunoglobulin be prepared. With the rabbit antibody, these can be 1, 10 and

100 μg/ml agarose, but for the antigen, titrations must be performed against a known precipitating antiserum (for example human IgG for anti-measles virus, anti-polio virus or anti-diphtheria toxin activity) to determine an optimum range of concentrations for the antigen. It is essential that the protein incorporated into the agar should be purified, for example IgG for the rabbit anti-mouse immunoglobulin.

3. The antigen or antibody should be added at a low ratio, usually 100 μl per 10 ml agarose, to give the desired final concentration. Some antigens, such as foot-and-mouth disease virus, are susceptible to heating at 56 °C. It is advisable that such antigens should be added to the agarose immediately prior to dispensing on to the Petri dishes, glass plates or microscope slides.
4. Place the agarose on 3 cm Petri dishes, glass plates or microscope slides as for the DID (§4.1.4(i)).
5. Allow to set, then punch 2–3 mm diameter wells separated by a distance which will give 8 wells per microscope slide; remove the agarose plugs.
6. Fill some wells with a standard solution of IgG of known concentration, and the others with the hybridoma supernatants (if the MAb concentration in the supernatants is suspected to be weak, a sample may be added to the well, allowed to diffuse into the agarose and more sample then applied). The standard solution should be normal mouse IgG when assaying hybridoma supernatants for mouse IgG, or IgG specific for the antigen incorporated into the agarose (if affinity purified IgG specific for the antigen is used, a direct estimation of antibody concenration in the hybridoma supernatant may be made).
7. Leave in a humid box for 4 h at 37 °C, and then transfer to 4 °C for 48 h. Certain IgG concentrations may form visible bands after the 4 h incubation, but it is recommended that the full 48 h incubation be performed.
8. Measure the diameter of the precipitin rings, which should give an estimation of MAb concentration in the hybridoma supernatant when compared to the reference standards.
9. If the rings are not distinct, soak the slides in 1 % tannic acid (will give a temporary increase in resolution) or stain with Coomassie blue R as described for DID in §4.1.4 (ii). Alternatively use radiolabelled rabbit anti-mouse immunoglobulin. The radiolabelled protein may be detected by drying the gels as for the Coomassie blue R and exposing to X-ray film. This is probably the most sensitive of all of these methods, since it will detect very low levels of radioactive decay by simply prolonging the time of exposure of the slide to the X-ray film or using fluorography enhancement.

4.1.6. *Radial haemolysis (RH)*

This is a combination of SRID and the PFC assay to be described below (§4.1.11). The procedure is identical to SRID except that the agarose is held at 45 °C and the antigen or antibody is replaced with erythrocytes coated with antigen or antibody as described above (Tables 4.8–4.10). The lower holding temperature is to prevent lysis of the erythrocytes. In general, the procedure is:

1. Dispense the agarose in aliquots of the appropriate volume for one Petri dish, glass plate or microscope slide and hold at 45 °C in a water bath.
2. Wash the sensitised rbc three times in balanced salt solution (Table 4.11) and resuspend to 6.6% (v/v) in the balanced salt solution.
3. Add the 6.6% (v/v) rbc suspension to the agarose aliquots at the ratio of 1 volume rbc : 10 volumes agarose.
4. Mix the rbc and agarose well, and place quickly on to the Petri dishes, glass plates or slides to prevent rbc lysis. The method of spreading the agarose is as detailed under DID in §4.1.4 (i).
5. When the agarose has set, cut wells, add samples to the wells and incubate as for SRID (§4.1.5.(i)).
6. After 4 h at 37 °C an antiserum specific for the MAb is poured over the gel (a 1 : 20 dilution is used and enough added to cover the gel).
7. Incubate for 90 min at 37 °C, and then add a 1 : 20 dilution of guinea pig or rabbit complement (absorbed with rbc to remove direct haemolytic activity) for a further 90 min at 37 °C.
8. Rings of haemolysis should be observed when a reaction similar to that shown in Fig. 4.11 has occurred.

The haemolytic methods for enhancing the visualisation of antibody–antigen interactions in a gel matrix is not the only means by which detection of MAb by precipitation in gels can be manipulated; there are also the immunoelectrophoresis systems. These are used (i) to force antibody and/or antigen through a gel system by altering the electrical potential, and thus increase the efficiency of the visible precipitation reactions; (ii) to separate the components of an antiserum or antigen, to characterise in more detail, at the molecular level, the antigen–antibody reaction; (iii) to enhance the formation of large aggregates of immune complexes (especially useful when the antibody and antigen move in opposite directions under a particular electrical charge shift, or one antigen or antibody moves faster than the other).

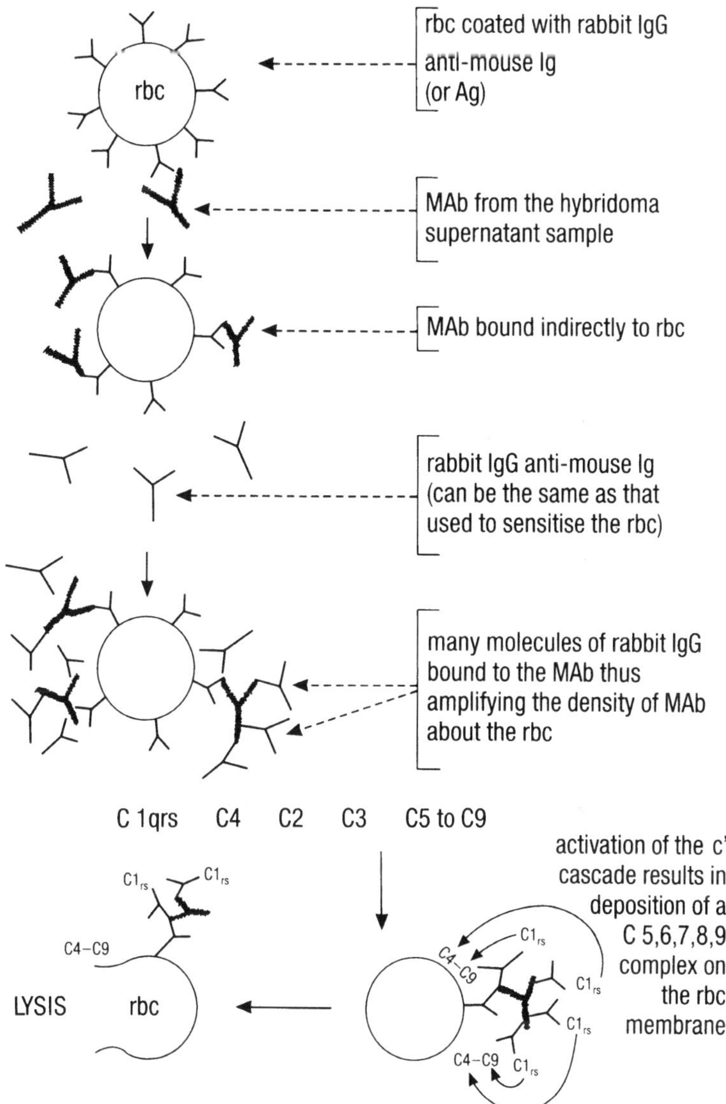

Fig. 4.11. The mechanism by which antibody, and then complement (C1qrs, C2, C3, C4, C5–C9), reacting with sensitised erythrocytes (rbc), can produce lysis and thus a visible reaction in the radial haemolysis assay.

4.1.7. *Immunoelectrophoresis (IEP)*

IEP is a combination of immunodiffusion (as in DID) and electrophoresis. As with DID, the MAb and antigen are permitted to diffuse towards one another and form an immunoprecipitate, but in IEP the antigen has been electrophoresed to separate it into the constituent components before the immunodiffusion step. A good example of the effectiveness of the procedure is shown by electrophoresing an antiserum and immunodiffusing an antispecies immunoglobulin against this. Fig. 4.12 shows such an example. Human antiserum is placed in the well and electrophoresed with the potential difference (+ and − poles) as shown by the + and − on the figure. Rabbit IgG prepared against human serum proteins is then placed in the trough and immunodiffused as for DID. A series of precipitin bands occur where specific antibody in the rabbit IgG reacts with the respective human serum protein. The position of this band depends on the electrophoresis characteristics of the human serum protein.

This is the simplest form of immunoelectrophoresis, and as such can be easily applied to separate the different constituent proteins of an antigen. It has been used for many substances including sera, yeast, bacteria, viruses, and cell membranes. However, the field of immunoelectrophoresis is a large and varied one. Adaptations of the basic IEP are often required to obtain a more qualitative and/or quantitative result.

When IEP is used with MAb, it is often to characterise the antigenic specificity of the MAb and not to screen hybridoma supernatants. Hence, since IEP is not a suitable screening technique but more an analytical tool of the characteristics of MAb prepared in large quantities, only the three techniques most applicable to hybridoma technology will be discussed. These are (i) crossed IEP (CIEP), (ii) counter-current IEP (CCIEP) and (iii) 'Laurell rocket' IEP (LRIEP). For further information on the other techniques, the reader should consult Williams & Chase (21).

(i) Crossed IEP (CIEP)

Many biological materials, in particular bacteria and viruses, can be

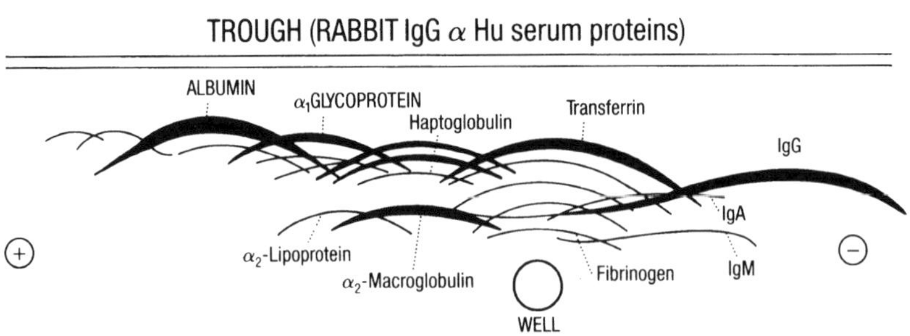

Fig. 4.12. Pattern of precipitation arcs seen with the immunoelectrophoresis of human serum, where the human serum is placed into the well and the proteins electrophoresed into agarose. The position of these proteins is then detected through the immunodiffusion of rabbit IgG specific for human serum proteins placed in a trough alongside the agarose.

applied to electrophoretic analysis of their constituent proteins. Some of these proteins may be attributed a function using mutants in that particular protein. They can also be analysed serologically, whereby antigenic functions such as the induction of an immuno-protective response can be identified. Two closely related isolates may have proteins difficult to distinguish by electrophoresis, but the additional scrutiny of IEP may detect more subtle antigenic differences.

It is for this antigenic analysis of proteins that CIEP can be used (22). CIEP is a two-dimensional electrophoresis system. The first dimension separates the antigen into constituent proteins, usually on a slab of gel of either polyacrylamide base (see below) or the agarose used in the second dimension.

Strips of these first dimension separations are cut from the slab and placed on a fresh glass electrophoresis plate, to which is then applied the agarose for the second dimension. Instead of running antibody against antigen by immunodiffusion (as with DID), one reagent can be run into a gel impregnated with the second reagent (as in SRID). This is what occurs with LRIEP. However, to speed up the process and sharpen the resolution (and the quantitative potential) of the system, the separated antigenic proteins are electrophoresed into the agarose containing the antibody (Fig. 4.13).

This technique does have certain limitations. The antigenic proteins must possess an electrophoretic mobility which differs significantly from that of the antibody in order that it can interact with antibody in the agarose and form visible precipitates in the second dimension. Thus, immunoglobulins could not be separated in a first dimension and then be expected to precipitate with anti-immunoglobulin in the second dimension. Furthermore, the MAb used in the second dimension must be of

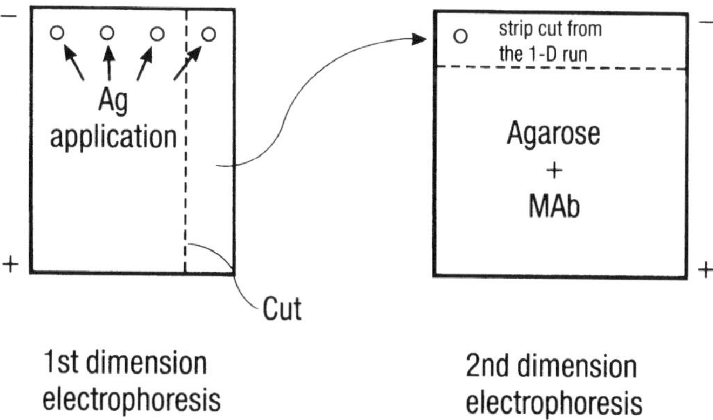

Fig. 4.13. The principle of the method of crossed immunoelectrophoresis (CIEP); see text for details.

high concentration and capable of recognising the denatured proteins obtained in the first dimension (some MAb react only with conformational determinants found on the intact 'native' antigen). If the precipitation reaction is weak, it can be enhanced by using radiolabelled antigen, as described in §4.1.5(i), step 9.

In order to perform CIEP, specialised equipment is required, namely an electrophoresis tank and power packs (can be obtained from several commercial sources), and 8 cm or 10 cm × 10 cm glass electrophoresis plates. The tank should be one which permits the electrophoresis to be performed on a water-cooled surface. With such equipment, the following procedure can be used.

1. An electrophoresis plate is covered with agarose as for DID, and 2 mm diameter wells cut 2.5 cm from the negative end.
2. To each well 6 μl antigen (in a denaturing buffer such as Laemmli buffer (23) if this is required to separate the constituent proteins) are applied. A sample of blue dextran or bromophenol blue marker dye is included such that the extent of the electrophoresis can be monitored. Certain manipulations are now performed which are general to most electrophoretic procedures which use 'electrophoresis tanks'. These tanks consist of two reservoirs, in which is placed the same barbitone buffer used to prepare the 2% agarose gel, separated by the water-cooled 'surface'. The plates are placed on this 'surface' and wicks of absorbent cloth or paper pre-soaked in barbitone buffer hung from the edge of the plates – covering the agarose gel to a depth of 3–8 mm – into the barbitone buffer in the reservoirs. The system is now ready for running.
3. An alternative to the use of agarose in the first dimension is the polyacrylamide gel electrophoresis (PAGE) system. Probably the most widely used procedure is that described by Laemmli (23), which can be performed in a flat-bed or upright electrophoresis apparatus (commercially available from companies such as LKB, Pharmacia and Bio-Rad Ltd). Modifications of this are often made for different antigens, e.g. the use of 0.5 M urea; polyacrylamide at 7.5%, 10%, 12.5%, 15%; or mixtures of these (gradient gels). The relevant publications should be consulted for each antigen, or different modifications tested to obtain the desired separations.
4. Electrophoresis is performed at 10 V/cm (8 mA/slide) for 60 min, or until the blue marker dye (marks the electrophoresis front) has reached 2.5 cm from the positive end.
5. A 1.5 cm wide strip is cut as shown in Fig. 4.13, carefully removed

under water to facilitate 'floating it off', and the second plate brought underneath to accommodate the strip.

6. The uncovered area of the plate is dried, and agarose containing the MAb (100 μl MAb – 1 μg, 10 μg or 100 μg – per 10 ml agarose) applied as described for SRID (§4.1.5.(i)). Care should be taken that the edge of this agarose meets the edge of the first dimension strip, but does not run over it.
7. Electrophorese at 2–2.5 V/cm for 22 h using the plate and electrophoresis set-up described in step 2. When the second dimension run is complete, the gels are washed in 0.9% saline to remove unprecipitated proteins, and dried and stained as described in §4.1.4(ii). This is a step applicable to all electrophoresis procedures.

Under conditions where the antigen migrates faster than the MAb, migration proceeds until the antigen is totally precipitated by the MAb in the agarose (if the MAb is reactive against the antigen). The precipitin bands appear as discrete, sometimes overlapping peaks, as shown in Fig. 4.14(*a*) where an antigen has been separated into components i, ii, iii, iv, v and vi. These would normally be antigenic polypeptides, glycoproteins or lipoproteins. More usual, however, is the situation shown in Fig. 4.14(*b*) where the MAb can precipitate only one of the components of the antigen.

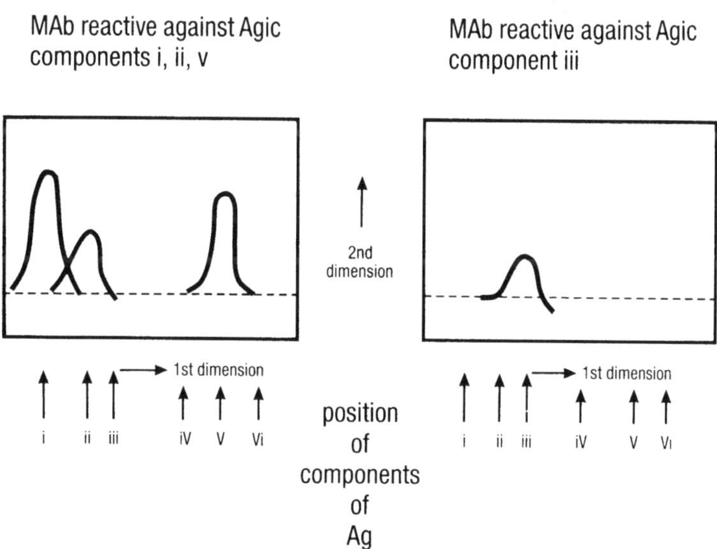

Fig. 4.14. Two possible patterns of precipitin lines which occur in CIEP analysis of MAb reactivity; see text for details.

(ii) Counter-current IEP (CCIEP)
As CIEP is the electrophoretic equivalent of SRID, counter-current immunoelectrophoresis (CCIEP) is the electrophoresis equivalent of DID. Instead of separated components of an antigen being electrophoresed in a second dimension into agar containing antibody, the antigen, or isolated components, and antibody are electrophoresed towards one another. This is most readily achieved when the antigen constituents migrate under electrophoresis towards the anode more rapidly than the antibody. The effectiveness of this will vary under different buffering conditions. When the antigen and antibody migrate in opposite directions, the procedure is given its alternative name, cross-over IEP. As with all IEP procedures, if the antigen and antibody can combine in the correct proportions a precipitate will form which cannot migrate any further.

Fig. 4.15 shows how a CCIEP plate is designed. Plates of agarose gel in barbitone buffer are prepared as above, and electrophoresed using the apparatus and procedure described for crossed IEP. Two wells are punched (as for DID) and antibody (or MAb) placed in well A (nearest the anode). Negatively charged antigen or electrophoretically separated antigenic components are placed in well B (nearest the cathode). The more negatively charged the antigen or component, the better the migration towards the anode. If the antigen is too positively charged, migration will be towards the cathode; if the antibody is relatively more positively charged and is used at the correct concentration a precipitate between antigen and antibody may still form (towards the cathode side of well B). The shape (concave or convex) of the precipitin band, whether it is to the cathode side of well B or between wells A and B, depends on the relative concentrations of the antigen and antibody.

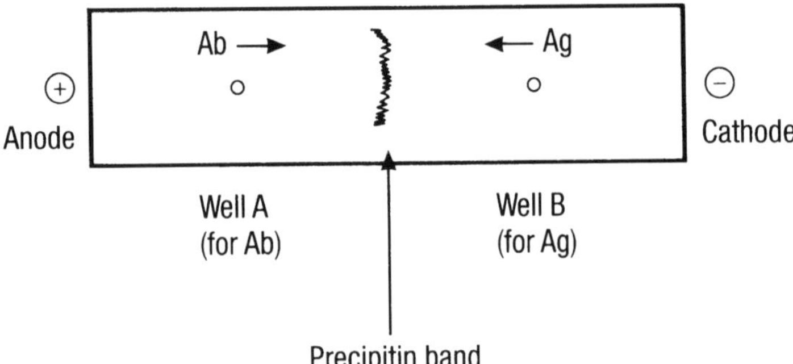

Fig. 4.15. The plate design and principle of the counter-current IEP (CCIEP) See text for details.

(iii) 'Laurell rocket' IEP (LRIEP)

This is a variation of crossed IEP in which only one-dimensional electrophoresis is performed. The method was originally developed from the report by Laurell (24). Agarose is prepared and antibody added as described for crossed IEP (§4.1.7.(i)). Plates are poured and wells punched as shown in Fig. 4.16(*a*).

As with the other IEP procedures, the more negatively charged the antigen is, the greater the resolution of precipitin arcs. Into the wells are placed different antigen preparations, components or dilutions, and electrophoresis performed as for CIEP: 8 mA/slide, 5–10 V/cm, 1–5 h (2 h is often optimal). Depending on the concentrations of antibody and antigen, and length of run, an arc of precipitation forms as shown in Fig. 4.16(*b*).

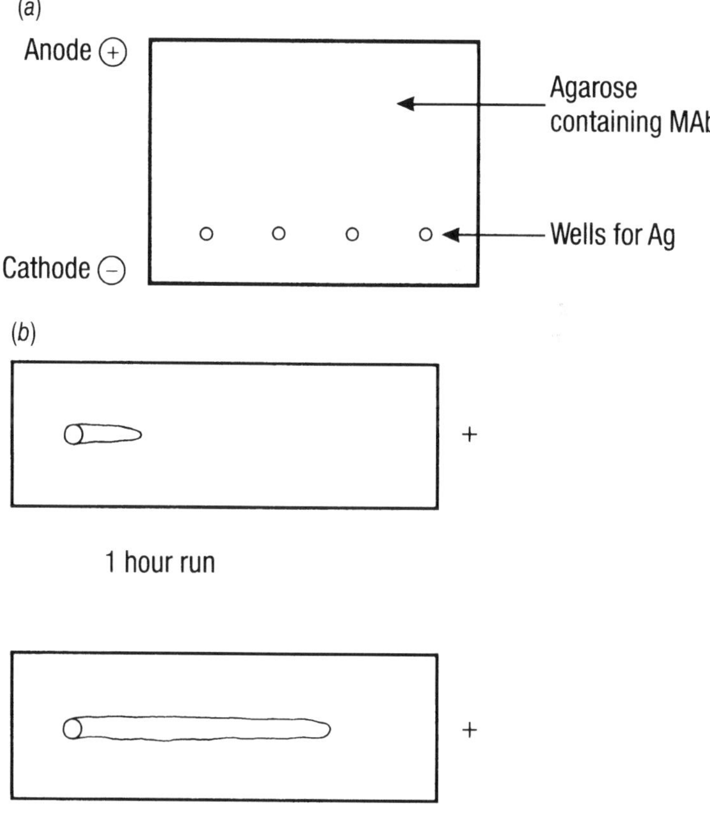

Fig. 4.16. 'Laurell rocket' IEP. (*a*) Plate design; (*b*) time-dependence of the formation of the precipitin arc or 'rocket'.

With some samples, a 5 h run may be required to give total precipitation of the antigen. Shorter runs given smaller precipitin arcs. As the electrophoresis continues, the precipitations redissolve as antigen reaches excess and a new precipitin line forms at the new point of equivalence. This continues until all the antigen applied is precipitated, at which point the precipitin arc is stabilised. Unprecipitated protein can be removed by washing in 0.9% (w/v) saline, and the slides are dried and stained as described in §4.1.4.(ii).

The analytic procedures so far discussed – immunoassays, immunodiffusions and immunoelectrophoresis – are general procedures to detect MAb in hybridoma supernatants and the reactivity of that MAb against a wide range of antigen. There are other procedures which are designed to detect the hybridoma cell secreting the MAb. These use sensitised erythrocytes, prepared as described for the passive haemagglutination and radial haemolysis assays (§§4.1.3 and 4.1.6). The procedures can be divided into those which use an agglutination of sensitised erythrocytes and hybridoma cells, and those which use lysis of the sensitised erythrocytes by the hybridoma cell product. The 'agglutination' procedures are haemadsorption, direct antiglobulin rosetting reaction and indirect antiglobulin rosetting reaction. The 'haemolysis' procedures are the Jerne plaque-forming cell assay and replica plate assay (although this can also make use of ELISA or RIA).

4.1.8. *Haemadsorption (rosette formation)*

The principle of haemadsorption (HAd) in the context of hybridoma technology relies on cells, which are secreting antibody, expressing immunoglobulin molecules on the cell surface. These immunoglobulin molecules will react with the antigen for which they are specific, or with rabbit IgG anti-mouse immunoglobulin. If that antigen or rabbit IgG is linked to erythrocytes by the sensitisation procedures of §4.1.3.(i), these erythrocytes will also be 'bound' to the hybridoma cell. Thus, hybridoma cells which are secreting antibody specific for antigen 'X' will bind erythrocytes sensitised with the antigen or anti-mouse immunoglobulin: that is, they will haemadsorb appropriately sensitised erythrocytes. However, the secretion of antibody by the hybridoma is in a dynamic state, and thus the cell surface immunoglobulin of the hybridoma cell must be maintained on the cell surface for the haemadsorption (HAd) process to be visible. Otherwise, the erythrocytes which bind to the hybridoma cell would soon be shed into the medium by the secretion of the antibody molecules to which they are bound. Two methods are suitable for converting the dynamic state of the hybridoma cell to a static state ideal for HAd. Firstly, if the hybridoma cells are not required in a viable state (for example, if a sample is removed from a hybridoma culture for testing), the cells can be fixed with 4% (w/v) *p*-formaldehyde in PBS for 15 min at room temperature (subsequently washed five times in PBS), or pretreated with 20 mM sodium azide in PBS (in this latter case, all steps of the HAd procedure would have to be performed in the presence of 20 mM sodium azide). Secondly, if viable hybridoma cells must be maintained, the cells should be pre-cooled to 4 °C and all processes in the HAd assay performed at 4 °C. After the numbers of haemadsorbing cells are counted, the cultures can be returned to 37 °C, at which temperature the erythrocytes will soon be shed from the surface of the hybridoma cells.

(i) HAd procedure

1. Sensitised rbc are gently centrifuged to remove large aggregates.
2. The remaining rbc are washed three times by centrifugation (150 *g* for 10 min at 4 °C), and resuspended in PBS to give 2–3 $\times 10^8$ rbc/ml.
3. Wash hybridoma cells as for the rbc, and resuspend to give 2–3 $\times 10^7$ cells/ml (or as many as the density of cells in the sample under test will allow). Controls should be non-secreting myeloma cells or hybridoma cells (negative) and a hybridoma or lymphocyte population known to be carrying the appropriate immunoglobulin molecules on their cell surface (if available).
4. Mix 0.1 ml aliquots of hybridoma cells with 0.1 ml sensitised rbc.
5. Incubate by rotating at 30 r.p.m. for 15 min at 4 °C.
6. Centrifuge at 150 *g* for 10 min at 4 °C.
7. Dilute sample to give 10^6, 10^5 or 10^4 hybridoma cells/ml.
8. Apply to a microscope or haemocytometer slide and count the percentage of cells with more than three rbc adsorbed out of a total of 1000 hybridoma cells counted over five different fields. Clumped rbc or rbc–hybridoma aggregates (rosettes) containing more than a single hybridoma cell should be ignored. Visualisation of the hybridoma cell may be enhanced by incubating the rosettes with fluorescein diacetate or acridine orange for live cells, or with Giemsa stain for fixed cells. (Unfortunately, acridine orange is mutagenic, which may influence the phenotypic characteristics of the hybridomas should they be required after the HAd procedure.)

   If only live cells are to be tested for their ability to rosette sensitised rbc, the fluorescein diacetate or acridine orange staining should be incorporated into the procedure, and an expendable aliquot of cells should be taken from the hybridoma culture. These staining procedures are to be found in Mischel & Shiigi (25).

4.1.9. *Direct anti-globulin rosette reaction (DARR)*

This is a variation of the HAd technique in which erythrocytes sensitised with, for example, rabbit IgG anti-mouse immunoglobulin are used. Much of the developmental work has been provided by Coombs, Binns and co-workers (8–12). Fig. 4.17 shows diagrammatically how the reaction is accomplished. In order to increase the sensitivity of the system, the rabbit IgG anti-mouse immunoglobulin is affinity purified by absorption to, followed by elution from, a 'mouse immunoglobulin affinity column': mouse immunoglobulin linked to Sepharose 4B or Ultragel ACA 40 by cyanogen bromide or glutaraldehyde bridges respectively. The erythrocyte of choice is donkey, although trypsin-treated bovine or ovine erythrocytes will suffice (this point applies to all tests utilising sensitised erythrocytes).

The procedure is as follows.

1. Equal aliquots (usually 50 or 100 μl) of washed hybridoma cells in RPMI 1640 (ideally at 2×10^6 cells/ml) and 1% (v/v) sensitised rbc are mixed and centrifuged at 225 *g* for 5 min at 4 °C.
2. Leave for longer than 1 h, or overnight, at 4 °C.
3. Gently resuspend the mixtures and count the rosetted cells as for the HAd procedure. Controls should also be as shown for HAd.

4.1.10. *Indirect anti-globulin rosette reaction (IARR)*

This is the DARR with an amplifying intermediate step. For example, surface immunoglobulin on hybridoma cells will bind rabbit IgG anti-mouse immunoglobulin, and this can be detected using rbc sensitised

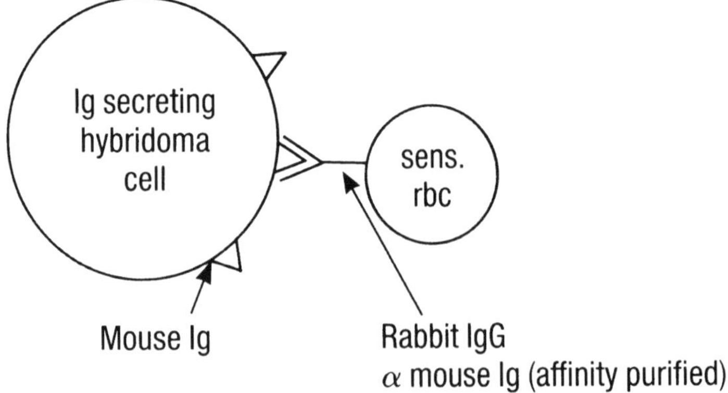

Fig. 4.17. Direct anti-globulin rosetting reaction (DARR); the principle of the reaction between the sensitised erythrocyte (sens. rbc) and the antibody (Ig)-secreting hybridoma cell (α, anti).

with affinity-purified sheep IgG anti-rabbit immunoglobulin Fc (Fig. 4.18).

The test uses 50 μl of hybridoma cells at 10^7/ml (or as many as possible), incubated with 50 μl of a pre-determined dilution (by titration to find maximum binding against 10^7 hybridomas or lymphocytes known to bear cell surface immunoglobulin) of rabbit IgG anti-mouse immunoglobulin on ice for 30–60 min. The cells are washed four times (250 *g* for 10 min at 4 °C), diluted to 2.5×10^6/ml (or as high a density as possible), and centrifuged with rbc sensitised with IgG specific for the Fc portion of rabbit IgG. This reaction with the sensitised rbc is as described for DARR; the counting of rosettes is again as described for HAd.

Both DARR and IARR can be taken one step further. In addition to being a screening system, they are also an enrichment procedure for hybridoma cells carrying surface immunoglobulin (or immunoglobulin reactive against a particular antigen if the rbc are sensitised with that antigen). After rosetting, the cells can be applied to a Ficoll–Hypaque gradient: 12 parts of 14% (w/v) Ficoll type 400 (relative molecular weight 400 000) are mixed with 5 parts 32.8% (w/v) Hypaque (sterilise by membrane filitration) to give a density of 1.09 g/cm^3 and an osmolarity of 280–308 mOsm. Place 4 ml Ficoll–Hypaque in a 16 mm × 125 mm polycarbonate tube and gently layer onto the surface a maximum of 5 ml of rosette suspension. Centrifuge at 2000 *g* for 20 min at 20 °C with rapid acceleration. The pellet contains rbc, rosetted cells, dead cells and cell debris. Resuspend the pellet in the 0.83% (w/v) NH_4Cl solution used when preparing splenocytes for fusion. This will lyse the rbc after 5 min at room temperature. Centrifuge and wash (twice) the hybridoma cells.

This purification procedure can also be applied to the splenocyte

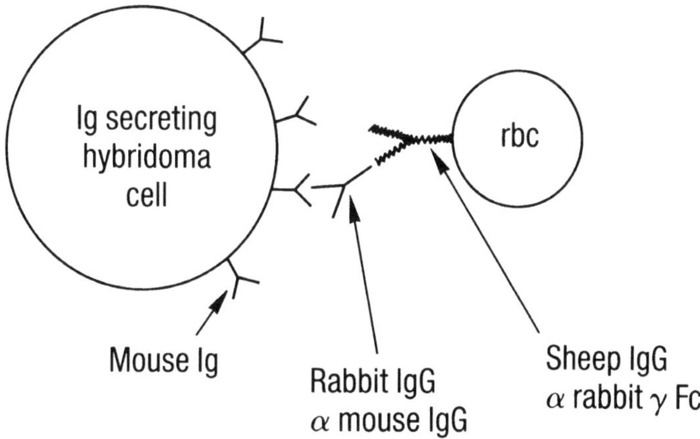

Fig. 4.18. The principle of the indirect anti-globulin rosetting reaction (IARR).

population which is to be used for fusion, to enrich either for all B lymphocytes and lymphoblasts or for those lymphocytes and lymphoblasts which carry receptors for the antigen of choice.

As a screening assay for antibody-secreting hybridoma cells, the rosetting procedures can be taken one step further. Instead of looking for rbc adsorbed to hybridomas, the secreted product (the MAb) of the hybridoma can be detected through induced lysis of rbc to which the MAb has bound. This is a combination of rosetting reactions and the radial haemolysis test, and is termed the haemolytic plaque assay (developed originally by Jerne & Nordin (26)).

4.1.11. *Haemolytic plaque assay (HPA or PFC assay)*

This was originally developed by Jerne & Nordin (26) in Petri dishes, but now many variations on both the procedure and the plates or dishes used are available (25). The technique which will be described here is the 'slide method' (27).

The principle is a variation on the radial haemolysis assay (§4.1.6). With the HPA, there are no wells cut in the agarose containing sensitised rbc. Instead, lymphocytes or hybridoma cells are incorporated into the agarose matrix at the same time as the sensitised rbc are added. It is a very sensitive technique, capable of detecting 10^3–10^6 antibody molecules released by a single cell into the adjacent agarose medium. These antibodies bind to the anti-immunoglobulin or antigen on the rbc in that vicinity, and are detected by adding free anti-immunoglobulin antibody (binds to the hybridoma or lymphocyte antibody now on the rbc) and complement (is activated by the Fc of the anti-immunoglobulin antibody bound by the hybridoma or lymphocyte antibody) which creates the visual effect of lysis. Since the reaction is performed in a gel, the diffusion of the hybridoma or lymphocyte antibody, and the movement of cells, is restricted. Hence, small zones of lysis – plaques – occur around each hybridoma cell which secretes the appropriate antibody. If that antibody is IgM, the direct fixation of complement by this is often adequate to lyse the rbc. With IgG, the number of molecules bound to the rbc must be amplified to permit the complement to effect visual lysis. However, not all IgM- or IgG-producing cells will form plaques if the density of binding to the rbc is too low (the rbc can repair a certain degree of complement-mediated lysis) or if the IgG is the wrong isotype (mouse IgG_1 is poor at fixing complement).

(i) HPA procedure (slide method)

1. Sensitise rbc using one of the methods described in Tables 4.8 to 4.10.
2. Add agarose to deionised water to give 1% w/v and boil in a water bath until 'dissolved' (melted and absorbed into the

water); measure out 0.25 ml volumes and place in a 45 °C water bath.

3. Add 0.25 ml of two times concentrated BSS (twice the concentration of each constituent of the balanced salt solution shown in Table 4.11) to each agarose aliquot (at 45 °C).
4. Pre-warm the sensitised rbc and hybridoma cell or lymphocyte suspension in a 37 °C water bath.
5. Dilute the rbc to 6.6% (v/v) in BSS.
6. Warm the microscope slide by passing through a bunsen flame until it can just be held on the back of the hand without discomfort; place on a levelled surface.
7. Add 50 μl of the 6.6% rbc suspension to each 0.5 ml aliquot of agarose/BSS. Mix rapidly; add 10–50 μl hybridoma cells, containing 10, 10^2, 10^3, 10^4, or 10^5 cells (with lymphocytes, use 10^3, 10^4, 10^5, 10^6 or 10^7 cells); again mix well and immediately pour onto one slide per aliquot using a pre-warmed (through a bunsen flame) 1 ml pipette and a circular dispensing motion as described in §4.1.4(i), point 3.
8. Allow to set.
9. For the detection of IgM-secreting hybridoma cells, add enough of a 1 : 20 dilution of rabbit complement (absorbed beforehand with rbc of the species used in the assay to remove any lytic activity against these) to cover the agarose, and incubate for 3 h at 37 °C (an additional overnight incubation at 4 °C may also be desirable) in a humidified box.
10. For the detection of IgG-secreting in addition to IgM-secreting cells, after step 8, incubate the slides at 37 °C for 90 min in a humidified box; cover the agarose as in step 9 with a 1 : 10 dilution of rabbit IgG anti-mouse IgG mixed with an equal volume of 1 : 10 rabbit complement (pre-absorbed with rbc as in step 9); incubate for 90 min at 37 °C (or overnight at 4 °C and then 60 min at 37 °C).
11. After incubation, dip slides in 0.9% (w/v) aqueous saline and drain off excess saline using paper towelling.
12. Small areas of lysis (plaques) can be observed using dark-ground illumination or a strong white light shining from the side of the slide.
13. To verify that the plaques are due to antibody secreted by the hybridoma cell or lymphocyte, the plaques can be viewed microscopically; this should reveal a hybridoma cell or lymphocyte at the centre of a true plaque.

4.1.12. *Replica plate assay (RPA)*

A variation of the HPA technique is to plate onto samples of the hybridoma cells filter discs impregnated with antigen-sensitised rbc. This is the replica plate assay (RPA) (28). The filter discs (Millipore cellulose acetate, or cellulose nitrate – nitrocellulose, 47 mm discs) are sensitised as follows.

1. Mark with a dot to show one face.
2. Drop over 0.9% (w/v) aqueous NaCl and impregnate with the saline (1 s); turn over and impregnate the other side.
3. Place, free side up, on a dry glass plate.
4. Overlay with 1.5 ml 0.25% (v/v) suspension of sensitised rbc. Leave for 30 min at room temperature to allow the rbc to settle.
5. Remove fluid and place filter on to new dry glass plate.
6. Air-dry (30–60 min).
7. Before they are completely dry, dislodge to prevent sticking to the plate.
8. Repeat steps 2–4 inclusive, but using 10% (v/v) aqueous foetal calf serum or bovine serum albumin in place of the NaCl and sensitised rbc; this will block any uncoated sites.

The discs can be placed on to semi-solid agar in which hybridoma cells are growing (being cloned; see §4.2.3). If a hybridoma colony is producing antibody, this will react with the sensitised rbc. Since the disc was marked before placing on to the agar containing the hybridomas, the antibody-secreting hybridomas can be identified within the agar.

In addition to the assay procedures mentioned so far, there are others which utilise certain functional properties of the antigen against which the MAb were raised. Bacteria, viruses and monocellular parasites fall into this character of antigen. It is impracticable to attempt to review all of these assay procedures, but the principles of many can be shown under five major headings:

(1) MAb inhibition of agglutination of certain species of rbc by the parasite.
(2) MAb inhibition of lysis of certain species of rbc by the parasite.
(3) MAb inhibition of the capacity of the parasite to function, for example, as in the infection of a host cell.
(4) Opsonisation to give MAb–parasite complexes.
(5) Immunofluorescent staining of MAb reacted with the parasite or intracellular inclusions of the parasite in the host cell which they infect.

4.1.13. *Haemagglutination inhibition (HAI)*

Certain parasites carry antigenic determinants on their surface which will react with certain species of erythrocyte. For example, influenza virus and measles virus are composed of a protein – nucleic acid core enveloped in a lipid-based membrane through which project glycoprotein 'spikes'. A proportion of these glycoproteins carry erythrocyte-binding sites for chicken erythrocytes (influenza virus) or rhesus monkey erythrocytes (measles virus). These glycoproteins are termed haemagglutinins. Antibody against these haemagglutinins can inhibit the haemagglutination (HA); that is, they are haemagglutination inhibition (HAI) antibodies. To test if MAb are HAI, first titrate the antigen against the correct species of erythrocyte. Dilute the antigen to 8 HA units and retitrate to check the dilution factor. Mix 8 HA units of antigen with dilutions of MAb and incubate at 37 °C for 30 min. Add erythrocytes and incubate as for the HA assay. The HAI titre of the MAb is the highest dilution of the MAb which inhibits HA by the antigen. It should be noted that a negative HAI may reflect too low a concentration of MAb, and a higher concentration of the antibody may indeed be HAI. This is because a minimum of 10^6 erythrocytes are required in an HA lattice to be visible as agglutination. Therefore, a minimum of 10^6-1 antigen particles are required. Since 8 HA units have to be used in the HAI test, and each antigen particle will carry multiple copies of the haemagglutinin, a large number of MAb molecules will be required to inhibit HA.

This is a general description of the procedure; the HA and HAI test conditions vary considerably for different antigens. Even different viruses, or isolates of viruses, require or can require different test conditions. For example, some isolates of measles virus will haemagglutinate rhesus monkey erythrocytes in PBS, but other isolates require the additional presence of ammonium sulphate. It is therefore impracticable to give detailed procedures for HA and HAI. Should the HAI test be a suitable assay for either screening hybridoma cultures or identifying the epitopes with which the MAb react, the relevant reports of the procedure for a particular antigen should be consulted.

4.1.14. *Haemolysis inhibition (HLI)*

Another glycoprotein on measles virus can effect a lysis of the erythrocyte with which the virus has agglutinated. Haemolysis (HL) is a more unique property of certain parasites, notably certain members of the Paramyxoviridae viruses and certain members of the Togavirus group. Measles virus and parainfluenza virus are representative of the first group. After HA, further incubation at 37 °C results in lysis of the erythrocyte if HL activity is present. A MAb specific for HL inhibition (HLI) should be capable of inhibiting HL without affecting HA. As with HAI, the procedural details of the test reported for a particular antigen should be consulted.

4.1.15. *Neutralisation*

Viruses, certain bacteria and protozoa, and certain multicellular parasites are obligate intracellular parasites (with protozoa and multicellular parasites this may be for only part of their life cycle). As such, they possess antigenic determinants through which they bind to the host cell. These are the 'cell-binding epitopes' essential for the infectivity of the parasite. MAb which bind at, or near enough to sterically hinder the function of, this epitope are said to 'neutralise' parasite infectivity.

The assay system uses the test conditions for determining the infectivity titre of the parasite. As a general rule, 50–100 infectivity units are mixed with dilutions of MAb and incubated for 30–60 minutes at 37 °C or 40 °C (depending on the parasite). The mixtures are then titrated in the appropriate assay system to determine if the MAb has reduced the number of infectivity units of the parasite. The neutralisation titre is determined and expressed differently for different parasites, and the appropriate reports should therefore be consulted.

Again, however, failure of the MAb to neutralise the parasite may reflect too low a concentration of the MAb, since more than one antibody molecule per parasite particle is required to neutralise, and this quantity will be higher for a low-affinity MAb than for a high-affinity MAb. In addition, synergistic reactions between two or more MAb, or MAb with auxiliary factors such as complement, may be necessary to neutralise parasites (29).

4.1.16. *Opsonisation*

This is not a recommended assay procedure, but may be used to link the *in vitro* binding of MAb with antigen to the *in vivo* immune response. Opsonisation was originally reported with respect to the enhancement of phagocytosis of complement-coated bacteria. The phenomenon will occur with a wide range of antibody and antigen, the antibody–antigen complex being bound by a receptor for the antibody Fc on the cell membrane of the phagocytic cell. Hence, using a culture of phagocytic cells, such as peritoneal exudate (the same cells as used for feeder cells; §3.7.3), and antigen linked to erythrocytes or radioactively or enzymically labelled, MAb reactivity against the antigen may be measured by detecting MAb–antigen complexes associated with phagocytic cells. Expertise is required in this area, and for this reason no further details of the procedure will be given. Learning the methodology involved is best achieved at the bench in a laboratory experienced in the techniques.

4.1.17. *Immunofluorescence*

The principle of this method is shown in Fig. 4.19. The antigen may be a bacterium, protozoan or multicellular parasite which can be viewed under high power magnification by UV light microscopy, or a host cell infected with a virus, intracellular bacterium, protozoan or multicellular

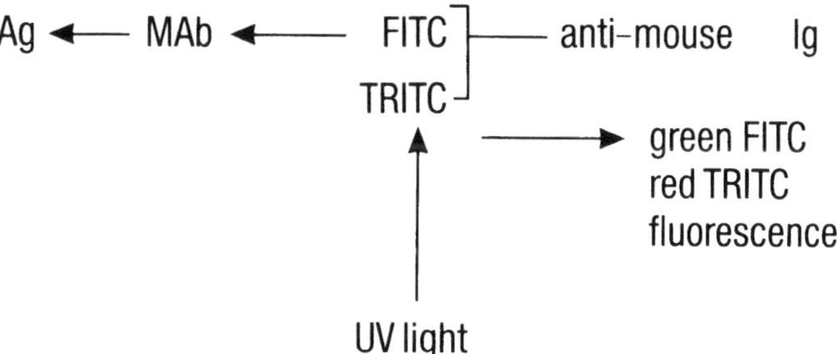

Fig. 4.19. The principle of the indirect immunofluorescence assay in which the reaction between antigen and MAb is detected using FITC or TRITC conjugated anti-mouse immunoglobulin.

parasite. Using the intact organism will reveal where the MAb binds, and hence where on the organism resides the epitope against which the MAb reacts. With the infected cells, 'factories' of parasite antigens can be identified, as can the stages and intracellular location of the parasite life cycle from an antigenic viewpoint.

The procedure uses either free antigen or antigen in association with infected host cells. If the parasite or infected cell is unfixed (living), the antibody will not penetrate and thus will only react with antigens on the surface. To permit antibody to enter the parasite or infected cell and react with antigens or antigenic determinants therein, a fixation procedure is used. The fixative agents in most common use are methanol, ethanol, glutaraldehyde, acetone, formaldehyde and *p*-formaldehyde. These can have a variable denaturation effect on different antigens, approximately in the order shown. It is recommended that a 4% (w/v) solution of *p*-formaldehyde in PBS be used as a fixative in most cases.

Dilutions of MAb in PBS are reacted with the antigen preparation for 30–60 min at 37 °C or overnight at 4 °C. The preparation is washed three times, and a pre-determined dilution of conjugated anti-mouse immunoglobulin in PBS is reacted for 30–45 min at 37 °C or 30–60 min at 4 °C (too long an incubation at this stage can result in some non-specific binding of the conjugate). The anti-mouse immunoglobulin is an IgG preparation conjugated with either fluorescein isothiocyanate (FITC), tetramethyl rhodamine isothiocyanate (TRITC) or Texas Red. The inexperienced should go to an established laboratory to learn these conjugation procedures, or purchase commercial conjugates. The commercial preparations can usually be used at 1 : 50 to 1 : 200 dilution.

After the conjugate has reacted, the preparations are washed three times. They can then be mounted in glycerol–saline on microscope slides (the infected cells may be grown on coverslips, which can be mounted on a drop of glycerol–saline on a microscope slide), and viewed microscopically under UV light illumination. If the MAb has reacted, it can be visualised by the subsequently bound anti-mouse immunoglobulin, showing as a green colour for FITC conjugates and red for TRITC and Texas Red conjugates.

Immunofluorescence can also be used to determine reactivity of MAb against cellular antigens such as the 'cell membrane antigenic determinants' (CMAD) of lymphocytes. In fact, the major assay procedures for detecting MAb against lymphocyte CMAD are RIA and immunofluorescence. The RIA uses a liquid phase system in which lymphocytes are incubated in suspension with MAb followed by iodinated rabbit-anti-mouse immunoglobulin (Fig. 4.20). Alternatively, the anti-mouse immunoglobulin may be conjugated with an enzyme or FITC/TRITC, and an ELISA or immunofluorescence assay performed. The incubation times are as shown in the appropriate sections on ELISA, RIA and here for immunofluorescence. To obtain further details on assays for MAb against cellular antigens, the review by Kennett *et al.* (30) is recommended.

In this context of lymphocyte antigens, there is one area of immunoassay which deserves mention. It is not used to detect lymphocyte antigens, but to determine lymphocyte function. As such, it can be used to identify lymphocyte subsets, or epitopes on parasites involved in the function of some of these subsets. These are the *in vitro* lymphocyte assays.

4.1.18. In vitro *lymphocyte assays*

These can be used to identify helper or suppressor lymphocyte activity, and antibody-dependent or independent cellular cytotoxicity reactions. The assays can be applied to determine the specificity of a MAb, but are less useful as hybridoma screening tests. For the latter reason, the assays will only be described briefly. More detailed descriptions can be found in Mishel & Shiigi (25) and Hudson & Hay (13). The success of the assays relies on an efficient protocol for the culturing of lymphocytes *in vitro* (25, 27, 31).

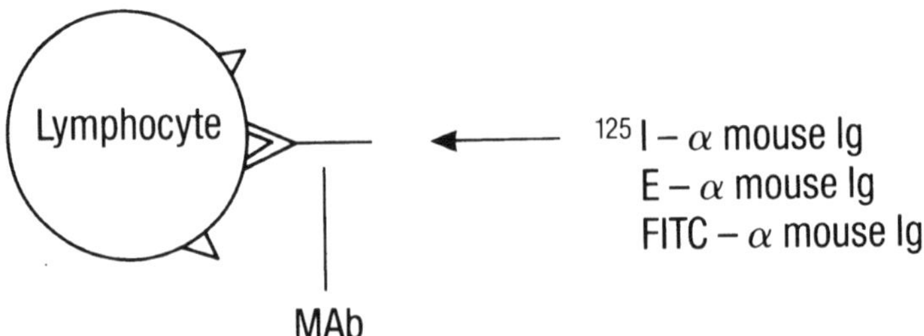

Fig. 4.20. The principle of the reactions involved in the RIA used for the detection of cell membrane antigenic determinants (CMAD).

The assays for helper or suppressor factors, and cytotoxic T lymphocytes (CTL) can also be used for screening T cell hybridomas or T lymphocyte clones, and to detect antibodies against the factors or these cells. If the test MAb are incubated with T lymphocyte supernatants, they may 'neutralise' the activity of T cell factors present in these supernatants. The MAb can then be characterised in terms of whether the factors had helper or suppressor factor activity. If the MAb are incubated with the cells and not their factors (MAb + rabbit anti-mouse immunoglobulin + complement can lyse the cells; MAb immobilised on to a plastic surface can 'pan' out cells for which it is specific; rbc sensitised with MAb can be used to remove cells for which the MAb is specific using centrifugation on Ficoll–Hypaque gradients), the presence or absence of T lymphocyte helper or suppressor activity can again be determined. The assays for factors are cultures of mononuclear cells (lymphocytes plus monocytes) stimulated with antigen. In this manner, antigen will be presented by the monocytes and stimulate the T lymphocytes to produce their factors. Helper factors are detected by using other lymphocyte cultures depleted of T cells. Here, the B cells will only differentiate into antibody-producing cells (after antigen stimulation) in the presence of helper factors. For T lymphocyte suppressor factors, a complete lymphocyte culture *in vitro* is used, and either T cell or B cell blastogenesis (antigen-driven) can be compared in the presence and absence of the proposed suppressor substances. If suppressor factors are present in the test material, then the functioning of the T_h lymphocytes will be impaired, and both T and B lymphocyte blastogenesis will be affected.

Similarly, MAb specific for CTL (T_c lymphocytes) can be used to remove these cells from a particular culture. The presence or absence of CTL activity can then be tested by either a mixed lymphocyte reaction (MLR) or cell-mediated cytolysis (CMC). The MLR can use lymphocytes from allogeneically distinct animals, which are identical at H2K/D*; for example, lymphocytes from C3H/HeJ and DBA/2 mice. A stronger MLR can be generated using H2K/D distinct species of lymphocytes, but this will not detect the effector progeny of CTL (CTL are H2-restricted). If one species of cells is irradiated (the stimulator cells) the other species of cells (the responder cells) undergo a blastogenic response since they recognise allogeneic determinants on the stimulator cells. The converse cannot occur, because only one population of cells (the responders) is living. This test will in fact detect both CTL and DTH (delayed-type hypersensitivity) type lymphocytes. The CMC assay will detect only CTL.

*H2 is the major histocompatibility complex (MHC) of the mouse (equivalent to HLA in humans); H2K and H2D are the two major loci coding for the so-called 'transplantation antigens'. Differences at H2K and/or H2D can occur between species, resulting in the expression of different transplantation or class I MHC antigens.

The CMC again uses cells which have antigenic differences but are H2K/D identical, because, as already mentioned, the CTL are H2K/D restricted. Usually a tumour cell line (target) and responder (effector) cells from the same species of animal are employed; for example P815Y mastocytoma cells and DBA/2 lymphocytes. The effectors will respond against the tumour antigens of the target cells under H2K/D restriction, the process being detected through lysis of the targets. This lysis can be estimated by increased uptake of Trypan blue by the attached tumour cell targets, or by release of radioactive chromium (^{51}Cr) from targets. (These targets were prepared previously by incubating with ^{51}Cr for 40 minutes at 37 °C followed by ^{51}Cr-free medium for 30 min on ice.) As an alternative to the use of a tumour cell target, PHA (phytohaemagglutinin, T cell mitogen) stimulated allogeneic but H2K/D identical T cell targets may be used.

Antibody-mediated cellular cytotoxicity (ADCC) is similar to CTL activity, except that the cells react against antibody which has bound to antigen on the target cell. In addition, the dominant effector cell type varies between animal species: lymphocytes in humans, monocytes in mice and polymorphs in domestic animals. MAb can be used as the antibody mediator (specific for the target cell) or to remove the effector cell as for the MLR and CMC assays. Otherwise, the assay is similar to the CMC: ^{51}Cr-labelled targets (not necessarily H2K/D identical to the effector cells) are incubated with antibody and the effector cell preparation for 18 h at 37 °C. Supernatants are then tested for ^{51}Cr release from the targets.

4.1.19. *Other assays*

There are numerous other assays which can be employed to screen hybridoma supernatants, but more particularly to determine reactivity of the MAb. Kennett *et al.* (30) and Houba *et al.* (32) have reviewed many of these, notably the polyacrylamide gel electrophoresis (PAGE) and isoelectric focusing (IEF). These procedures are notable for two reasons. Firstly, the specificity of MAb for a particular protein of an antigen is determined, either by immunoprecipitation of the antigen with the MAb followed by PAGE or IEF analysis, or by the crossed immunoelectrophoresis procedure given in §4.1.7(i). The basic PAGE and IEF procedures for use with immunoprecipitations are shown in Tables 4.12 and 4.13; the immunoprecipitation method is shown in Fig. 4.21. Secondly, the chain composition of the MAb can be determined, that is, whether the heavy and light chains were derived from splenocyte genes, or whether one or more were derived from myeloma cell genes (§2.4). Cells (2×10^5) are pelleted and resuspended in 0.2 ml leucine-free

Table 4.12. *Polyacrylamide gel electrophoresis as used with immunoprecipitation*

1. Prepare antigen in RIPA buffer:
   2% (v/v) Triton X-100
   0.15 M NaCl
   0.6 M KCl
   5 mM Na_2-EDTA
   3 mM phenylmethylsulphonylfluoride
   1% trasylol–aprotinin
   2.5 mM iodoacetamide
   0.01 M Tris–HCl, pH 7.8
2. Mix 200 μl antigen with 20 μl of a 1 : 20 dilution of hybridoma ascites fluid.
3. Make up to 500 μl with RIPA buffer.
4. Incubate for 3 h on ice.
5. Add 80 μl of a 50% (v/v) suspension of *Staphylococcus aureus* protein A bound to Sepharose CL-4B in 0.01 M Tris–HCl–0.15 M NaCl, pH 8.0.
6. Incubate on ice for 1 h with frequent vortexing.
7. Centrifuge in an Eppendorf microfuge for 2 min at 10 000 r.p.m.
8. Wash five times with RIPA buffer, and once with 0.01 M Tris–HCl–0.15 M NaCl, pH 8.0.
9. Dry the beads and dissociate the immune complexes by adding 100 μl of sample buffer:
   3% (w/v) sodium dodecyl sulphate
   3% (v/v) 2-mercaptoethanol
   0.1% (w/v) Na_2-EDTA
   10% (v/v) glycerol
   0.0625 M Tris–H_3PO_4, pH 6.8
   0.002% (w/v) bromophenol blue
10. Incubate at 100 °C for 2 min.
11. Remove the beads by centrifugation (10 000 r.p.m. for 2 min).
12. The polyacrylamide separation gel depends on the characteristics of the proteins to be separated, but normally consists of either 7.5%, 10% or 12.5% (w/v) acrylamide and 0.20%, 0.27% or 0.34% (w/v) *N,N'*-methylenebis-acrylamide (bis-acrylamide).
13. Prepare stock solutions of
   A. 30% (w/v) acrylamide and 0.8% (w/v) bis-acrylamide in distilled water.
   B. 18.15 g Tris in 50 ml H_2O, adjusted to pH 8.9 with 1M HCl, made up to 100 ml with H_2O.
   C. 10% (w/v) sodium dodecyl sulphate in H_2O.
   D. 3.0 g Tris in final volume of 50 ml H_2O after adjusting pH to 6.8 with 0.33 M H_3PO_4.
   E. *Freshly* prepared 10% (w/v) ammonium persulphate in H_2O.
   F. 0.25% (w/v) Coomassie brilliant blue in 30% (v/v) methanol, 10% (v/v) glacial acetic acid in H_2O.
   G. 30% (v/v) methanol, 10% (v/v) glacial acetic acid in H_2O.
14. Prepare the gel by mixing the required volumes of A (for a 7.5% gel, 12.5 ml A + 24.325 ml H_2O; for a 10% gel, 16.7 ml A + 20.125 ml H_2O; for a 12.5% gel, 20.8 ml A + 16.025 ml H_2O) with 12.5 ml B, and then degassing.

Table 4.12. *(cont.)*

15. To the degassed solution add 0.5 ml C, 0.025 ml TEMED and 0.15 ml E.

16. Cast the gel *immediately* between glass electrophoresis plates (13 cm × 22 cm and with a gap of 0.15 cm; one of the plates has a 13 cm × 2 cm notch cut in the top edge). The plates – which are detergent-washed and dried – are placed together with 0.15 cm thick, 0.5 cm wide spacers between them, along the side edges, and held together with clamps. The edges are sealed from the outside by using melted 2% (w/v) agarose, and allowing this to set. The plates are then placed in a trough containing a small amount of gel solution, which is allowed to set (to seal the bottom edge). The gel is cast by pouring this in between the plates from the top, until it reaches 2.5 cm below the notch (the height of the combs to be used).

17. Gently overlayer the poured gel with solution A diluted 1 : 3 in water, in order to achieve an even surface.

18. Leave the casting for 20–30 min at room temperature, to allow the polymerisation to occur.

19. Remove the unpolymerised overlaying solution.

20. A comb with the desired size of channels is inserted in the space at the top of the gel.

21. Pour in the stacking gel until it reaches the top of the comb. This gel is 1 ml solution A + 2.5 ml solution D + 6.3 ml H_2O, degassed; 0.1 ml solution C, 0.005 ml TEMED and 0.1 ml E are added just before pouring.

22. After polymerisation, remove the comb and then remove the unit from the trough; the bottom of the plates are then cleaned of loose pieces of gel.

23. Place the unit in the electrophoresis tank; Vaseline is put around the notch, where it contacts the upper reservoir.

24. The upper and lower reservoirs are filled with electrode buffer: 3 g Tris + 14.4 g glycine + 10 ml solution C, made up to 1 l with H_2O and to pH 8.3.

25. Ensure that there are no air bubbles where the electrode buffer contacts the gel.

26. Apply samples (10–50 μl) to the slots made by the comb.

27. Connect the electrodes (upper: cathode, negative; lower: anode, positive).

28. Run at a constant voltage of 40 V until the bromophenol blue dye reaches the bottom of the gel.

29. Remove the gel unit and mark (in order to remember the orientation).

30. Remove the gel from between the glass plates under water, *carefully*.

31. Stain the gel for 20 min at room temperature with solution F.

32. Destain in solution G for at least 2 h at room temperature, with constant shaking.

33. Transfer on to a drying block or unit to which water-wettable Cellophane and then Whatman 3MM chromatography paper have already been applied.

34. Dry the gel onto the filter paper, following the instructions for use of the drying block.

Table 4.13. *Electrofocusing as used with immunoprecipitation*

1. Prepare antigen by immunoprecipitation as described in Table 4.12, steps 1–8.

2. Dry the immunoprecipitates and dissociate the immune complex (aliquots of 400 μl) as follows.

3. Add 143 μl 0.01 M Tris–H_3PO_4, pH 7.4, containing 1 mM EDTA.

4. Sonicate and then heat at 60 °C for 2 min.

5. Cool.

6. Add 5 μl of pancreatic ribonuclease in 0.01 M Tris–H_3PO_4, pH 7.4 and 1 mM EDTA (stock: 0.2 mg/ml).

7. Incubate at 37 °C for 1 h (MINIMUM).

8. Add 11 μl of a 1 : 1 NP40–2-mercaptoethanol solution.

9. Immediately add 143 μg ultra-pure urea.

10. Leave at 37 °C until the urea has dissolved and the sample has cleared.

11. Take stock gel which has been stored at −20 °C and heat in a 37 °C water bath until the urea has dissolved.

Stock gel: 315 g urea
19 g acrylamide
1 g bis-acrylamide
500 ml deionised water
Dissolve in a 37 °C water bath (takes a long time).
Stir in 30 g Amberlite MB-1 to remove residual ions.
Leave 10–30 min on a magnetic stirrer at room temperature.
Filter, divide into aliquots and store at −20 °C.

12. Prepare ampholines; the relative proportions of each ampholine will depend on the desired pH gradient in the gels. One example, as used for the separation of the virion proteins of foot-and-mouth disease virus, is

100 μl ampholine '2.5–4'
150 μl ampholine '4–6'
100 μl ampholine '5–7'
150 μl ampholine '3·5–10'
added to 9.5 ml gel stock.

This will separate the four virion proteins, leaving the VP1 at the source.

13. Add the ampholines to 9.5 ml gel stock.

14. Degas.

15. Add, to every 10 ml gel (9.5 ml gel stock + 500 μl ampholine mixture), 10 μl FRESHLY PREPARED 10% (w/v) ammonium persulphate in deionised water.

16. Add 7 μl TEMED.

17. Pour gels as for PAGE, or suck up to a 130 mm mark on gel tubes which are 2.5 mm internal diameter tubes cut to a length of 150 mm.

18. Leave between 3 and 18 h at 20–25 °C to set.

19. Mount gels into electrophoresis apparatus.

20. Remove any unpolymerised gel and apply between 3 and 20 μl of the immunoprecipitate preparation (steps 1–10).

Table 4.13. *(cont.)*

21. Overlay samples with 10 μl 8 M urea, 5% (v/v) NP40, 1% (v/v) ampholine '3.5–10'.
22. Carefully overlay this with 0.1 M H_3PO_4.
23. Apply the reservoir solutions:
    upper (anode): 0.1 M H_3PO_4
    lower (cathode): 0.2 M KOH.
24. Run the gels; voltage can be varied, but a useful protocol is:
    200 volts for 1 h
    400 volts for 4 h
    (600 volts for 2 h extra, if required to increase discrimination of the protein bands).
25. At the end of the run, remove slab gels from between glass plates as described in Table 4.12; for tube gels, insert a syringe needle between the gel and the tube wall. Inject a slow stream of water from a syringe. Do this alternately at each end of the gel in the tube, until the gel slips out.
26. Stain gels and dry as described in Table 4.12.

RPMI 1640 or Eagle's medium supplemented with 2–5% (v/v) foetal calf serum or horse serum and 5 μCi*/ml [^{14}C] leucine or 20 μCi/ml [^{3}H] leucine. The cultures are incubated overnight at 37 °C, and supernatants collected for assay by PAGE or IEF (33–35).

4.1.20. *Assay of MAb: summary*

The assays of MAb can be divided into two major groups: those for screening hybridoma supernatants for the presence of usable MAb and those for determining the characteristics of the reactivity of the MAb. Probably the most frequently used 'screening' assays are the immunoassay procedures ELISA and RIA, which detect the interaction of MAb with antigen using enzyme-labelled or ^{125}I-labelled anti-species immunoglobulin, or ^{125}I-labelled antigen. All antibody specificities may be detected by these assays, providing that a number of procedures are used to encompass the differential effect that different procedures can have on epitope expression by certain antigens.

MAb can also be detected through the precipitation of antigen. This requires a certain density of MAb on the surface of the antigen, and a large number of epitopes on the antigen to permit efficient lattice formation between antigen and antibody. Such assays are often performed in solid matrices like agarose, e.g. DID, SRID and RH. The time of such

* 1 Ci = 3.7×10^{10} Bq.

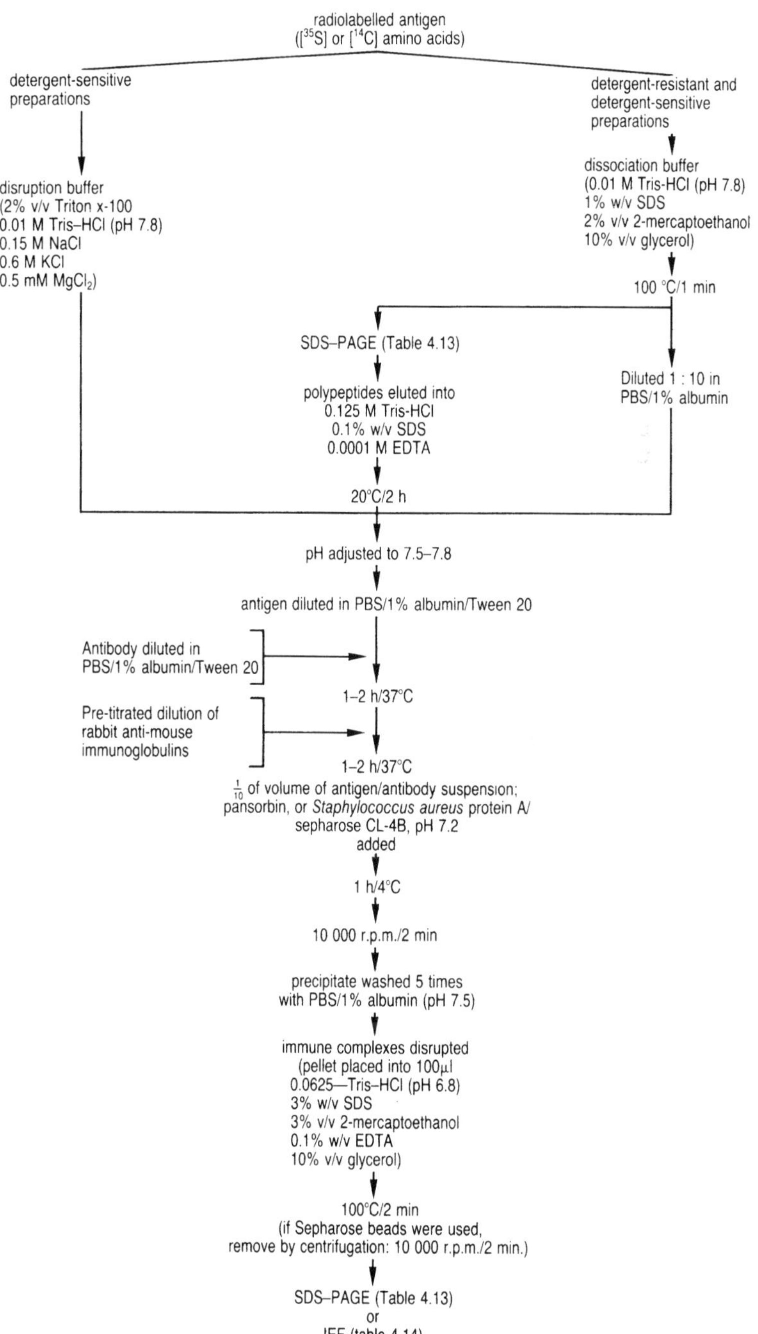

Fig. 4.21. Flow diagram of the immunoprecipitation reaction as used with SDS-PAGE (Table 4.13) and IEF (Table 4.14).

assays can be reduced by applying an electric potential across the gel: immunoelectrophoresis (IEP, CIEP, CCIEP, LRIEP). These IEP assays can also be linked to PAGE or IEF in which only electrophoretically separable proteins of the antigen are used.

As an alternative to the use of enzyme-labelled or ^{125}I–labelled material as in ELISA and RIA, erythrocytes of certain species may be sensitised with antigen or antibody and used in a number of assays: PHA, HAd, DARR, IARR, and Jerne PFC assay (HRA). These procedures are often more rapid than ELISA or RIA but can suffer from the drawback that not all antigens can be coupled efficiently to erythrocytes, and MAb molecules in the test sample are required to form lattices with PHA. The tests have the advantage in that they can directly detect antigen-specific antibody-secreting hybridoma cells.

Using certain antigens which can infect host cells or haemagglutinate (HA) erythrocytes, MAb can be used to inhibit such reactions (the neutralisation, HAI and HLI assays). The presence of the infectious agent within host cells can also be demonstrated by immunofluorescence, or through a modification of ELISA–RIA to identify cell-associated antigen.

Functional assays, such as the opsonisation assays, which utilise the capacity of phagocytic leukocytes to react with and engulf antigen–antibody complexes, may be performed. This test has greater value in determining the relative efficiency of MAb with particular epitope specificities at taking part in the immunological defence *in vivo*.

Thus, there are numerous assay procedures which will determine if a hybridoma is secreting antibody, and if so, what the epitope reactivity and other characteristics of the MAb are. With the initial screening, the assays are used only to detect antibody secretion in polyclonal cultures, in order that the positive clones may then be cloned. Since it is through the cloning that the hybridoma culture secreting a homogeneous population of antibody is produced, this method is essential for the generation of the usable product of hybridoma technology: the monoclonal antibody (MAb).

4.2. **Cloning**

The function of the cloning procedure is to isolate the different types of hybridoma cell within a particular culture. This will separate the antibody-producing hybridomas and permit the characterisation and assessment of their usefulness. Cloning relies on the isolation of single cells from which colonies develop, and thence monoclonal hybridoma cultures secreting a homogeneous (monoclonal) population of antibody. This isolation of individual cells can be achieved by using one of a number of cloning procedures currently in use, each with particular advantages and disadvantages. The major types of cloning in current use are (i) isolation of well separated colonies from the 'masterplates' (the plate into which the fusion mixture was originally placed); (ii) limit dilution cloning (initially the favoured procedure, but used less frequently now, although still with many advantages); (iii) cloning in semi-solid medium (sloppy agar) (now the most widely applied cloning method for B cell systems); (iv) micromanipulation of individual cells (the procedure favoured for cloning T lymphocytes, in particular cytotoxic T lymphocytes, CTL or T_c).

4.2.1. *Isolation of colonies from 'masterplates'*

With certain fusions, some 5–14 days after placing in 24 w plates, isolated colonies of growing hybridoma cells may be visible. A low density of growing hybridoma cells may develop in each well of the masterplate, by careful manipulation of the ratio of splenocytes : myeloma cells in the fusion mixture, the density of cells plated and the use of feeder cells. This will facilitate the easy distinction of colonies derived from single cells. By using a dissecting microscope and a microcapillary tube, cells from a colony may be transferred to another plate fed with feeder cells. This procedure is somewhat of a cross between cloning by limit dilution and cloning in semi-solid medium. As such, the procedure has several disadvantages.

(i) Plates must be carefully held motionless to prevent cell movement within each well. This is very difficult, and it is uncertain whether it can ever be achieved in modern incubator systems.

(ii) Viewing wells microscopically to identify wells with only a single colony cannot be reliable owing to the difficulty in accurately determining whether or not cells are present near the edge of wells.

(iii) If two cells are growing close to one another, the colony which arises is similar to a monoclonal one, since the liquid medium permits easy movement of the cells; as such, the shape of the colony cannot be a reliable indicator of monoclonality. In fact, what appears to be a monoclonal culture can arise from several cells.

(iv) McCullough *et al.* (36) compared different cloning methods and found isolation of colonies from the masterplate totally unsuitable. The colonies were not necessarily monoclonal, subsequent cloning was still essential (to the same degree as if no cloning had previously been attempted) and the cells were not adapted enough to *in vitro* growth to be successfully and consistently passaged even with feeder cells.

Thus, the disadvantages of this procedure far outweigh the advantages of ease of manipulation and rapidity at obtaining 'monoclonal' cultures after fusion. In this sense, the other major cloning procedures are more reliable at generating monoclonal hybridomas.

4.2.2. *Cloning by limit dilution*

The theory and practice of cloning cells (not just hybridoma cells) has been reviewed by Fazekas de St Groth (37). The basic limit dilution procedure is shown in Fig. 4.22. Successful cloning by this method

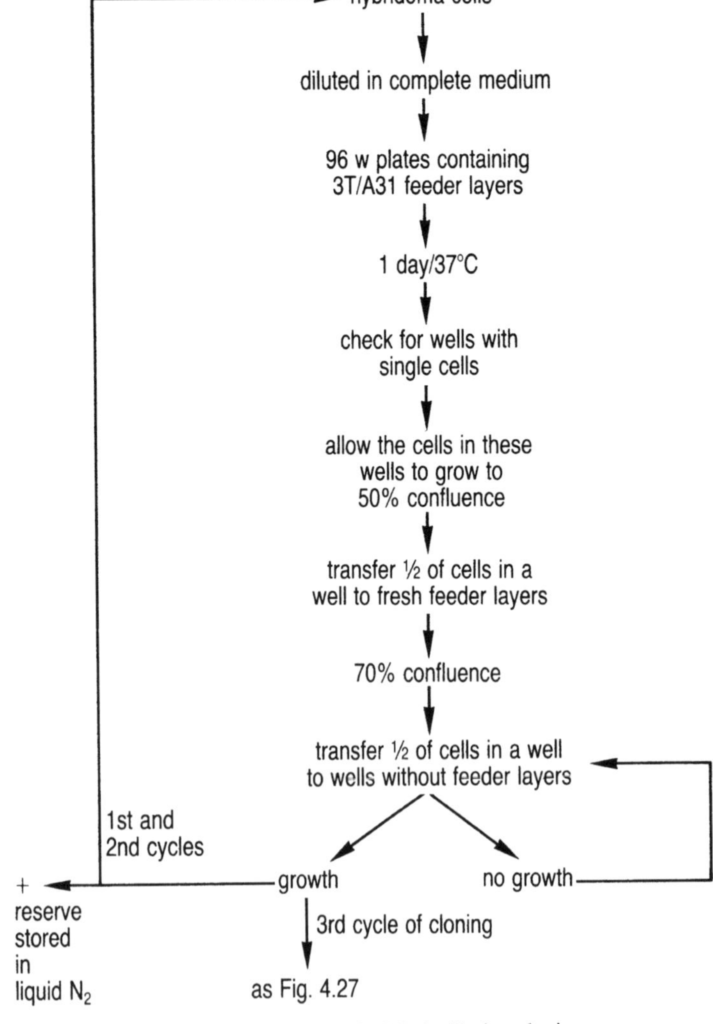

Fig. 4.22. Flow diagram of the method of limit-dilution cloning.

requires three basic ingredients: firstly, healthy hybridoma cells which have adapted to growth *in vitro*. This means cultures which have been 'weaned' off the feeder cells onto which the fusion mixture was plated, and shown capable of growth in the absence of such feeders. Those cultures which have been shown to secrete antibody (§4.1) should be taken into their exponential phase to a density of between 0.9 and 3.0 $\times 10^5$ cells/ml and at a viability of more than 95%. The cells are passaged 1 : 2 (that is, given a ½ dilution) and cultured for a further 24 h (this ensures the cells are in an active growth phase).

Secondly, the cloning is performed on plates conditioned with macrophage or mitomycin C-treated 3T3 feeder cells as described in §§3.7.3 and 3.7.5. The reasons for this are also explained in these sections. The plates used are either 96 well tissue-culture grade microtitre plates (96 w) or 60 well Terasaki plates (TSP).

Thirdly, the cloning medium is conditioned with 50% (v/v) medium from 72 h old cultures of myeloma cells. This medium is sterilised by filtration, mixed with an equal volume of RPMI 1640, and then foetal calf serum (FCS) and glutamine are added to a final concentration of 10% (v/v) and 2 mM respectively.

The hybridoma cells are diluted in conditioned medium to give 1 cell per 12 wells, added to the 'fed' plates and cultured for 6 h at 37 °C. This permits hybridoma cells to settle, and the wells can be viewed microscopically for the presence of round hybridoma cells (most of the feeder cells will be fibroblastic in appearance). Wells containing more than one cell are discarded, but this value should be low (0.3% by Poisson distribution). The other wells are incubated at 37 °C, and after 14–28 days growing cultures should be visible. When these cells cover about half the growing surface (50% confluent) they are passaged into the well of a 24 w plate conditioned with feeder cells. If the cells grow and secrete antibody, they are allowed to reach 70% confluence and then tested for independency of feeder cells. That is, half of the cells are passaged into a fresh well of a 24 w plate without feeder cells. If no growth is observed, the remaining cells in the 'fed' well are again cultured until they reach 70% confluence, when the whole procedure is tried again. When the hybridomas can grow in the absence of feeder cells, they are given one further passage and then recloned by the same limit dilution procedure using the criteria described above. This cloning procedure is performed a total of three times; each time, only antibody-secreting cultures are used.

(i) Advantages of limit dilution cloning (LDC)

The advantages of LDC are shown in Table 4.14. It is a relatively easy procedure to initiate, with dilution of cells, microscopic examination and subculture the only manipulations. Likewise, the recloning steps

Table 4.14. *Advantages and disadvantages of limiting dilution cloning*

Advantages	Disadvantages
initiation simple	uncertainty as to whether a well has a single cell
small number of manipulations	the large number of wells used are tedious to check microscopically for single cells
recloning straightforward (few intervening steps or subcultures)	difficult to see single cells on feeder layers
very large numbers of wells can be used	skewed distribution of probability of the number of cells/well from low concentrations of cells
large numbers of cultures can be cloned	several reclonings *always* necessary

are easily attained. Through the use of plates with large numbers of wells, a large number of cloning samples can be set up.

(ii) Disadvantages of LDC

These are also shown in Table 4.14, and far outweigh the advantages. Firstly, it is difficult to visualise cells at the edges of wells microscopically, and thus a well scored as having only one cell may in fact have more than one. Secondly, it is not feasible to accurately determine if each well of a large number – often hundreds – has a hybridoma cell. Staring down a microscope for long periods of time causes eye strain, and loss of concentration is often a problem. Thirdly, it may be difficult to discern a single hybridoma cell from some feeder cells, especially those of PEC, which often contain lymphocyte-like cells. Permitting the hybridoma cells to divide and produce a small colony of less than 10 cells is not necessarily the answer since two cells close together would produce a similar looking colony to one derived from a single cell. However, the probability of two hybridoma cells settling on to feeder cells in close proximity of one another (within fewer than 10 cell diameters) is low.

The greatest disadvantage of limit dilution cloning is the skewed distribution of colony growth from such a procedure (Fazekas de St Groth (37)). This complicates confident assessment of the probability of how many cells were originally in a well in which hybridoma cells grew after limit dilution cloning. If Poissonian distribution laws are applied, several of the reported successful limit dilution clonings could be taken as representing wells in which more than one cell were seeded (see McCullough *et al.* (36)). Conversely, since a skewed distribution is likely, these reports may indeed reflect wells seeded with single cells. Determining the degree of skew is, however, impracticable owing to the variability in culture characteristics between different hybridoma cultures, even those derived from the same fusion.

Most of these disadvantages are only minor drawbacks since one of the major rules of cloning is that recloning is essential; hence the three cycles of cloning shown in Fig. 4.22. If a hybridoma culture derived from a single limit dilution originated from two cells, it is highly probable that the subsequent two cycles would separate these. Limit dilution passage can also be incorporated into other cloning procedures in which the initial cloning used a method other than limit dilutions, such as cloning in semi-solid medium.

4.2.3. *Cloning in semi-solid medium*

As with limit dilution cloning, the success of cloning in semi-solid medium relies on the presence of a feeder cell layer. This can either be in the form of a pre-formed monolayer of PEC or mitomycin C-treated 3T3 cells, or the feeder cells can be incorporated into the semi-solid medium containing the hybridoma cells. In the former, the feeder cell layer is established at 2×10^4 cells/ml three to seven days before applying the hybridoma cells. With the latter procedure, 2×10^4 PEC or mitomycin C-treated 3T3 cells/ml, or 10^6 splenocytes or thymocytes/ml (final concentration) are mixed with the hybridoma cells in the semi-solid medium.

The semi-solid medium is one in which cells can easily divide and expand through this support to produce a viable colony, without permitting cells to break away and establish a more dispersed series of hybridoma cells. These media again use RPMI 1640–10% (v/v) FCS–2 mM glutamine supplemented with 50% (v/v) conditioned medium (the conditioned medium can either be the medium from a 72 h old culture of myeloma cells or that from the 5–7 day old feeder layer if that is the choice of feeding). The semi-solid nature of the medium is provided by either agar or methyl cellulose. Agarose (indubiose), bacto-agar and agar Noble have all been used; certain batches of the latter can in fact be used without the prerequisite for a feeder layer, although this is an exception rather than a rule. McCullough *et al.* (36), using pre-formed PEC and 3T3 cell feeder layers, compared these agars as sources of semi-solid medium, and found the agar Noble to be superior. They concluded that this may be due to the lower degree of purity of this compared with the other agars, related to the level of mitogenic substances present. However, they also noted that methyl cellulose-based semi-solid media were superior to the agar-based ones with respect to hybridoma cloning. A similar conclusion was also formed by Davis *et al.* (38) who used feeder cells (thymocytes) incorporated into the cloning medium. Both groups found that the medium based on DMEM was also optimal, but disagreed as to the efficiency of RPMI 1640-based media. McCullough *et al.* (36) concluded that this may reflect the different feeder cell systems used by the two groups. DMEM may be a more appropriate medium for culturing lymphocytes and thymocytes, but RPMI 1640 is apparently superior for the culturing of PEC and 3T3 cells. Since it is the success of the growth and feeding potential of the feeder cells which ultimately determines the success of the cloning, this may be the reason for the conflicting conclusions over the usefulness of DMEM and RPMI 1640 media made by the two groups. This could also explain why McCullough *et al.* (36) found that RPMI 1640, and not DMEM, was the more successful medium for culturing hybridoma cells. However, taking all of the information available, the optimal cloning medium with universal application is probably as shown in Table 4.15.

The preparation of the methyl cellulose must be done well in advance of the cloning. Into a 25–30 ml glass bottle weigh 0.4 g methyl cellulose (4000 cp). Carefully layer on 5 ml distilled water without disturbing the powder, which should remain submerged. Autoclave at 15 lbf/in^2 for 15 min. Add 5 ml ×2 concentrated medium and mix with a pipette. Leave at 4 °C with daily inversions for at least 5 days, by which time the medium and gelled methyl cellulose (gels after 24 h at 4 °C) should have mixed. Add 5 ml conditioned medium followed by 5 ml hybridoma cells (400, 200, 100 cells/ml) in complete culture medium. Mix vigorously by inversion. The preparation is quite viscous and air bubbles form, but these do not apparently harm the cells and are lost within 5–10 min. Owing to the viscosity, it is preferable if a pipette-aid is used to assist the dispensing. The hybridoma cell – methyl cellulose mixture is then plated, either with feeder cells incorporated or on to monolayers of feeder cells, in multi-well plates at the rate of 1 ml/well of 24 w dish, 1.5 ml/well of 12 w dish or 2 ml/well of 6 w dish. The cloning procedure is completed as shown in Fig. 4.23.

When colonies have developed to the appropriate size, they are isolated with a Pasteur pipette and transferred into wells of a 96 w plate or 24 w plate containing feeder layers. Growth is erratic between different colonies, but when those which do grow reach 50% confluence, they are tested for specific antibody production. Positive cultures are incubated until they reach 70% confluence (50% with a 96 w plate), and half the cells are transferred to a well of a 24 w plate without feeders (with feeders if from a 96 w plate, and when this reaches 70% confluence, half the cells are transferred to a feederless plate). If no growth is observed, the remaining cells are cultured and given one more subculture with fresh feeder layers. If necessary, the procedure is repeated until the hybridoma cells can be cultured in the absence of feeders. When this is attained, the cells are expanded by one further passage, and a small portion used for recloning while the remainder are stored in liquid

Table 4.15. *Composition of an effective semi-solid medium for the cloning of hybridoma cells over feeder layers*

1 vol. 4% (w/v) methyl cellulose in H_2O
1 vol. ×2 concentrated DMEM† – 20% (v/v) FCS–4 mM glutamine, or ×2 concentrated IDMEM–4 mM glutamine
1 vol. conditioned medium (10% v/v FCS–2 mM glutamine)
1 vol. hybridoma cells suspended in DMEM–10% (v/v) FCS–2 mM glutamine or IDMEM–2 mM glutamine.

Note:
†GMEM or RPMI 1640 medium can be used in place of DMEM; all media should contain HEPES to 20 mM final concentration, and 7.5% (w/v) sodium bicarbonate as buffering agents.

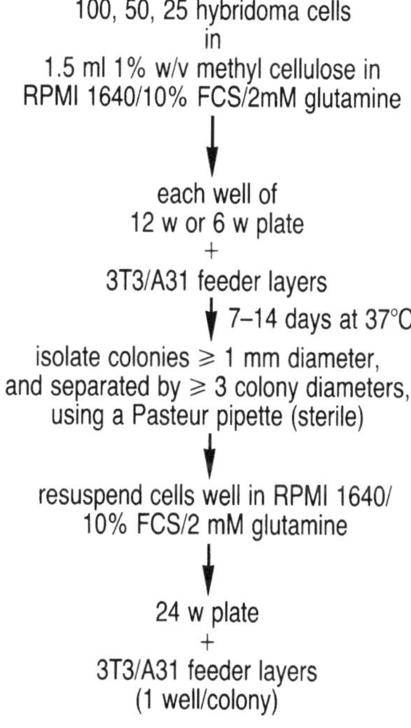

Fig. 4.23. Flow diagram of the method for cloning in semi-solid methyl cellulose-based medium over 3T3/A31 feeder cells.

nitrogen as a precaution. This recloning can use either the semi-solid medium method, or that of limit dilution. Only one repeat cloning by the former procedure appears necessary, but two of the latter are required, since it is easier to perform limiting dilution passage than limit dilution cloning. That is, the cells are diluted, and the highest dilution

Table 4.16. *Advantages and disadvantages of cloning in semi-solid medium*

Advantages	Disadvantages
consistency of successful cloning	accuracy of determining monoclonality low if too many colonies develop
easy to see colony development	several reagents required
as colonies develop, cells stay together owing to the semi-solid nature of the medium	semi-solid medium has to be prepared well in advance
feeder layers can be incorporated into the medium	recloning often desirable
easy to isolate colonies	
high success of isolation of colonies	
easily recloned	
antibody production can be determined easily before colony isolation	
cloning rapid	

(lowest concentration of cells originally) which yields antibody-secreting hybridomas is expanded to 50% confluence and given a second limit dilution passage. Eventually, the recloned hybridoma cells are expanded and stored in liquid nitrogen.

(i) Advantages of cloning in semi-solid medium

The advantages and disadvantages of this method are shown in Table 4.16. The major advantage is the consistency of successful cloning. When 3T3 cells are used as feeder cells, well-separated colonies of hybridoma cells develop (separated by 5 nominal colony diameters, or one colony per microscope field using ×10 eyepieces and ×10 objective). Macrophage or splenocyte feeder cells can be as efficient at supporting the growth of hybridoma colonies, but they show high variability in this property (Table 4.17).

Thymocyte or splenocyte feeder cells may be easily incorporated into the semi-solid matrix simply by adding them at 10^5–10^6 cells/ml to the diluted hybridoma cells before mixing with the equal volume of 2% (w/v) methyl cellulose (for example). Again, however, these feeder cells can be inconsistent at supporting hybridoma cell growth, and thus a 'suspension feeder' of 3T3 cells should again prove the optimum.

Cloning by semi-solid agar also has the advantage that well-developed colonies can be seen easily by the naked eye, especially when viewed under indirect light or dark-ground illumination. This has an additional

Table 4.17. *Relative efficacy of different feeder sources at supporting the growth of hybridoma cells during cloning in methyl cellulose overlay*[1]

Expt	Feeder source[2]	Hybridomas added/well	Number of wells	Number of colonies: total	$\bar{x}$well	SD/well
1	none	25–100	12	0	—	—
	ECGS	25–100	24	0	—	—
	mϕ (17 d)	100	8	2	0.25	0.7
		50	8	0	—	—
		25	8	2	0.25	0.7
	mϕ (17 d)	100	4	0	—	—
	[+ECGS]	50	4	0	—	—
		25	4	3	1	1.7
	mϕ (9 d)	100	8	269	34	18.7
		50	8	157	20	8.0
		25	8	25	3.1	2.2
	mϕ (9 d)	100	4	151	38	4.9
	[+ECGS]	50	4	89	22	5.6
		25	4	47	12	2.8
	3T3/A31 (9 d)	100	4	233	58	19
		50	4	152	38	28
		25	4	20	5	4.7
	3T3/A31 (9 d)	100	4	39	9.8	9.5
	[+ECGS]	50	4	93	23	16
		25	4	9	2.3	2.6
2	none	25–100	12	0	—	—
	ECGS	25–100	12	1	0.13	0.36
	mϕ (8 d)	100	8	111	14	6.0
		50	8	39	4.9	2.5
		25	8	7	0.88	0.64
	mϕ (8 d)	100	8	5	0.6	0.9
	[+ECGS]	50	8	7	0.88	1.1
		25	8	9	1.1	0.8
	3T3/A31 (7 d)	100	8	282	35	7.0
		50	8	133	16	5.0
		25	8	60	7.5	3.0
	3T3/A31 (7 d)	100	8	103	13	4.6
	[+ECGS]	50	8	34	4.2	2.5
		25	8	11	1.4	0.7
	3T3/A31 (24 h)	100	8	84	21	6.0
		50	8	34	11	6.5
		25	8	13	4.3	1.2

Source: [1]From Butcher *et al.* (39).
Note:
[2] *ECGS, endothelial cell growth supplement; mϕ, peritoneal exudate macrophages; (17 d), (9 d), (8 d), (7 d), (24 h), time in days (d) or hours (h) of the culture of the feeder layers before being used for the cloning.*

advantage in that it restrains the operator from cloning until the colonies are easily visible. At this time, that is when the colonies are 1–2 mm in diameter, they can be removed using a sterile Pasteur pipette. Again no microscopic aid is required and the removal of the colony is readily visualised. Furthermore, if such colonies are transferred to liquid medium over feeder cells in a 24 w plate, a high rate of success for culturing and propagating these hybridoma colonies is ensured.

Once isolated, these colonies can easily be recloned in semi-solid medium, or given two cycles of limit dilution passage to ensure that if the colony was derived from more than one cell, the end product will probably be derived from only a single cell. The full cloning cycle is shown in Fig. 4.24.

The final advantage of this method of cloning is that the growing colonies can be assayed for specific antibody before picking. This uses the replica plate assay described in §4.1.12.

Cloning (and recloning) using the semi-solid matrix procedure is rapid, the first colonies usually being picked after 7–10 days, and recloned after a further 4–7 days. Thus, a usable cloned or recloned hybridoma culture can be obtained after 3–5 weeks. The incorporation of the replica plate assay means that only useful colonies will be manipulated.

(ii) Disadvantages of cloning in semi-solid medium

This method does not suffer from the disadvantages of LDC in which single cells in wells cannot be confidently identified. However, the two methods are similar in that a colony in a semi-solid medium may have derived from one, two, or possibly three cells. If the hybridoma cells are well mixed, and only a few colonies develop in each well, it is likely that each has derived from a single cell. However, to be confident of this, the colony is recloned or passaged twice at limiting dilution as for LDC.

The other drawback is that this procedure requires more reagents: 24 w, 12 w and 6 w plates, normal strength medium, 2× strength medium, 4× strength agar support (if this is methyl cellulose it can be mixed with the 2× strength medium to be ready for use), sterile Pasteur pipettes. The use of methyl cellulose poses an additional problem due to its viscosity and slow mixing. It has to be prepared about 7 days in advance (as described on page 248).

However, cloning and recloning in a semi-solid support has proved to be very successful, and using the procedure based around 3T3/A31 cell feeder layers and methyl cellulose supports we have generated thousands of hybridoma colonies in our laboratory. It is this method of cloning which is recommended for routine use. Only when very accurate isolation of single hybridoma cells is required, for example with clonal

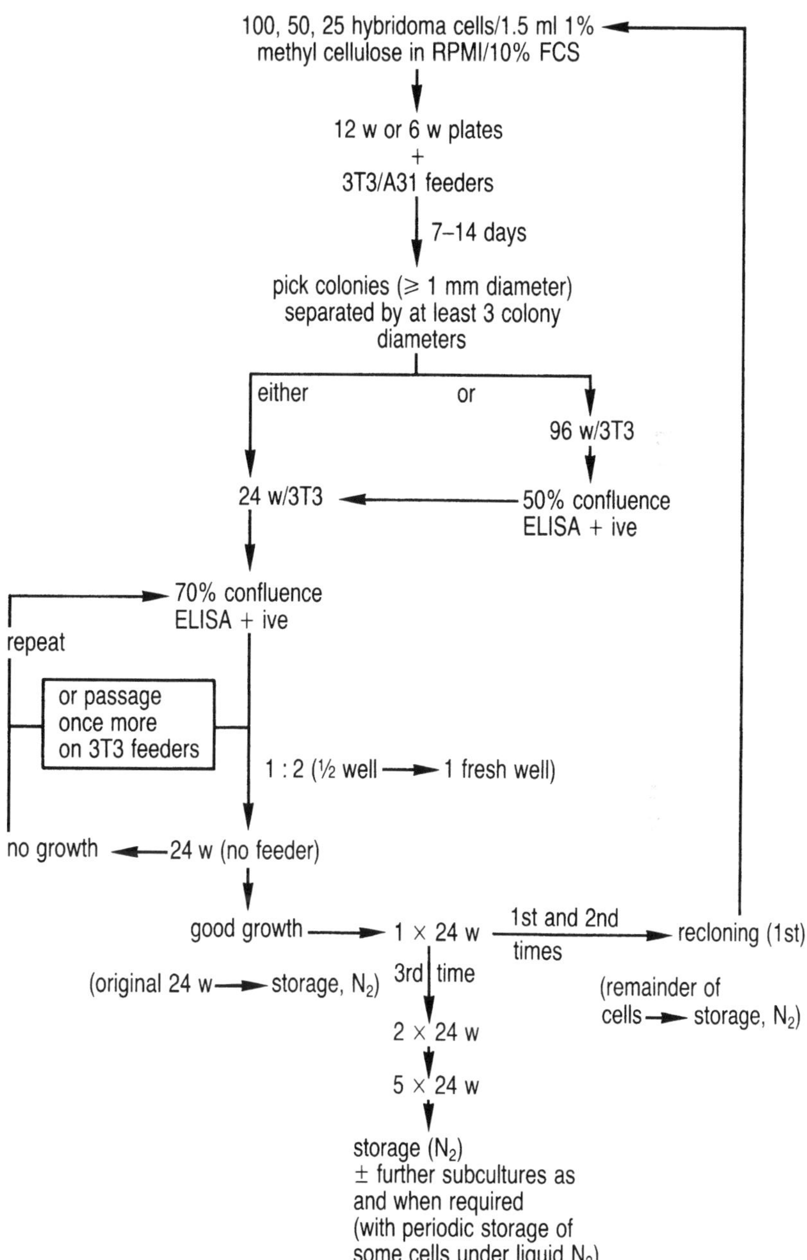

Fig. 4.24. The full cloning and culturing procedure for the method of cloning in methyl cellulose-based medium; 24W/3T3 and 96W/3T3, 24 w plates and 96 w plates, respectively, carrying 3T3/A31 cell feeder layers; N_2, liquid nitrogen cryogenic system.

analysis of cell populations and their products, should another procedure – micromanipulation – be considered. Normally this is not necessary, since the conventional passage of cloned hybridoma cells will result in a heterogeneous population of cells; heterogeneous with respect to the relative degrees of growth and synthesis of their product, but homogeneous in the 'specificity' of that product.

4.2.4. *Micromanipulation*

This method, when properly used, is the only procedure for the confident and consistent isolation of colonies which have been derived from a single cell. The reason for this is that micromanipulation isolates single cells. In order to achieve this, the scheme in Fig. 4.25 is followed. Hybridoma cell lines which have been 'weaned off' feeder cells are placed in liquid medium in the wells of a 6 w plate at 3×10^4 cells/ml (2 ml/well). The plates are incubated at 37 °C until small colonies of cells (seen microscopically) develop. This will ensure that any cells which are micromanipulated will be in an exponential phase of growth. A small colony or loose group of cells is removed by using a Pasteur pipette (the manipulation being most easily achieved under low power magnification of a binocular inverted microscope). The cells are dispersed in 5 ml of medium in a 5 cm Petri dish. Only small colonies or loose groups of cells should be used such that a small number of cells (fewer than 100) will be taken, and all, or at least most, of these are actually growing. With the cells dispersed in the Petri dish, single cells should be very easily discerned. These are then picked individually. From this, it can be seen that the further apart adjacent cells are, then the easier it will be to pick an isolated cell. This 'picking' can be done with a fine-bore Pasteur pipette, one which has been drawn out in a bunsen burner flame. For accuracy, however, a 10 μl capillary tube or melting-point tube should be used. These should be sterilised at 180 °C for 3 h. The manipulation is performed as follows.

1. Attach a length of silicone tubing (sterilised by autoclaving) to one end of a microcapillary tube with the other end in the user's mouth.
2. Hold the tongue against this end of the tubing.
3. Place the microcapillary into the cell suspension in the Petri dish, next to a single cell (viewed under the binocular inverted microscope).
4. Relax the tongue to allow the cell with 10 μl of medium to enter the capillary.
5. Place the capillary into fresh medium in the well of a 24-well or 96-well plate seeded with 10^5 mitomycin C-treated feeder cells/ml.

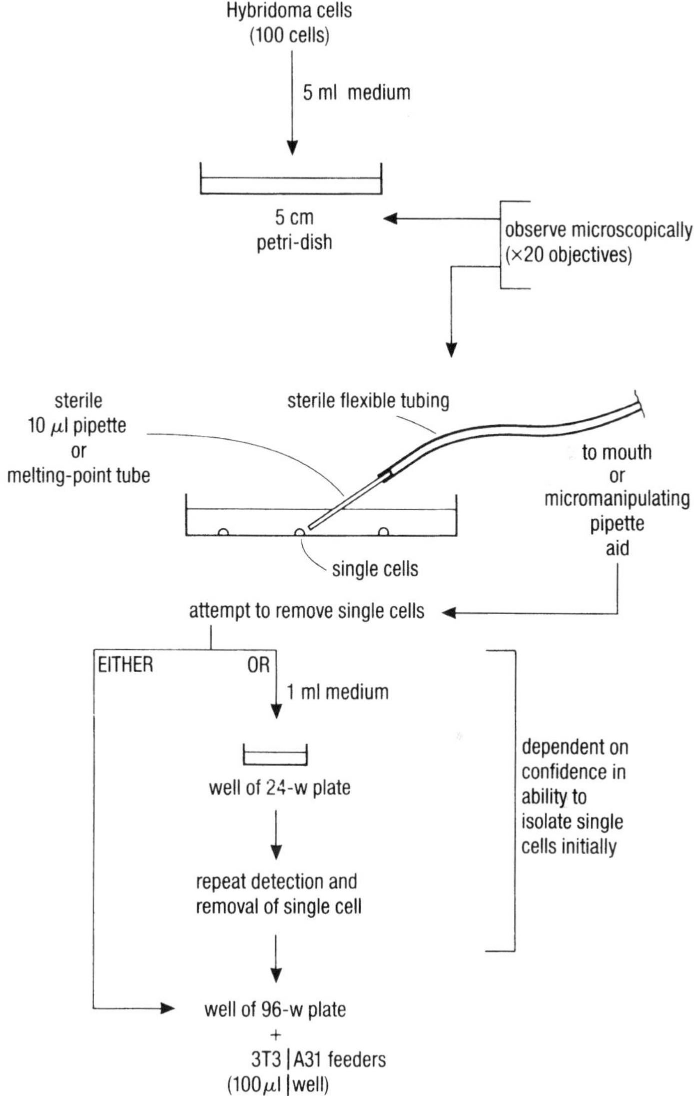

Fig. 4.25. Flow diagram of the method of cell cloning by micromanipulation.

By placing the microcapillary against the edge of the well and gently blowing the 10 μl volume out until air bubbles just form, the micromanipulated cell can be successfully transferred to the well. Since the air bubbles form at the edge of the well and are few in number, little damage is caused to the cell. (A hand-operated device for use with specially marketed micromanipulation capillaries is sold by Arnold R. Horwell Ltd.)

It is advisable that the medium in the wells has been incubated in the humidified CO_2 incubator in order to establish the correct pH. If buffered with HEPES and bicarbonate, this should maintain the pH throughout the micromanipulation. However, if the pH does start to rise, then the plate should be replaced in the incubator, even if only a few cells have been micromanipulated. It is better to have a large number of plates each containing only a small number of wells with micromanipulated cells but in medium which was maintained at the correct pH, than to have a few plates in which all the wells contain micromanipulated cells but in medium which underwent considerable (from the viewpoint of the cell) pH and temperature changes.

The micromanipulated cells are incubated as for hybridoma cultures and the other cloning procedures. After about 10–14 days, colonies should be seen easily under the microscope, and subculture should be possible after a further 5–14 days. These time periods will depend on the characteristics of the cell which has been isolated; different hybridoma cells can have very variable mean generation times. When subculture is possible, the cells (which are producing antibody) should be transferred to fresh wells containing feeder cells, as shown in Fig. 4.24, for subculturing of colonies isolated from 'methyl cellulose cloning'. The only difference between this figure and subculture of micromanipulated cells is that recloning of the latter should be unnecessary because a single cell was isolated originally, and any cell line which developed from this should be monoclonal.

(i) Advantages of micromanipulation

The advantages and disadvantages of micromanipulation are shown in Table 4.18. The major advantage is that mentioned above: clones which develop will have arisen from single cells and as such should not require recloning. Therefore, confidence in the monoclonality of both the hybridoma cells and their secreted antibody is high. It should be remembered, however, that some clones will require periodic recloning owing to a high mutation rate or an imbalance in the chromosomes and cellular division rates. This is not necessary for all clones – some may be continuously cultured for over a year without recloning – but no general rule can be applied and each clone has to be treated separately with the requirements for recloning determined on culture.

(ii) Disadvantages of micromanipulation

The disadvantages are, firstly, that the cells are being manipulated considerably and this may be detrimental to their successful propagation. Secondly, the procedure is very time-consuming and rather tedious. From this comes the disadvantage that the longer a procedure takes and the more manipulations are involved, the greater the risk of fungal, yeast

Table 4.18. *Advantages and disadvantages of micromanipulation*

Advantages	Disadvantages
clones can be most easily identified as arising from single cells	many manipulations
high confidence in monoclonality	time-consuming
recloning *not* always necessary	relatively tedious
certain hybridomas can be selected at the outset (e.g. those which have been rosetted or tagged with antigen to identify specific-antibody secretors)	risks of contamination are higher
easy to isolate colonies if growth occurs in the culture	microscopic work may be tiring
	requires practice

or bacterial contamination. Finally, a microscope is an essential piece of apparatus for this procedure, and the time spent using this may prove disadvantageous for some workers who find microscope work tiring on the eyes.

Micromanipulation does require substantial practice, but the advantage of producing cell lines which can confidently be termed monoclonal far outweighs any minor disadvantages the procedure has. The disadvantages are termed minor since they concern the capacity of the worker to use the procedure and not on the reliability of the procedure itself. Although micromanipulation is highly recommended, it must be left up to the individual to decide if this or one of the other procedures is most practical to use and the most appropriate for the generation of monoclonal hybridomas of the desired specificity.

4.3. **Cloning immediately after fusion**

The generation and successful propagation of monoclonal hybridoma cell lines is a time-consuming procedure. One method which would help to shorten the programme would be cloning the cells immediately after fusion, as opposed to waiting until the polyclonal cultures had been expanded. The disadvantage is that the cells would not have recovered from the fusion and adapted to growth independent of feeder cells; that is, they would not be in a state to benefit as much from the feeder cells. For this reason, cloning of certain fusion mixtures will not be as successful as others. Hybridomas generated against foot-and-mouth disease virus are difficult to clone immediately after fusion, whereas such clonings of hybridomas generated against rinderpest virus and pig thymocytes are relatively successful (R.N. Butcher & K.C. McCullough, unpublished data). Owing to the advantages which cloning immediately after fusion can offer, it is recommended that it should be attempted to see if it is a viable proposition for cloning a particular hybridoma series. There are three possible alternative procedures which may give success.

4.3.1. *Cloning with pre-formed feeder cells*

This procedure is basically the same as that described in §4.2.3. Either peritoneal exudate cells, mitomycin C-treated 3T3/A31 cells or splenocytes are used at 2×10^4 cells/ml as feeder layers. The 3T3/A31 cells are again the most successful (39). The fusion ratio can vary from 10 splenocytes : 1 myeloma cell to 1 : 1, depending on the efficiency of the immunogen used to generate the splenocytes. A ratio of 1 : 1 is adequate when potent immunogens were used (this ratio was used when rinderpest virus or pig thymocytes were the immunogen). The medium in which the fusion mixture is plated is the methyl cellulose cloning medium described in Table 4.15, except that the DMEM or IDMEM is replaced by HAT-containing DMEM or IDMEM. The fusion mixture is plated out in this cloning medium at the same density as after a conventional fusion procedure, that is, the equivalent of the 10^5 myeloma cells/ml. The rest of the procedure is as for the cloning in §4.2.3, although colony development may take longer, the efficiency will be lower and it may take a number of passages of the subsequently derived clones on feeder layers before they can be 'weaned off'.

4.3.2. *Cloning with adjacent feeder cells*

The difference between this procedure and that of §4.3.1. is that the feeder cells – peritoneal exudate cells, mitomycin C-treated 3T3/A31 cells or splenocytes – are mixed with the fusion mixture before plating in the semi-solid medium. The cell densities are as in §4.3.1. Davis *et al.* (36) successfully used thymocyte feeder cells in this procedure, but the 3T3/A31 cells were found to be the most consistently successful feeder layer by McCullough and co-workers (39). When splenocytes stimulated with a relatively poor immunogen are used, this cloning procedure is often more successful than that of §4.3.1. This is probably because the hybridomas are closer to the feeder cells and hence under greater influence of their diffusion gradient of growth-promoting stimuli.

4.3.3. *Cloning using a feeder cell–hybridoma 'monolayer'*

The cells in the fusion mixture and the feeder layer are brought into close proximity by plating the fusion mixture in liquid medium into wells containing the feeders as in a conventional fusion procedure. Normally, the aminopterin would be added to the liquid medium after 24 h. This manipulation is again used with this procedure, but at the 24 h point, most of the medium is removed, taking care not to disturb the cells which are on the feeder layer. It is replaced by the HAT–methyl cellulose–DMEM cloning medium described in §4.3.1. The remainder of the procedure is as in §4.3.1. This method has the advantage over that in §4.3.2 of a much closer contact between hybridoma and feeder. Additional advantages are also conferred through the 24 h delay in the addition of aminopterin (see §3.8.1).

4.3.4. *The 'fusion/cloning' procedure (Fig. 4.26) (40)*

1. The Balb/c hybridoma cell line SP2/0, which has myeloma cell-like characteristics, NS0, NS653, or NS1 myeloma cells are fused with splenocytes from Balb/c mice immunised with the antigen of choice. Fusion is performed at a ratio of 5 splenocytes : 1 myeloma cell, using 50% (v/v) PEG as described in §2.6.2. The PEG is added over 1–2 min at 4 °C, and the treated cells are left at 4 °C for a further 1–2 minutes before diluting with 20 ml pre-warmed (37 °C) serum-free medium. The treated cell suspension is then incubated at 37 °C for 15 min, centrifuged at 200 *g* for 8 min and resuspended in medium according to the cloning procedure below.
2. The fusion mixture is resuspended in GMEM supplemented with 2 mM glutamine, 10% (v/v) foetal calf serum (complete medium), 1×10^{-4} M hypoxanthine and 1.6×10^{-5} M thymidine (HT medium) to give 3×10^6 cells/ml. This cell suspension is plated on to mitomycin C-treated 3T3/A31 cell feeder layers in 75 cm^2 flasks at 30 ml/flask, and incubated for 24 h at 37 °C.
3. Aminopterin is then added from a 10× preparation in HT medium to give a final concentration of 4×10^{-7} M. The cultures are incubated at 37 °C for a further 2–4 days (this variation in time does not appear to influence the efficacy of the procedure).
4. The cells are then resuspended in the medium and washed three times using HT medium and centrifugation at 250 *g* for 5 min, before resuspending in half of the original volume of 2× HT medium (HT medium in which the concentrations of hypoxanthine and thymidine are doubled).
5. This cell suspension is completely mixed with an equal volume of 2% (w/v) methyl cellulose in complete medium. The methyl cellulose is prepared in advance in 10 ml volumes (for convenience) as follows: 0.2 g methyl cellulose (Sigma, 4000 centipoise) is placed in a glass 'universal' (20 ml) bottle; 5 ml of deionised water is carefully added so as not to disturb the methyl cellulose;

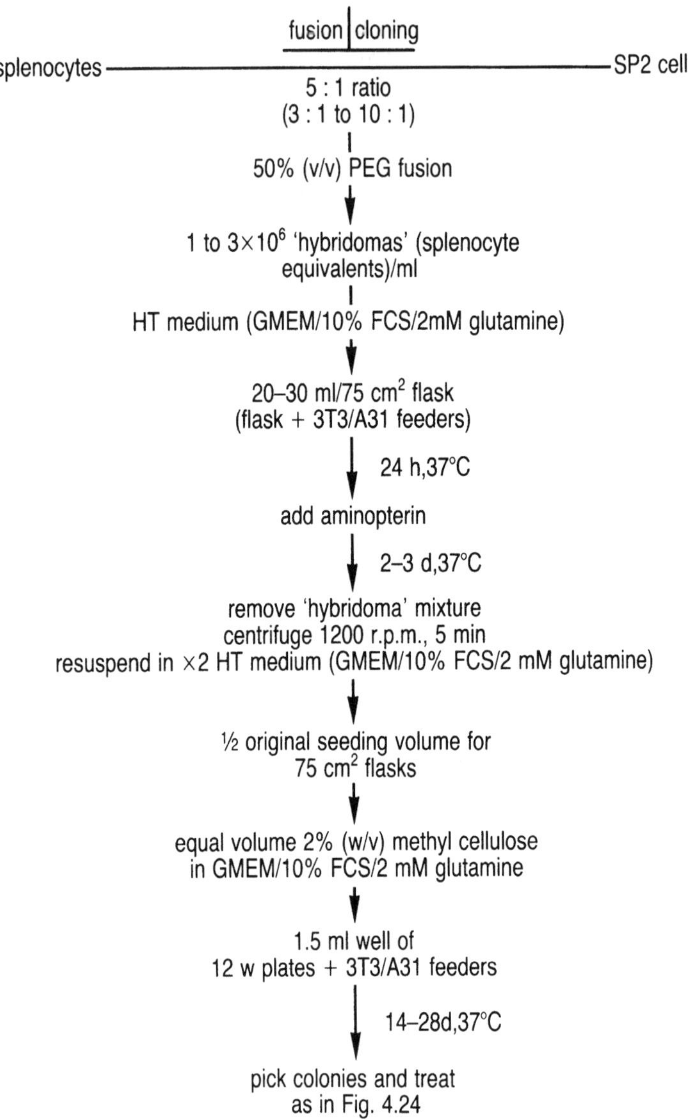

Fig. 4.26. Flow diagram of the joint 'fusion–cloning' procedure . See text for further details.

the bottles are autoclaved (15 lbf/in^2 for 15 min) and then left at 4 °C for at least 24 h; 5 ml of 2× strength complete medium (2× concentrated media plus 20% (v/v) FCS and 4 mM glutamine) is added and the bottles inverted and stored at 4 °C for at least 3 days.

6. The cells in the methyl cellulose are plated on to 3T3/A31 feeder layers in the wells of 12-well plates, at 1.5 ml/well. These plates are incubated at 37 °C for 7 days.
7. The cultures are then observed for the development of colonies, visible by eye. The remainder of the procedure is as described for the growth and isolation of colonies in semi-solid medium in §4.2.3., except for the following.
8. Colonies are isolated from the methyl cellulose overlay into wells of 96 w or 24 w plates containing 3T3/A31 feeder layers and HAT medium. The use of HAT medium permits selection against any colonies in which the cells have lost aminopterin resistance, which usually is associated with loss of antibody synthesis or secretion.
9. When the cells cover 50% (for wells of 96 w plates) or 70% (for wells of 24 plates) of the well surface, half of the cells are transferred into fresh wells (with or without feeder layers). The medium is now changed to HT medium, and the culturing protocol is similar to that described for uncloned hybridomas. The method of culture is described in §4.5 and Fig. 4.27.

4.4. **Determination of monoclonality**

Many of the assay procedures described in §4.1 can be used to ascertain if a cloned hybridoma culture is secreting a single species ('monoclonal') of antibody. However, there are four methods which are most often used.

Firstly, the kinetics of reaction between the antigen and specific antibody is determined. The ratio of bound to free antibody is plotted against free antibody, from which it is possible to identify the reaction of a single antibody molecule which will be of a single affinity (seen from the slope of the graph). However, with complex antigens, especially microorganisms and cells, a single antibody may have different affinities for different constituents of the antigen mixture. Thus, the antigen would also have to be cloned. In addition, two antibodies may have the same affinity for different epitopes on a complex antigen. Analysis of such a culture supernatant would give the impression of a single antibody molecule. Hence, determination of monoclonality by kinetic analysis has some drawbacks. More appropriate methods would look at the antibody composition of a hybridoma culture.

One such method is the analysis of the proposed monoclonal antibody preparation by PAGE and IEF as described in §4.1.19. Fuller details of the procedures have been given by Kohler (33, 34) and Trinchieri (35). The procedure uses antibody labelled *in vivo* with ^{35}S or ^{3}H. The light and heavy chains are then separated and run on PAGE or IEF gels,

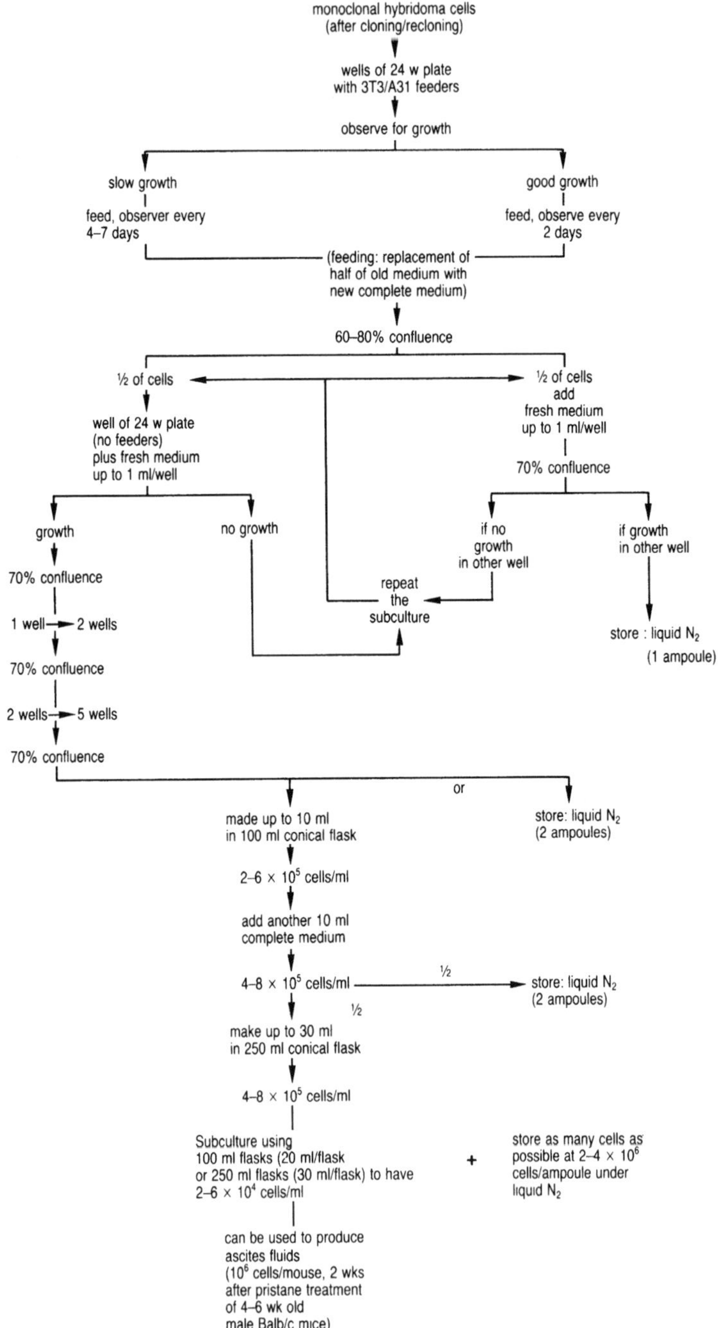

Fig. 4.27. Full details of the culturing of hybridoma cells after cloning.

which separate them according to their molecular mass and charge. It is the heavy chains which are analysed most closely. Some hybrids using NS1 cells will secrete antibody containing one splenocyte light chain and one NS1 cell MOPC light chain. Therefore, two light chains would be seen with such antibodies. If two heavy chains were seen, however, this would signify mixtures of antibodies and probable non-monoclonality. The exceptions would be with certain hybrids using P3–X63–Ag8 myeloma cells in which the MOPC heavy chain would be present. This can be easily identified in a gel system by running a labelled lysate from unfused P3–X63–Ag8 cells in a parallel channel. The other exception is the hybridoma which secretes two antibody molecules of different isotype. These will therefore differ in their heavy chains, but the antibodies from such dual-secreting hybridomas may have identical light chains. Thus, only one light chain should be found, or two chains of which one can be identified as the MOPC light chain when NS1 or P3–X63–Ag8 myeloma cells were used in the fusion. Otherwise, the hybridomas would be classified as non-monoclonal.

The third method of analysis follows the same rules for determining monoclonality as does analysis by PAGE–IEF. This is the analysis of the amino acid sequence of the antibody. Such procedures are very involved and require considerable expertise; they are therefore not recommended for the routine determination of monoclonality. If amino acid sequences are done on hybridoma antibodies, then determination of monoclonality will be a secondary bonus.

The most reliable, and relatively easy, method for monoclonality is the procedure of recloning. This does not actually determine monoclonality, but increases the probability of having a monoclonal culture such that it is unlikely to have two or more cells of different specificity present in a culture, providing the correct cloning protocol is followed. The cloning–recloning procedure shown in Fig. 4.24, as applied to cloning in semi-solid medium or by micromanipulation, is one which should fulfil these requirements.

4.5. Culturing of monoclonal antibody-secreting hybridoma cell lines

The culturing protocol for monoclonal hybridomas is basically the same as for polyclonal cultures (§3.8.2), and is shown in Fig. 4.27. Basically, clones are 'weaned off' feeder cells, and when this is successful they are recloned or propagated and recloned. Another 'weaning' follows, and the cells are expanded and stored in liquid nitrogen. Further expansion of the cells will be used to produce large volumes of the secreted antibody, or to inject Balb/c mice for the generation of ascites tumours.

4.6. Summary

The successful isolation of monoclonal antibody-secreting hybridomas relies on the ability to detect efficiently, and at an early stage, the production of antibody of the desired specificity, and on an efficient method of cloning. Detection of the hybridoma antibody can use a number of different assay systems, depending on the characteristics of the antibody which are being sought. This topic has been dealt with in detail in §4.1 (4.1.1–4.1.19), and summarised in §4.1.20.

The different methods of cloning were detailed in §§4.2 and 4.3, where consideration of their efficiency was also made. From the different methods of cloning, micromanipulation of single cells is the most accurate, but also the most tedious and not the most efficient at producing colonies. Cloning by limit dilution or in semi-solid medium is less tedious, and the latter may have certain advantages over the method of limit dilution, with respect to rapidity and efficiency of cloning. An adaptation is the 'fusion–cloning' method where cells are cloned immediately after fusion. The objective of cloning is to ensure the monoclonality of the hybridomas. For this to be performed immediately after fusion enhances the efficiency of the whole methodology. Nevertheless, aminopterin can present a problem when using semi-solid media, since hypoxanthine is more rapidly depleted than the aminopterin under such conditions. Thus, recently fused hybridomas are cultured in liquid HT media, aminopterin is added after 24 h, and after a further 2–3 days of incubation the cells are removed from the HAT medium, resuspended in semi-solid (methyl cellulose based) HT media, and cultured in 24-well plates until colonies develop.

Colonies of hybridomas are always isolated into liquid medium and tested as soon as possible (most often either by sandwich ELISA for the presence of mouse immunoglobulin, or by a mixture of ELISA, e.g. the TULIP ELISA (41), for the presence of antigen-specific antibody).

During all of these procedures for cloning, feeder layers are used, but when colonies are growing in liquid medium they are weaned off the feeders as described in §3.8.2.

Ultimately, cloned hybridomas can be grown *in vivo* as ascites tumours. Male Balb/c mice of 6–7 weeks of age (treated 2 weeks previously with 0.5 ml Pristane per mouse intraperitoneally) are inoculated with 10^6 cells per mouse. Within 2–4 weeks thereafter, ascites tumours normally develop. The fluid of these can be clarified and, if deemed necessary, treated to purify the antibody (normally between 1 and 10 mg/ml of antibody). However, it may be considered easier to prepare and purify the antibody from tissue culture supernatants. Tens or hundreds of litres of such supernatants can be produced, often in serum-free conditions, and concentration procedures can yield milligrams per millilitre of antibody. This aspect of hybridoma technology will be dealt with in detail in Chapter 5.

5 The large-scale production of monoclonal antibodies *in vitro*

5.1. Introduction

There are two pressing reasons for producing large quantities of monoclonal antibodies by *in vitro* technologies. The first is associated with the problems of the presently popular alternative route: that of using mice and rats to produce ascites fluids from the inherently carcinogenic effects of inoculating them with a monoclonal antibody-producing hybridoma. This route has five major problems:

(i) it is costly in manpower and facilities;
(ii) the materials produced, although present in high concentration (2–10 mg/ml) are contaminated with other immunoglobulins, plasma proteins (70–80%) and other possibly infectious adventitious agents;
(iii) there is a growing movement in modern societies to cause the minimum discomfort to those animals which are of value nutritionally, scientifically and technically;
(iv) there is a lack of reproducibility; and
(v) it is not possible to produce human antibodies in rodent bodies.

The more positive reasons for looking towards *in vitro* technologies are:

(i) the ability to scale up such cultures and thus to be able to satisfy requirements for kilogram or hundred to thousand kilogram (1, 2) quantities of pure antibody for a variety of therapeutic and preparative purposes; and
(ii) the exploitation of the potential of animal cell systems for the more efficient production of antibodies by using very dense suspensions of animals cells.

The difference between the rodent and tank methods can be illustrated by presenting the alternative systems necessary to produce 1 kg of antibody (Table 5.1). The size of the tank culture for such a production (5000 l) is well within current practice for animal cell cultures; lymphoblastoid interferon is presently produced commercially from mammalian cells in 8000 l volumes (3, 4). The housing and processing of 40 000 animals, on the other hand, is a tedious and labour-intensive activity.

There is therefore a clear need to move from the presently reliable

Table 5.1. *Quantitative comparison of rodent and tank methods for the production of 1 kg of pure antibody*

Assumptions

1 Concentration of antibody in ascites fluid: 5 mg/ ml

2 Volume of ascites fluid produced per animal: 10 ml

3 Impurity concentration: 20 mg/ml

4 Losses on purification of ascites fluids: 50%

5 Concentration of antibody produced in tank culture: 200 μg/ml

6 Amount of impurity in tank culture: negligible

Numbers of rodents needed therefore:

$$\frac{1000 \times 1000 \times 2}{10 \times 5} = 40\ 000$$

Size of culture required:

$$\frac{1000 \times 1000}{0.2 \times 1000} = 5000$$

ascites-type production system to a more technically suitable process. Although culture volume itself is not a major problem, there is little doubt that until recently the systems *in vitro* have proved more difficult to master and exploit than the counterparts *in vivo*. However, during the past five years (1983–1988), considerable progress has been made. It is the purpose of this chapter to describe that progress, to delineate the extent to which it falls short of present requirements and to indicate developments which could overcome those technical and biological limitations. In this description of present systems, and projection into new ones, four different types of culture system will be discussed. The first, which is least used but which could have considerable potential, is that based on exploiting the producing cells as attached to the surface of a supporting substratum. The second method, which although it has been described has not yet achieved its promised performance, involves holding the producing cells within a gel or semi-solid matrix; this method can be developed further to a third variation which traps cells within a chamber and provides for their nutrition by the manipulation of external fluids. The fourth option is that based on growing and exploiting the hybridoma cells in deep tank fermenters in a homogeneous culture. This last method has many variants which can be roughly divided into those which use a rotating device to effect homogeneity (evenness of cell distribution throughout the culture volume) and the alternative methods founded on the use of bubbles of air or gas as the suspending and distributing force. For each such system the factors of (i) cell biology and cell selection; (ii) medium composition during the growth of cells and the production of antibody (which could be the same or different); and (iii) the process used to achieve optimal productivity of the system as a whole, are also considered.

5.2. The cell population

The hybridoma cell, formed from the union of two diploid cells, will, over a number of cell doublings, consolidate the number of chromosomes which find a place in the reproduction machinery. Once this process has occurred, providing external factors do not obtrude on the normal growth and replication cycle of the cell, a near-stable cell line can result. It should be noted that to go from a single cell to a 1000 l culture with 10^6 cells/ml there will have had to have been about 40 reproduction cycles to make the trillion (10^{12}) cells.

Cultivation of hybridomas at this scale has recently been reported. It is thought practicable as one company has installed two such 1000 l fermenters for this purpose (1, 3). Cultures of the 100 l size (requiring the original cell and its progeny to have undergone some 35 cycles of cell division) are relatively commonplace and can be 'done to order'. Indeed, techniques of hybridoma production and isolation have so improved that the generation of stable antibody-producing lines is at present the rule rather than the exception (5). The productivity of such cell populations also seems to be rated at roughly the same levels in each individual laboratory. For example, van Wezel (6) quoted productivities of 10–40 μg/ml from 2×10^6 cells/ml for most of the cell lines which pass through his hands. Birch also used figures of 40–50 μg/ml, and more recently 40–500 μg/ml from about the same cell concentrations. Such figures are in a similar range to the productivities which were quoted by Merten *et al.* (7) where the range of productivities indicated was between 1 and 300 μg/ml from similar cell concentrations. However, in spite of such reports, cells have been known to lose their productivities with continual passaging (1), in which case recourse to frozen cell reserves laid down during the early passages of the cell lines is often sufficient to overcome the problem. Alternatively, it is practicable to reclone the cells of the poorly producing populations and recover from them cells with high productivities. This has been achieved for hybridomas; although some workers feel the need to repeat this procedure regularly (8), others reclone only on recovery (5). A similar procedure has been used to recover cell lines productive of discriminating strains of foot-and-mouth disease virus (9).

There is little doubt that cell lines vary in their antibody productivity (10). Merten *et al.* (7) have recognised a type of hybridoma which seems to have lost the negative feedback control of antibody production which inhibits antibody production in a similar but different cell line. The difference in productivity of such cells can be between 100 μg/ml and 0.1 μg/ml, so it is well worth while effecting pragmatic searches for new and more productive cell lines. The limitations of such search procedures will become apparent when the increase in yield per number of cell lines tested drops to zero.

When a plateau of productivity by the search technique is reached, it is probable that further attempts to manipulate the genetic composition of the cell could also be of value. For instance, it is clearly practicable to fuse hybridoma cells together and examine the resultant clones for higher productivities (11). Alternatively, the isolation of chromosomes from one hybridoma population and their micro-injection into the nucleus of another hybridoma cell offers the prospect of direct genetic engineering. A less crude method could involve the isolation of mRNA from a highly productive hybridoma and from it making the cDNA for re-injection back into either a hybridoma or indeed any other animal or eukaryotic cell line which could have some desirable characteristic, such as acceptability by a regulatory agency or growth on serum-free medium (but see below). Attempts to achieve such aims in engineered yeasts have shown the possibility of the approach but so far at levels which are orders of magnitude lower than comparable animal cell systems (12).

5.3. Culture media

The culture media for the large-scale production of monoclonal antibodies are presently far from optimal. Media which have been in use for some time such as Roswell Park Memorial Institute 1640 (RPMI 1640) or Eagle's Medium (or one of its many variants, such as Dulbecco's modification of Eagle's medium (DMEM)) with additional and varied supplements seem to work well. Table 5.2 presents a listing of the components of a number of such media (13, 14). The medium situation is further complicated by such requirements as (i) the need to grow the hybridoma cells so that they do not lose the ability to excrete antibody, (ii) the need to use a medium for antibody production which has few proteins which co-purify with the antibody end product (such as the antibody fractions of added mature animal sera), (iii) the need for a medium which is inexpensive and which does not rely on commodities which, if used excessively, can lead to a market scarcity with a consequent substantial increase in price (for example, foetal calf serum), (iv) the need for a medium which can be made consistently to the same biological performance specification, (v) the need to be free of exogenous biological contaminants, and (vi) a medium which promotes, to the maximal extent, the generation of product.

Table 5.2. *Common media used for large-scale production of hybridoma cells*

Figures are given in milligrams per litre.

Constituents	medium[1]			
	1	2	3	4
Amino acids				
L-Arg HCl	126	105	84	200
L-Cys Na_2	28	30	83	59
L-Gln	292	294	584	300
L-His HCl H_2O	42	42	30	15
L-Ile	52	52	42	50
L-Leu	52	52	105	50
L-Lys HCl	73	72	105	40
L-Met	15	15	146	15
L-Phe	33	32	66	15
L-Thr	48	48	95	20
L-Try	20	20	16	5
L-Tyr	45	47	104	24
L-Val	47	46	94	20
L-Ala			25	
L-Asn			28	56
L-Asp			30	20
L-Glu			75	20
L-Gly			30	10
L-Pro			40	20
L-Ser			42	30
L-HO-Pro				20
Glutathione				1
Vitamins				
D-Ca pantothenate	1.0	1.0	4.0	0.25
choline chloride	1.0	1.0	4.0	3.0
folic acid	1.0	1.0	4.0	1.0
inositol	2.0	2.0	7.2	35.0
nicotinamide	1.0	1.0	4.0	1.0
pyridoxal HCl	1.0	1.0	4.0	
riboflavin	0.1	0.1	0.4	0.2
thiamine HCl	1.0	1.0	4.0	1.0
biotin			0.013	0.3
B_{12}			0.013	0.005
P-aminobenzoic acid				1.0
pyridoxine				1.0

Table 5.2. *(cont.)*

Constituents	medium[1] 1	2	3	4
Salts				
$CaCl_2.2H_2O$	185		218	
KCl	400	400	330	400
KH_2PO_4	40			
$MgSO_4.7H_2O$	200	242	200	100
NaCl	8000	6500	4505	6000
$NaHCO_3$	350	2000	2520	2000
$NaH_2PO_4.2H_2O$	1583	1500	141	
Na_2HPO_4	47			
$CaNO_3$				69
KNO_3			0.076	
NaSe			0.017	
HEPES			5962	
Carbohydrates				
glucose	1000	2000	4500	2000
Na pyruvate			110	
Phenol red	17	10	15	5
Others				
transferrin			1	
BSA			400	
lecithin			100	

Note:
[1] Media: 1, MEM (Hanks Salts); 2, Dulbecco's modification; 3, Iscove's modification of Dulbecco's; 4, RPMI 1640.

5.3.1. *Hybridoma isolation media* (see also chapter 2)

In the development of a manufacturing process for the production of monoclonal antibodies from *in vitro* cell cultures, the cells may be exposed to a number of media in series. In the first instance the media used are selective media which contain inhibitors such as aminopterin, which prevents the growth of those myeloma cells which have not fused to a lymphocyte with a competent capability to use the 'recovery' pathway for nucleotide biosynthesis. Such media may be enriched by the addition of 'conditioned media' which are normally added in a 1 : 1 (v/v) ratio and are prepared by processing (centrifugal clarification) the supernatant medium derived from a culture of a rapidly growing myeloma, fibroblastic or epithelial cell line. Alternative arrangements for providing undefined growth factors depend on the use of feeder cells, which are killed by irradiation or mitomycin C if they are capable of growth in culture; if the feeder cell does not normally replicate in culture (peritoneal macrophages or blood lymphocytes) the added cell is not expected to survive (see §3.7). When the hybrid-forming cell systems are sufficiently concentrated, the cells which do not survive the hybridisation process die and can provide the necessary growth materials (*sui generis*).

5.3.2. *Hybridoma establishment media* (see also Chapter 2)

The use of feeder cells and/or conditioned medium of any sort is a tedious requirement, so the 'adaptation' of the hybrids to more conventional medium is desirable. This is often achieved by formulating media with significant proportions of foetal calf serum (from 10% to 50%). As the foetal serum contains low concentrations of antibody molecules the detection of the antibody products of these culture fluids bathing newly formed hybrid cells is facilitated. Such cultures range in size between 0.1 ml and 10 ml. At this stage in the development the cultures are tested for productivity, growth potential and 'major cell seed stocks' which can be characterised or defined and stored over liquid nitrogen. However, it is clear that practicable manufacturing processes which rely on the use of media with substantial concentrations of foetal calf serum are not only undesirable from considerations of cost but also because they present a source of virological and mycoplasmal contaminants. (Sera from mature animals are, when they are protected from the ingress of exogenous organisms, relatively free of contaminants as the fully developed immune system of the adult will normally have eliminated the contaminating organism, at least from free circulation in the blood.) By the end of the establishment phase the hybridoma cells grow loosely attached to a surface in medium which contains up to 10% of foetal calf serum or an alternative adult serum from bovines or equines. The detachment of such cells from the supporting substratum is achieved by gentle agitation of the growth vessel.

5.3.3. *Intermediate phase media*

The phase between the establishment of the hybridoma cells and their use in large-scale (over 1 l in volume) cultures may be termed intermediate. The two factors which demand most attention at this stage are those of adapting the cells to growth in free suspension in a simple version of a stirred tank reactor (STR) or air-agitated reactor (air-lift reactor, ALR) and the design of a medium with the lowest protein levels consonant with the maintenance of cell growth and antibody production capability.

The cultivation of hybridomas in suspension cultures requires that the cells perform well in a detached mode, that they withstand the hydrodynamic effects introduced by liquid shear forces and the additional effects resulting from the introduction of air via a bubbling system. Although it is well recognised that it is possible to scale up cell cultures to the 100–200 l scale while relying on surface oxygenation (using oxygen gas and higher reactor back pressures) (15) or alternatively to use bioreactors which provide oxygen to the medium by passing the oxygenating gas (oxygen or air) through a thin-walled silicone or polypropylene tube immersed in the culture (16–19) such methods become less practicable with reactors of 1000 l and 10 000 l in volume, a scale-up operation which presently constitutes the level of technical capability in the commercial domain. The effects of bubbling derive from a combination of several factors. In the development of a foam both the denaturation of serum proteins and damage to the cells (from unspecified causes) can result. Were foam formation to be depressed, as by the use of an antifoam agent (an aqueous emulsion of polydimethylsiloxane at a final dilution of 1:10 000) or by use of a caged aerator (J.P. Whiteside, personal communication) the impact shock waves caused by bubble breakages could still be implicated in cell damage (20). To overcome such effects media are either supplemented with a polyol such as Pluronic F68, (a co-polymer of polyoxyethylene and polyoxypropylene), methyl cellulose or dextrans of various molecular weights, or more serum is added to the medium. This latter response is clearly counter-productive in view of the basic need to use low-protein and better defined media for large-scale production (20).

Recent work shows that it is possible to adapt or 'harden' hybridoma cells to the environment of the antibody production vessel. Such hardened cells would be characterised by their ability to grow with minimal levels (0.5–2%) of an inexpensive serum (adult bovine or more generally calf or newborn calf serum). Although a defined procedure of 'weaning' cells from their dependence on high levels of sera rich in growth factors has not yet been established, a number of guidelines are becoming discernible (21). Working from the hypothesis that all cells are capable of producing their own growth-promoting factors if suitably stimulated, the careful and progressive removal of exogenous growth factors allows the cell to adapt to the new conditions by expressing hitherto dormant genes. Therefore, the weaning or coaxing exercise has to be effected carefully. Starting from cultures which grow well to moderate cell densities (1×10^6 to 5×10^6 cells/ml) the serum used for the passage which begins the weaning process is reduced to half its usual level. It is then important to allow the cells to adjust to the new level and for them to re-establish their previous growth rates and cell concentrations at the end of the growth cycle. In any event, even were this to happen at the first such passage, further attempts to reduce the serum concentration should not be made for at least three further passages or, for more reliable results, a further five passages. Subsequent reductions in serum concentrations should recognise the increased difficulty the cells experience and the number of passages at the new, lower, serum level should be increased to ensure that the cells have effectively adapted their growth capabilities to the lower serum levels. By using such techniques it has been found to be relatively simple to reduce serum levels to between 0.5 and 2% and still retain reliable growth and production characteristics. The elimination of the serum altogether requires more than the simple adaptation process described.

5.3.4. *Serum-free media*

A recent review of reviews by Lambert & Birch (14) classifies serum-free media into three groups. The Type I serum-free media are those rare media which are chemically defined insofar as one can define the purity of the individual medium components. One such medium has been used to grow an established mouse hybridoma cell line as an attached monolayer (22). This medium is based on a 1 : 1 mixture of Ham's F12 medium with that of Iscove & Melchers. To this medium is added progesterone, α-thioglycerol and an additional 18 trace elements. Antibody productivities of between 50 and 150 μg/ml during 100 days in culture were reported.

The Type II media are defined as serum-free media with protein supplements. Although such supplements have names they are rarely, if at all, pure, nor in some cases are they defined in terms of the availability of knowledge on their primary structure (e.g. transferrin). The protein supplements commonly used are mixtures of 2–5 materials from the following list: insulin, epidermal growth factor, transferrin, albumin, fibronectin, platelet-derived growth factor, thrombin, casein, hydrocortisone, oleic acid, cholesterol, ethanolamine and ascorbic acid (1). The addition of such materials will provide an effective medium generally low in total protein content but which is often as expensive as, or more expensive than, a medium based on a low-level addition of foetal calf serum. However, the use of such materials as supplements to very low serum levels (less than 1%) could provide a useful stepping stone in the weaning process whereby cells can be grown free of both serum and protein supplement.

The high cost of such supplements can be obviated by the use of less well-defined additions; such formulations constitute Type III media. Low cost additives such as bovine colostrum peptone, milk, lactalbumin hydrolysate, yeast extract and egg yolk emulsion have been used in animal cell cultures in general, although such media have not been reported as having a role for the growth of hybridoma cells.

There are, however, a number of commercially available media which are serum-free but whose cost approaches, if not exceeds, that of standard serum-supplemented media (D. Billig (Pharmacia), personal communication). One such medium whose formulation has been partly disclosed is that offered by K.C. Biologicals (23). This medium contains transferrin, fetuin, serum albumin with other 'essential nutrients', vitamins and fatty acids, resulting in a protein level equivalent to a 0.5% foetal calf serum medium. Two media marketed under the names HB101 and HB102 (NEN Products, Boston, USA) are on offer but are not recommended for operation at cell counts in excess of 1×10^6/ml. From the considerations above it is unlikely that investigators will be able to adapt a cell line growing on a serum-containing medium to a serum-free medium in one step. It is clear that a weaning or adaptation process will be necessary. There is therefore a need to determine whether any particular medium formulation is advantageous or whether success in growing cells serum-free is more dependent on how the cells are adapted to the low-protein medium.

5.3.5. *Alternative approaches to medium formulation*

The provision of alternatives to serum is a quest many have adopted. Collaborative Research (USA) formulated a powder called Nu-Serum; AMF Incorporated (USA) have developed a process which produces serum more reliably free from endotoxin contamination (24). Workers at Bioresponse have used bovine lymph, continuously expressed by a tethered animal, as a source of growth factors in addition to, or in substitution for more conventional serum (23). Yet there is little doubt that although the empirical approach to a serum-free medium has yielded much of value and will continue on its present course for some time to come, the pivotal breakthrough to the practical exploitation of an understanding of the molecular parameters which control growth has yet to be made. The end product of such investigations would be a chemically defined medium with specified additives which realiably and cheaply control the growth, maintenance in a non-growing state and productivity of animal cells in large-scale cultures.

5.3.6. *Relationship between cell growth and antibody production*

The question which is often asked is 'are antibody molecules excreted by growing and dividing cells or by cells which have ceased to grow and divide and are "senescent"?' As yet a definitive study which answers this question has not been reported. While there have been many demonstrations that as cultures increase in cell number the concentration of antibody in the supernatant fluids increases commensurately whether such cultures be batch, fed batch or continuous (24–27) there is, as yet, scant information published indicating whether it is the dividing or stationary cells which are producing the antibodies. However, work by P. Hayter in the author's laboratory has clearly demonstrated that, in the synchronised culture, antibody production is associated with the G1 phase of the cell cycle and shuts down almost completely when the cells are synthesising their DNA and proceeding through to cell replication (P. Hayter, N. Kirkby and R.E. Spier, unpublished data, 1987). Graphs typical of such cultures are presented in Fig. 5.1 (*a–c*). Under normal mass culture conditions it is difficult to distinguish between the productivity of cells which are actively dividing, and thereby maintaining the population, and cells which have ceased to divide and which could have devoted their energies to antibody production as such cultures contain variable proportions of both cell types. The work with systems exploiting bundles of capillaries wherein the cells are held in the extracapillary space and the nutrients circulate through the lumen of the capillaries (see §5.3.7. below) should answer such questions, for in such systems it is possible to retain cellular activity for many (15–20) weeks with cells held at concentrations of 2–4 × 10^8/ml of extracapillary volume. It is not clear whether such cells are all equally viable or whether there is a constant turnover of viable cells caused by the death and disappearance rate equalling the rate of replacement. Indeed, such cells are provided with serum-free medium after the second or third week of exposure to such conditions, which, even if it did not decrease cell replication entirely, would decrease the rate of new cell production.

In view of these uncertainties it would be unwise to classify the generation of antibodies by cells in culture as the production of 'secondary metabolites', although the major antibody-producing cell in the body, the plasma cell, is a terminal cell which has differentiated for the specific function of antibody production. The elimination of this uncertainty is crucial to the development of such systems. The present guidelines indicate that more antibody can be produced from more cells, but they do not indicate whether it is conducive to higher productivities to have the cells continuously grow, divide and die, or whether a cell culture system in which all the cells are maintained alive, but not dividing or even increasing in size, would be more productive.

5.3.7. *Culture techniques for the large-scale production of monoclonal antibodies from hybridoma cell lines*

Animal cells have been used on a large scale for the production of viral vaccines (28). Present practice for the production of foot-and-mouth disease (FMD) vaccines typically involves stirred tank reactors of between 5000 and 10 000 l in operating volume. Other vaccines for human

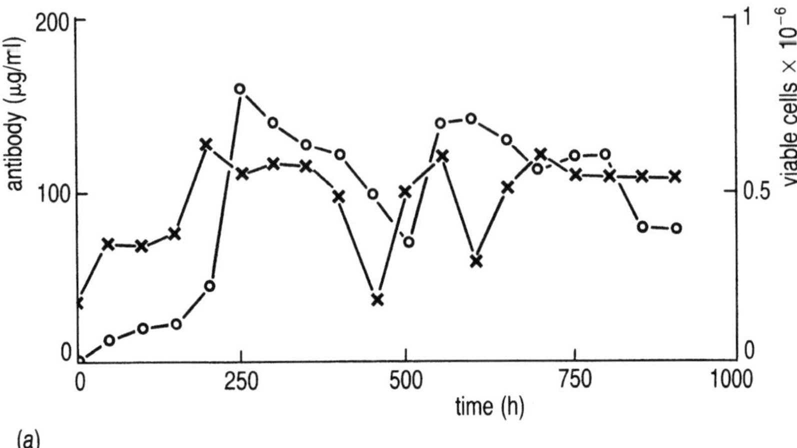

(*a*)

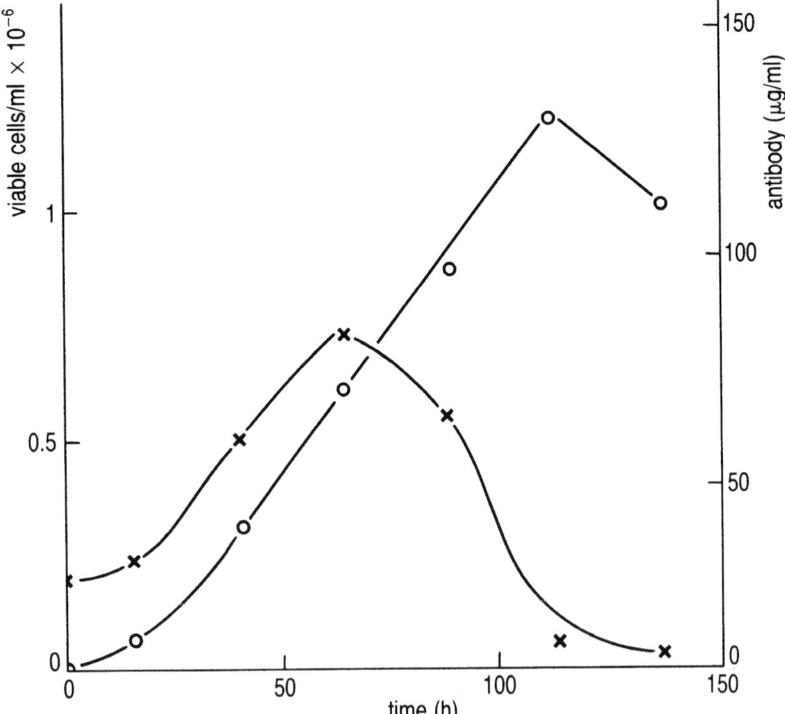

(*b*)

Fig. 5.1. Cell concentration and antibody levels from suspension cell systems run as (*a*) continuous culture, (*b*) batch culture and (*c*) synchronised culture. (Symbols: crosses, viable cells; open circles, antibody.) (*d*) Antibody production as a function of growth rate; the straight line indicates the linear regression function.

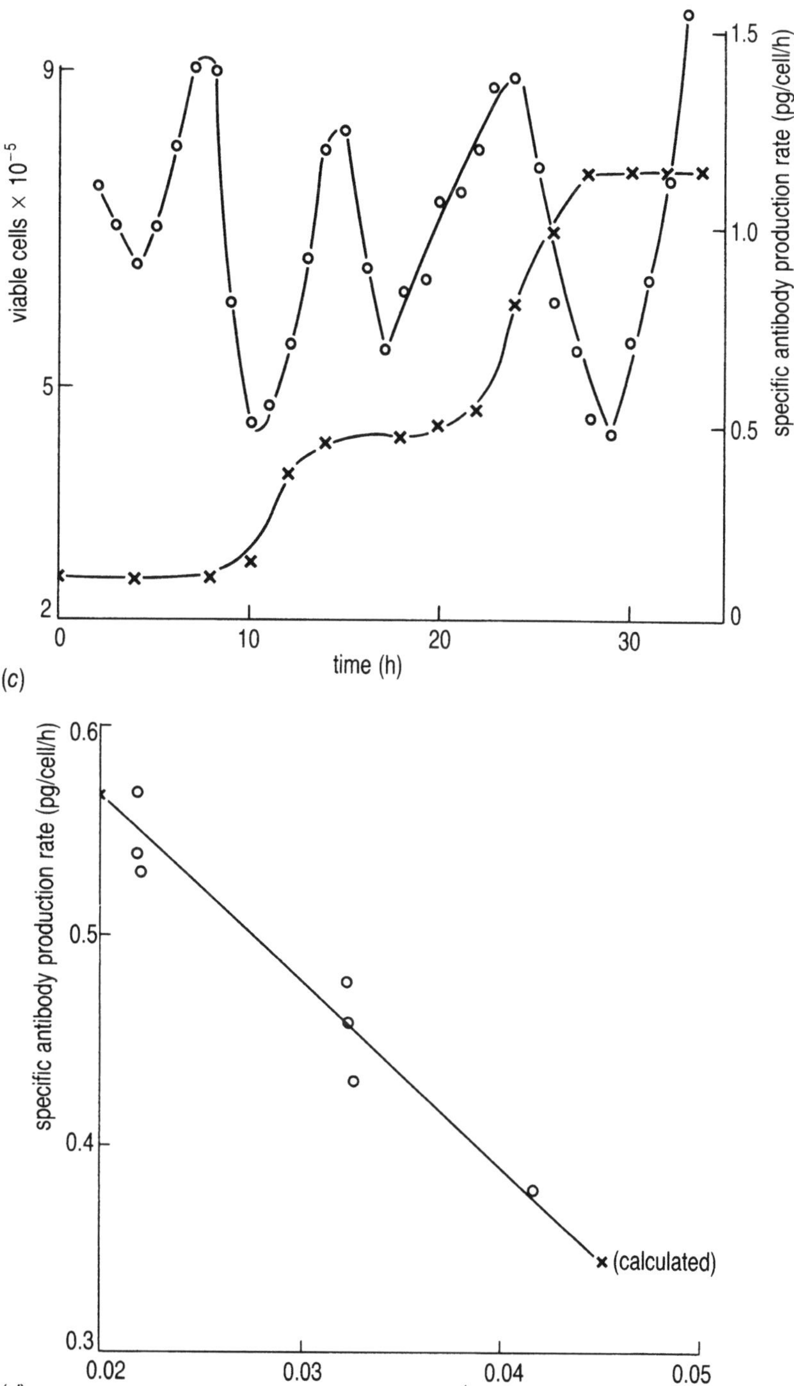

9
5
2
viable cells × 10⁻⁵
1.5
1.0
0.5
0
specific antibody production rate (pg/cell/h)
0
10
20
30
time (h)
(c)
0.6
0.5
0.4
0.3
specific antibody production rate (pg/cell/h)
(calculated)
0.02
0.03
0.04
0.05
growth rate (h⁻¹)
(d)

and veterinary uses (Polio (29) or Marek's (30)) are made from surface-attached cells and the scale of operations is generally between 100 and 1000 l of medium volume per unit process reactor system. The later development of processes for the production of α-(lymphoblastoid) interferon and β-(fibroblastic) interferon from animal cells in culture have used similar technologies to the systems used for virus vaccines (4). Hence the mammalian cell system for α-interferon has been scaled up to 8000 l in a stirred tank reactor system (31) while in Japan it is reported that cells adhering to microcarriers are producing β-interferon at unit scales of operation of greater than 5000 l (4). The two examples quoted (viral vaccines and interferon) differ significantly in that nucleic acid transcription is necessarily required for virus production while the emphasis in the production of the proteinaceous interferon is on the super-induction of mRNA formation (by transcription) followed by an inhibition of further nucleic-acid-dependent reactions and an enhancement of translation activity for protein formation.

The production of antibody molecules is not dependent on DNA transcription to RNA as is required for some virus replication; rather, the rate of formation of mRNA is probably the prime determinant of the role of product generation. Once the cell has been provided with its complement of mRNA all other biosynthetic reactions are, from a producer's viewpoint, superfluous. Under ideal conditions the biosynthetic systems of the cell would be provided with a mixture of amino acids and then coupled to a readily metabolisable energy source and allowed to manufacture the required (antibody) end product. Clearly 'cell' growth and nucleic acid (DNA) replication is not only unnecessary but undesirable. Therefore, a technical objective would be to realise the theoretical maximum productivities from cell systems maintained specifically for antibody product formation.

5.3.8. *Overview of present techniques*

To obtain maximal productivities, workers in a number of laboratories have used a wide variety of alternative techniques. Indeed, so wide is this variety that it is difficult to evaluate the relative performance of the various systems. Examples of these alternatives are:

- a modified STR with a shaft fitted with a spin filter as originally described by Himmelfarb *et al.* (32) and used by van Wezel in four different modes of operation (24);
- the development of the air-lift system redesigned for animal cells by Katinger (33) to scales of 100 and 1000 l by Birch (1, 34);
- systems based on surface adherent cells attached to microcarriers (35) or glass discs (25);

cells entrapped within the matrix of agarose gel beads held in suspension in an air-lift reactor (27);
the use of a capillary bundle reactor with cells confined to the extracapillary space (37);
reactors based on holding cells sandwiched between two membranes while perfusing nutrient fluids between alternate films (MBR Bioreactor Ltd, Wetziken, Switzerland);
cells encapsulated in a small polylysine–polyornithine based hollow microspheres maintained in suspension in an STR (38–41).

Thus in order to approach this array of possibilities with a view to determining which of the systems offers the greatest prospects for that development which will make it the predominant technical approach to producing monoclonal antibodies from hybridoma cells, it is necessary to form an appreciation of the range of conditions and the nature of the situation in which animal cells work most effectively. Such a model situation can be found in an examination of the state of the environment presented to animal cells *in vivo*. For this reason data will be presented below on the environment supplied by living whole animals (man) to some of the cells in selected tissues.

5.3.9. *Environments surrounding animal cells* in vivo

The external world to an animal cell *in situ* consists of an aqueous fluid within which materials essential for or injurious to that cell may be found. Nutrients (materials which are required for growth and maintenance of the cell; when serving that function they are altered or consumed irreversibly) and waste products of metabolism discharged from the cell co-exist in the fluids bathing the cell. The cell is therefore exposed to supplies of amino acids (the essential ones), sugars, fatty acids, inorganic ions, co-factors and oxygen (see §5.3). In return lactic acid, amines, carbon dioxide and excreted proteinaceous materials are exocytosed or leave the cell by diffusion. The regulation of cell metabolism *in vivo* may not depend solely on the availability of nutrients whose concentration limits cellular performance nor upon the build-up of toxic materials. Rather, the sum of all the environmental parameters, in conjunction with the way in which the cell has been treated during the course of its existence as an individual unit, determines which genes are expressed and the extent of such expression.

The examination of the situation *in vivo* will, however, indicate what is possible. For example, with regard to molecular oxygen, which is distributed from the blood by diffusion, it should be possible to determine the maximum depth of cells which can be served by a particular supply system. This will have implications for the design of equipment which attempts to provide oxygen to cells at their maximum density (concen-

Table 5.3. *Blood flow through defined organs*

Organ	Blood flow (ml blood/100 g organ/min)
Thyroid	560
Kidney	150
Liver	150
Heart	100
Intestine	70
Brain	65
Spleen	40
Stomach	25
Hand	7–12
Finger	15–40
Muscle	1–2.5

Note:
Average blood flow through organ: 100 ml/100 g organ/min (± 50 ml)
Source: Adapted from Tables 27 and 29 of Bell *et al.* (43), p. 504.

trations in excess of 10^9 cells for cells 10 μm in diameter), a density which is equalled, if not exceeded, in tissues.

5.3.9.1. *Cells in tissues* in vivo *require similar amounts of oxygen to cells in bioreactors* in vitro

The oxygen demand of cells *in vivo* may best be obtained by calculation from the figures as presented in the tables below. In Table 5.3 the blood flow through selected organs is presented. The range of flows is considerable: from 2 ml per 100 g organ per minute for muscle to 500 ml per 100 g organ per minute for the thyroid. Most organs have a blood flow of between 50 and 150 ml per 100 g organ per minute; for the purposes of calculation a value of 100 may be most suitable. From the differences in the degree of saturation of arterial and venous blood in conjunction with the rate of flow of blood through 100 g of an organ it is possible to calculate the total oxygen demand of that 100 g of tissue and hence the oxygen used per cell of tissue (Table 5.4*a*).

5.3.9.2. *Oxygen can diffuse through many cell diameters before oxygen limitation becomes apparent*

There are two approaches to determine the 'maximum allowable distance' between a cell and its source of oxygen. The most simple procedure

Table 5.4. (a) *Oxygen demand of a theoretical cell in a theoretical organ*

1. Arterial blood contains 19 ml oxygen/100 ml blood (43, p.528).
2. Venous blood contains 10.6 ml oxygen/100 ml blood (43, p.528); therefore on average 8.4 ml oxygen is removed on passage of 100 ml of blood through an organ.
   This is equivalent to $(8.4 \times 32)/(22.5 \times 1000) = 0.012$ g oxygen.
3. Weight of a 10 μm diameter sphere of density 1 g/cm^3 = 5.2×10^{-10} g.
4. Assume that the cells are close packed without intracellular spaces.
5. Number of cells per 100 g of organ is
   $100/(5.2 \times 10^{-10}) = 2 \times 10^{11}$.
6. Assume an organ is irrigated with 100 ml of blood per minute.
7. Each cell uses $0.012/(2 \times 10^{11})$ g oxygen/min
   $= 6 \times 10^{-14}$ g oxygen/cell/min or 3.6×10^{-12} g oxygen/cell/h.
8. Most cells would fall in the range $1.8–5.4 \times 10^{-12}$ g/cell/h; this figure is comparable to the figures found for cell culture systems (range of values for lymphoid cells is $1.3–1.6 \times 10^{-12}$ g oxygen/cell/h (18); range of values for other cells is $1.6–11 \times 10^{-12}$ g oxygen/cell/h).

(b) *Calculation of the mean distance of a body cell from a capillary*

1. Assume total body weight is 100 kg.
2. The body retains 40% of its weight as intracellular water (96, p.523).
3. Animal cells contain between 80 and 85% water (97) (say 82%).
4. Therefore the weight of cellular material in a 100 kg body will be $40/0.82 = 48.780$ kg.
5. The blood volume of a 100 kg body is about 7 kg (98, p.554).
6. 6.75% of the blood is found in the capillaries (98, p.554).
7. The average capillary diameter is about 10 μm (between 9 μm and 15–20 μm) (99).
8. The total capillary surface area is therefore:
   $$\frac{7000 \times 6.75 = 2\pi \times 5 \times 10^{-4}}{100 \times \pi \times (5 \times 10^{-1})^2} \qquad = 1.9 \times 10^{6}\ \text{cm}^2.$$
9. The thickness of the film of cells spread out over the surface area of the capillaries is $48\,780/1.9 \times 10^6 = 256$ μm or 21 cell diameters (taking cells to be 12 μm in diameter).

would be to examine fixed and stained tissues microscopically and determine the number of cell diameters between nearest-neighbour capillaries. Krogh's 1919 summary (42) of observations on the spacing of capillaries in muscle reports that in guinea pig resting muscle there are

Table 5.5. *Calculation of the number of layers of cells supportable by 1 ml of culture fluid (oxygen diffusivity not considered)*

Assumptions

1 Cell density: 5×10^5 cells/cm^2 (10^8/200 cm^2/h).
2 Assume cells adopt the form of a cube of side 12 μm.
3 Oxygen demand per cell: 3×10^{-12} g O_2/cell/h or 8.3×10^{-16} g/cell/s (18).
4 Amount of oxygen dissolved in 1 ml of medium 7×10^{-6} g.

Calculation

(*a*) Total oxygen demand/cm^2 for 1 layer for 1 s = $5 \times 10^5 \times 8.3 \times 10^{-16}$ g O_2.
(*b*) Total number of such layers supportable by 1 ml of water
= $7 \times 10^6/(5 \times 10^5 \times 8.3 \times 10^{-16})$ = 16 867 layers.

Note:
This calculation assumed that the *rate* at which oxygen can diffuse is not a limiting factor.

200 capillaries/mm^2 whereas in active muscle this figure could rise to 2500 capillaries/mm^2 (43, p.528). The former situation leads to 5–6 cell diameters between adjacent capillaries (assuming a capillary diameter of 5 μm) while in the active muscle the distance allows for 1–2 cell diameters (in both cases, for the purposes of calculation, the capillaries were considered to occupy positions defined by a regular matrix). An alternative method is to consider that all the cells of the body are layered onto a membrane which has the surface area of the capillary system of the body. Table 5.4*b* presents data showing that, were all the cells of the body to be spread out over the combined surface area of all the capillaries, the thickness of the layer would be some 250 μm or 21 cells of 12 μm diameter. Such a consideration indicates a possible limiting dimension for equipment which seeks to provide cells with nutrients and remove the products of metabolism. The guideline principle would be to design equipment where each cell is either within 250 μm of its supplies or the cells are periodically moved to a position less than that distance away from their nutrient and discharge exchange points.

5.3.9.3. *Model systems which can be used to calculate the number of layers of cells which can be supported by a source of dissolved oxygen*

A simple calculation which did not take into account the time required for oxygen diffusion would show that it is possible to support some 17 000 layers of cells 12 μm in diameter; a cell sheet 20 cm thick (Table 5.5). However, when the rate at which oxygen diffuses (the diffusivity of oxygen) is brought into consideration, along with the fact that some of the oxygen is removed from the diffusing material as it passes through

Table 5.6. *Computation of the number of layers of cells supportable by 1 ml of culture fluid when the diffusivity of oxygen is taken into account and the oxygen consumption of the cells is included*

Additional assumptions

1 Diffusivity of oxygen at 37°C in water is 2.5×10^{-5} cm^2/s.

Program

```
100  OX DEM = 4.1 E−10          oxygen demand (5 × 10^-5
                                × 8.3 × 10^-16)
110  DIFCO = 2.5 E−5            (diffusion coefficient of
                                oxygen in water)
120  LAYTH = 1 E−3              (thickness of cell sheet)
130  DISOX = 7 E−6              (dissolved oxygen concentration
                                in water)
150  T1 = (OXDEM × LAYTH)/(DIFCO * DISOX)
               (T1 = time taken for oxygen to move to
                     the top of the first layer)
160  T=T+T1
170  DISOX = DISOX − OXDEM
175  N = 2                      (for second layer of cells)
180  TA2 = OXDEM * N * LAYTH
185  TB2 = DIFCO * DISOX
190  T2 =TA2/TB2
195  T=T+T2
200  PRINT" ";N:" ";T
205  IF T>1 THEN END
210  DISOX = DISOX − OXDEM
220  N = N + 1
230  GOTO 180
```

Running this program gives N = 29 layers for T = 1 s.

each succeeding layer, the extent to which oxygen can diffuse can be calculated (Fig. 5.2).

These iterative calculations are most readily effected by a computer; Table 5.6 presents a program in BASIC (BBCB Microcomputer, Acorn) which calculates that in a time of 1 s it is possible to provide oxygen to some 30 layers of cells before time (but not oxygen) runs out, Such a figure is comparable to the 21 layers of cubic cells 12 μm per side, as in Table 5.4*b* and the previous section. Again, such figures are well within the range of observations on the growth of cancer tissues, which form cell masses whose cells lie between 100 μm (44, 45) and 2000 μm (46) away from a source of nutrient (blood vessel). Such distances are equivalent to 8–160 cell diameters. That it is possible to derive such a wide

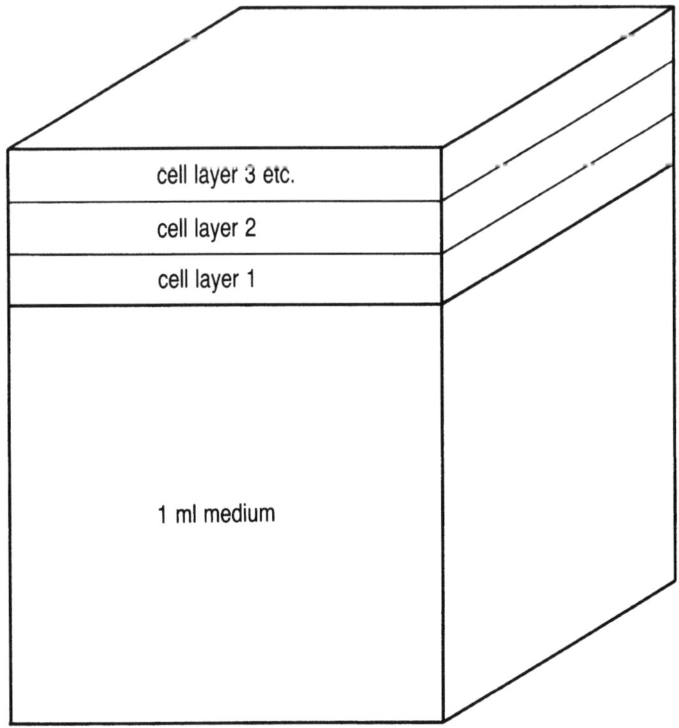

Fig. 5.2. Model used to calculate the number of layers of cells that can be supported nutritionally.

range of figures from the published literature complies with the wide range of oxygen demands expressed by various organs (see Table 5.3).

It can be concluded from such research that animal cells can be accommodated with regard to their oxygen demand when they form clumps or layers such that the cells furthest from the source of oxygen are not more than a few tens of cells away from the source of that nutrient; it is assumed that the nutrient source is saturated with oxygen at 7×10^6 g/l for the purposes of these projections. Further detailed calculations on the degree to which oxygen can diffuse into a mass of cells is presented in a recent review by Murdin *et al.* (47).

5.3.9.4. *Interim conclusion*

Cells *in vivo* exist in densely packed masses. It is now possible to duplicate such conditions *in vitro*. However, it would be foolhardy to proceed to an all-out commitment to such systems without a review of the advantages and disadvantages which are inherent in such dense systems as they are transferred onto the production shop floor.

5.4. A survey of the advantages and disadvantages of techniques based on dense cell systems

It is clearly necessary to first define what is meant by a 'dense cell system'; it then becomes possible to proceed to a discussion of the merits and demerits of such operations.

5.4.1. *What are dense cell cultures?*

Conventional animal cell cultures used for the production of viruses for vaccines function well at cell concentrations in the range 5×10^5–5×10^6 cells/ml culture fluid (however that is applied; as in a single medium or a perfusion system). By contrast, if we assume that a cell of 10 μm diameter is a solid non-deforming sphere, then 10^9 will pack into a 1 cm^3 space. Were the spheres to be deformable, then about twice that number would fit into the same volume. It should be noted that the deformable animal cell can be configured at biomass densities greater than those which can be achieved by cells which cannot be so deformed owing to their possession of a rigid cell wall (bacteria, yeasts, algae, etc.). For this reason it is possible that animal cells could offer process intensities greater than those achievable by micro-organisms bounded by non-deformable sheaths (which in themselves are non-productive and space-consuming). The equivalent figures for cells of 12 μm and 15 μm diameter are 6×10^8 and 3×10^8 for rigid spheres and 1×10^9 and 6×10^8 for deformable spheres, respectively. Hybridoma cells in suspended culture have a size range of between 7 and 15 μm in diameter (Fig. 5.3). This implies that maximum cell densities for deformable spheres could be in the range 6×10^9–6×10^8 (for cells 7 μm and 15 μm in diameter). From these considerations, and taking an 'average' cell size of 12 μm a dense hybridoma cell culture would be one in which the cell concentration was greater than 5×10^8 cells/ml of cell slurry. That is the number of cells per delineated volume (bounded either by (i) the membranes or sides of the reactor or (ii) membranes built round clusters of the cells; or (iii) the value defined by the edges of a morula of clumped cells or cells plus an enveloping or entrapping matrix).

5.4.2. *Some advantages of dense cell cultures*

A summary of the advantages and disadvantages of dense cell systems is presented in Table 5.7. It is assumed that the systems under consideration are unit process systems (i.e. ones in which scale-up is achieved by increasing the size of the equipment rather than the number of pieces of equipment). The first advantage, that of using less voluminous equipment, is to some extent negated by the requirement to use a particular volume of medium to obtain a defined number of cells (48), which means that equipment capable of containing the medium volume needed by the cells has to be on hand and that, whereas the cells could be contained

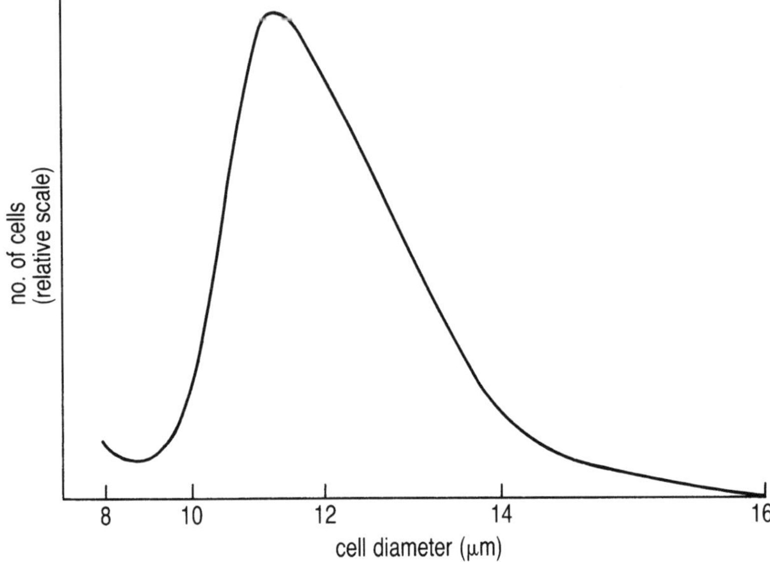

Fig. 5.3. Size range distribution of a growing hybridoma culture in the suspension mode.

in a chamber of 10 l volume, the medium needed to produce that number of cells (10^{13} at 10^9/ml) would occupy 10 000 l were it made at any one time (assuming a productivity of 10^6 cells per millilitre of medium).

The process intensity increase, resulting from the biomass being held within boundaries whose dimensions force the cells to be held at local concentrations of the order of 5×10^8/ml (see §5.4.1), enables the fluids bathing the cells to be separated from the biomass easily by decantation, simple filtration using large pore screens (200–600 μm or more) or by the use of a protected overflow device. There are considerable advantages to be obtained from producing a clear cell-free fluid from the bioreactor as the subsequent downstream procedures would be liable to fouling, contamination and blockage were particulate materials to emanate from the production vessel. In the event that it is not possible to eliminate cells and cell debris, filters based on bentonite or diatomaceous earth (fuller's earth) (49) or filters of defined hydrophilicity and hydrophobicity (50) can be used.

Although it is relatively simple to concentrate culture fluids by a factor of 10 times by using tangential membrane filtration systems (1, 51, 52), it is generally more effective to use starting materials which are already at the highest concentration. A tenfold increase in the concentration of such materials would, of course, concentrate contaminant materials, which could lead to yield reductions during the subsequent processing.

Table 5.7. *Advantages and disadvantages of dense cell systems*

Advantages	Disadvantages
smaller reactor volumes (and buildings) more concentrated product: easier separations higher recoveries smaller equipment for separations less energy for MAb, possibility of higher specific productivities for MAb, greater ease of obtaining serum-free operating systems: easier separations cheaper media more reproducible productivities run length increases fewer cell–medium separation problems biomass densities greater than those obtainable in prokaryotic systems	greater difficulties in scale-up: mass (oxygen) transfer problems more physically complex reactor designs equipment sterilisation problems higher degree of control necessary, adding to capital costs, complexity of operation and reliability of system some (not all) such systems require additional processing steps: cost of materials increases mechanical and contamination problems

A factor in the processing of proteins is that precipitations and phase separations are more efficient when the solutes to be separated are present at higher concentrations (53). Advantage may also be taken of the lower quantities of reagents required and the smaller, less energy-consuming equipment needed to achieve pure concentrated product.

With regard to the prospects of higher specific productivities when cells are held in dense cell systems, it is far from clear whether this advantage can be obtained. Little appropriate comparative investigatory work has been done and it is difficult to compare different cell lines operating under different physical and chemical conditions. Yet the specific productivity figures which are quoted (2) do indicate an increase in specific productivity with cell concentration, a fact which is not inconsonant with the theoretical considerations of §5.3.6 based on cells generating product rather than cellular biomass.

Following the early observations of Rein & Rubin in 1968 (54) that cells will only grow when planted above a minimum cell density, it is reasonable to project that cells at even higher concentrations are more likely to be able to grow and maintain themselves on less rich, and serum-free, media. The projection is borne out by the use of serum-free media for the cultivation of hybridoma cells in dialysis-type reactors (55) and in being able to maintain cells in the capillary reactor systems for extended periods of time using serum-free medium, with periodic boosts from a serum-containing medium (56). Clearly, the ability to operate monoclonal antibody-producing bioreactors with serum-free medium is a boon. The product separations are facilitated and the medium for all cell growth and/or maintenance is free from such materials at the onset. The media are less expensive as the serum (or serum supplement) often used may cost many times more than all the other ingredients put together. Furthermore, the omission of a material of biological origin enables a higher degree of control of the bioreactor performance, as a source of uncontrollable (and as yet unknown) elements in the reaction systems has been eliminated.

The consequences of many of the advantages discussed above are that run length increases with concomitant savings in labour, energy for sterilisations, and wastes. The more efficient use of capital equipment justifies the use of reliable, accurate and sophisticated control systems which in turn lead to increase in reactor performance. In addition, stable reaction conditions enable product targets to be forecasted and sales to be scheduled more reliably.

5.4.3. *Some disadvantages of dense cell cultures*

With systems operating at high concentrations the tolerances on reactor performance are more critical. The rates at which change occurs with cell concentrations some 500 times higher are more rapid in the same proportion. Furthermore, the cells are generally in contact with only a proportion of the culture medium at any one time so that the 'volume buffering' effect is not available. For these reasons the dense cell cultures provide quite difficult problems which have to be surmounted to achieve reliable performance.

The difficulties experienced in scale-up of dense cell cultures, which are not generally experienced with dilute cell cultures (up to 5×10^5 cells/ml) (stirred tank reactor, air-lift reactor with or without perfusion and cell recycle), derive from the more complex geometry of the bioreactors holding the cells, which in turn is derived from the requirement to provide the cells with nutrients (particularly oxygen) and to control the pH of the microenvironment of the cell. Note that the removal of lactic acid *per se* may not be as much of a necessity as the maintenance of the appropriate concentration of free hydrogen ions (35, 57).

The physically more complex designs are required to provide oxygen to all the cells in the reactor. The general approach has been to divide the cell mass up by the use of membranes, capillaries or microspheres, or by the formation of cellular masses in the form of agglomerates, surface- or bulk-captured masses or enmeshed cells. Such divisions or divisors require maintenance, cleaning, implementation and sterilisation; as a result of complex geometries and tight limitations on the maximum distance between the cell furthest away from the source of nutrient and that nutrient (a matter of some 0.05–0.5 mm) these processes present practical problems which generally do not decrease as the size of the equipment increases in the unit process mode of scale-up.

The gas and nutrient permeable divisors of the equipment used for dense cell cultures are often synthetic and not generally sterilisable by wet steam at 121 °C. Membranes of polysulphone–polyacrylonitrile (45), cellulosic materials (cellulose nitrate and cellulose acetate) (55, 58) and polylysine–polyornithine (41) are not heat-stable and have to be either formed sterile or sterilised by ethylene oxide or some other non-degrading but somewhat less reliable sterilant than wet steam at 121 °C (59, 60).

The more intensive process resulting from dense cell systems requires more careful control. It is often impossible to insert sensors into the cell-containing compartments, so the cells' conditions are generally inferred by measurement of pH and dissolved oxygen concentration at the points just as the oxygen-saturated (with air or oxygen gas) nutrient medium enters the reaction chamber and then again immediately after it exits from that chamber. The difference between these two readings reflects the nature of one of the nutrient gradients within the cell-containing chamber; this represents an overall gradient and does not relate to other gradients set up at the sub-millimetre dimensions. Clearly, medium circulation rates can be adjusted to decrease the overall gradients to a tolerable level yet such control requires reliable pumps, equipment that does not block on extended operations and control equipment which does not become unstable and hunt excessively for conditions defined by the operational set of control points required by the process operator. Again, the stability of analogue (and more recently, digital) equipment over periods of several months of continuous operation will provide a most testing challenge to any control system, particularly if that system is energised by an erratic (spiked) mains voltage or is in a situation which generates static voltages at low humidities or under other environmentally inhospitable conditions.

Although, as §5.4.2 has stressed, there are advantages to the downstream systems of dense cell cultures, some disadvantages also accrue. Broken particles provide effective blocking agents for clarifying filters; additional processes are required to release product from cell-containing compartments; cellular debris, cells and cell clumps block or foul columns used in purification systems; and it is possible that nucleic acid released from degenerate cells can alter fluid viscosities to levels where process scheduling becomes changed. Such disadvantages may be overcome by the application of appropriate techniques; each additional step, however, represents an increase in cost, a decrease in yield and an additional source of malfunctions.

5.5. The influence of controllable parameters on monoclonal antibody production by hybridoma cells in culture

There are relatively few controllable parameters which influence the production of monoclonal antibodies by hybridoma cell lines in culture. Some of the parameters which investigators have manipulated in attempts to enhance antibody yields are summarised in Table 5.8. It should, however, be noted that it is important to optimise the productivity of the cell before, or in parallel with, the optimisation of the parameters controlling the conditions in the culture (see §5.2).

5.5.1. *Physical factors*

The physical factors which are readily available for modulation are those of temperature, pH, dilution rate and hydrodynamic environment (the liquid shear forces pertaining at the location of the cell membrane).

(i) Hydrodynamics: There is little systematic work which defines the relationship between the hydrodynamic environment and the production of antibody in situations where the cell growth rate and percentage viability are held constant. Such experiments can be done in chemostat-type continuous cultures where pH, dissolved oxygen concentration and, most importantly, dilution rate can be held constant while the effect of changes in the hydrodynamic environment (r.p.m, impeller size, viscosity, configuration, etc.) can be studied. Apart from the observation that stirrer speeds in excess of 200 r.p.m. would have a detrimental effect on the cells (61), most investigators have operated their stirred tank reactors at stirrer speeds of between 10 r.p.m. (62) and 300 r.p.m. (J.P. Whiteside, personal communication) (62, 63). Again there have been few systematic attempts at determining the influence of the air–liquid interface forces on the viability and productivity of hybridoma cells. Although air-lift reactors are alleged to generate hydrodynamically benign environments of low shear stress (1), bubbles can be detrimental to hybridoma cells (20) as it seems that when the bubbles discharge into the headspace of the fermenter the cells in the area local to that action are subjected to much violent agitation. The effect of this disturbance can be mitigated by the use of low concentrations of the polyol Pluronic F68 (20).

(ii) Light: Workers have occasionally remarked on the influence of light on the growth and productivity of hybridoma cells (61, 62, 64). Growth media contain light-absorbing materials such as riboflavin and phenol red, yet light is not generally regarded as a problem in animal cell biotechnology (but see 65) as evidenced by the tens of thousands of

Table 5.8. *Parameters used to influence monoclonal antibody production from hybridoma cells in culture*

Temperature
pH
dilution rate (not growth rate)
hydrodynamic environment (± bubbles)
serum:
concentration
time of addition
exposure to light
glucose concentration
ammonia–ammonium equilibrium
glutamine concentration
lactic acid concentration
cell concentration
other chemical factors:
oleic acid
selenium
ethanolamine
steroids
Primatone
Pluronic polyol

roller-bottle cultures which are operated in virus vaccine-producing laboratories throughout the world. Large-volume cultures do not promote light penetration and industrial-scale cultures in metal vessels are not at risk. Light intensity is a factor as it can be demonstrated that hybridoma cells are seriously impaired in their growth when sited 1–2 ft† from a fluorescent light source but unaffected at a distance of 6 ft (S. Musgrave, personal communication).

(iii) Temperature: Although some experiments (27, 57) have been done at temperatures other than 37 °C, such experiments are relatively rare. The results showed that at 32 °C there was little change in the specific antibody production rate compared with that of cells growing at 37 °C (27), and that if the temperature is reduced as low as 28 °C the productivity of the culture halved and then increased almost linearly with temperature thereafter, returning to maximum production at 37 °C (57).

(iv) pH: Cells in culture are sensitive to external pH but the effect is not dramatic over a broad performance plateau between pH 6.8 and 7.6. Provided that cultures can be kept within such bounds, even though

† 1 ft = 12 in; 1 in = 2.54 cm.

there may be fluctuations on a major scale (± 0.4 pH units from 7.2), the cells appear to function normally. Precise control of pH so that a fluctuation of only ± 0.02 pH units is permitted does not seem to improve productivity significantly (61).

(v) Dilution rate and growth rate: By contrast with the parameters discussed above, those investigators who have used continuous cultures to study the physiology of the antibody production system from hybridoma cells have considered dilution rate (or growth rate, where cell numbers are held to be relatively constant) as a primary physical variable worthy of investigation. Birch *et al.* (1) and Subhash *et al.* (2) found little change in the amount of antibody produced per 10^6 cells when the growth rate varied between 0.01 and 0.04 h. It seems that cultures were not easy to maintain outside these conditions. This observation is borne out by the study by Himmler *et al.* (27) where the growth rate varied between 0.02 and 0.05 h with little correlation between growth rate and antibody production. Other workers (63) have tended to operate at flow rates of one reactor volume per day, i.e. with doubling times of 24 h or a growth rate of 0.0287 h. However, recent work in the author's laboratory has demonstrated a decrease in the specific productivity of antibody with increases in the dilution rate (P. Hayter, N. Kirkby & R.E. Spier, unpublished data) (Fig. 5.1*d*).

5.5.2. *Nutritional factors*

The nutritional factors can be most readily divided into those of metabolites whose biochemistry is relatively well understood and other materials which are either complex (serum) or whose role in antibody production, although seeming necessary, is not fully comprehended.

5.5.2.1. *Simple basic metabolites*

The metabolites which have received most attention are those of glucose and oxygen, followed by glutamine (and hence ammonia ± ammonium ions) and lactate.

(i) Glucose and lactate: Concepts, which have yet to be given firm experimental foundation, abound. For example, much of the glucose which disappears during cell cultivation can be accounted for as lactic acid produced (the conversion factors tend to be in the range 70–90%) (66, 67) and as the lactic acid produced decreases the pH of the medium, cell growth is retarded. However, where the pH is controlled, cells will thrive at quite high concentrations of sodium lactate (2.5–3 mg/ml) relative to the concentrations to which the cells are exposed in most culture situations (35, 68). Attempts to cut down lactate formation by controlled

feeding of glucose in a chemostat culture whose instantaneous glucose concentration was held below 0.01 g/l were successful in the sought-after aim but the cell growth was not substantially improved (66). An alternative approach using different carbohydrate feeds (fructose, galactose, pyruvate) (69, 70) has been tried many times, yet formulated culture media rely, virtually exclusively, on glucose as the primary source of carbohydrate. Fructose might, however, be a viable substitute for glucose in non-dividing cell cultures. In such cultures the rate of lactic acid production would be expected to be lowered (§5.3). More recently glutamine has been used as a primary carbon source (71, 72) but with little substantive success (see below) in terms of its use as a replacement for glucose in cell cultures.

Although it is necessary to recognise that each combination of cell–medium–bioreactor can be different, it is still useful to observe the rate of utilisation of glucose in relation to the volume of medium required to nurture the cells in the reactor. Two different situations should be considered: one in which cells are actively dividing and the total number of cells in the fixed volume of the bioreactor is increasing, and the other in which there is no net increase in cell number (although cells may be dividing, others are dying). In addition to the rate of cell division, the glucose consumption rate is markedly affected by the dissolved oxygen levels (73) (Table 5.9). Thus, while cells are growing and increasing in number, one gram of glucose can support $0.1–1.4 \times 10^9$ cells, whereas in 'static' culture the figure is increased tenfold to $2.0–12.9 \times 10^9$ cells/g of glucose consumed. Such figures should indicate that in 'static' cultures it should be practicable to use ⅓–⅒ of the medium one used to obtain the number of cells which are held viable but not increasing in cell number. These figures also define the amount of medium needed to maintain such cultures when the medium has been formulated to a specification which has the highest possible ratio of glucose to other medium components. Under such operating conditions, and assuming an 85% conversion of glucose to lactate, the buffering capacity of the medium and/or the efficacy of the pH control system become critical elements in the prosecution of successful cultures.

(ii) Glutamine and ammonia: The major problem with the use of glutamine as the major source of carbon is that it is excessively endowed with nitrogen. The ratio of carbon atoms to nitrogen atoms in animals is about 7.2 : 1 (calculated from data in (74)), whereas the equivalent ratio for glutamine is 2.5 : 1. The result is that cultures fed glutamine tend to build up higher concentrations of ammonia and ammonium ions in their supernatants. Opinions differ as to the concentration of ammonia–ammonium which retards cell growth or peformance. For example, BHK21 C13 cells grown in medium containing glutamine at

Table 5.9. *Cell numbers per gram of glucose consumed*

	Culture conditions			
Cell type	increasing cell no.	static cell no.	No. of cells/g glucose consumed ($\times 10^{-9}$)	Reference
BHK suspension			0.5–1.4	73
BHK monolayer	√		0.5–0.7	82
chick embryo fibroblasts	√		0.1–0.13	unpublished[1]
BHK 21 suspension	√		1.388	100
HeLa suspension	√		0.472	14 (by calc.)[2]
LS suspension	√		1.216	14 (by calc.)
WI-38 monolayer	√		0.12	14 (by calc.)
MRC-5 monolayer	√		0.144	14 (by calc.)
Bri-8 suspension (lymphoblastoid)	√		0.256	14 (by calc.)
hybridoma		√	12.9	35 (from Fig. 14 assuming 4.5 g/l at start)
hybridoma		√	6.3	68 (assuming 2 l culture vol.)
hybridoma		√	2.0	55

Source:
[1] J.P. Whiteside & R.E.S., unpublished observations.
√*Note:*
[2] By calculation; involves using a dry mass per cell of 600×10^{-12} g (97).

4 mM and with additional 2 mM ammonium chloride grew to over 75% of the cell concentration of the unsupplemented control (75). The amount of ammonia present in the supernatant in these experiments was 3 mM. Similar results were reported by Reuveney *et al.* (68); on the other hand, Hu *et al.* (66) found that adding ammonium to the culture at the 7 mM level was strongly inhibitory (50%) yet when the lactate concentration was increased by 3.0 mg/ml the effect of twice that ammonium concentration (6 mM) was only inhibitory by 20% compared with the case without additional lactate and additional ammonium. This result indicates that ammonium lactate was not particularly inhibitory. The effect of deliberate additions of ammonium lactate to cultures has not (at the time of writing) been reported, to the authors' knowledge. As yet the specific removal of ammonia from the cell culture has not been achieved in a way which has resulted in higher productivities of antibodies.

5.5.2.2. *Serum*

Most of the long-term perfused cultures have used low-serum or serum-free medium. Some such media have been supplemented with proprietary compositions; others have not. It is possible to generalise from observations of the literature (19, 56) that it often proves beneficial to periodically dose the cell cultures with a medium which contains a greater than normal serum concentration. It could be that when process parameters express a downturn (rate of utilisation of oxygen or glucose at constant medium flow rate) investigators 'boost' the system with a dose of serum-containing medium. The subtle and careful use of this operable parameter can result in the ability to hold dense cultures in the productive phase for periods of many months' duration. It would be reasonable to infer that the 'serum boost' was an enabling event leading to the maintenance of the level of cellular activity (the integral of cell number multiplied by the activity per cell).

5.5.2.3. *Other chemical components*

The addition of a widely diverse set of chemicals (Table 5.8) to media used for the growth and exploitation of hybridoma cells has proved in particular cases to be beneficial. Careful studies of the effects of different concentrations of such materials, either singly or in combination, leads to the formulation of a particular medium for a particular cell line. Sometimes different cell lines will benefit; at other times they will not receive any advantage. In any event the determination of the role of such materials as selenium, ethanolamine, and oleic acid as growth factors will keep cell biologists well engaged for some time to come.

5.6. The technologies used to produce large quantities of monoclonal antibodies from cells held in culture

The preceding sections have introduced many of the concepts which are presently under intensive examination by those microbial biotechnologists (engineers) whose job it is to exploit the monoclonal antibody-productive potential of hybridoma cells grown in culture. Meetings of the American Chemical Society in 1984, the European Society for Animal Cell Technology in 1982, 1984 and 1985 and the Hanover meeting (Biotechnology '85) all testify to the adage 'there is more than one way to skin a cat'. The job of the microbial biotechnologist is, however, not just to achieve a given level of performance but to design, build and operate a system such that other systems are rendered less competitive in terms of being less able to manufacture product at a lower cost, with a higher quality and with greater reliability and consistency. This challenge is not simple. Many biotechnologists have drawn up lists of what they perceive would be an ideal bioprocess system for the manufacture of monoclonal antibodies (1). An extended version of such a list is presented in Table 5.10. Were the data available, it would be possible to compose a matrix within which a number could be assigned to each parameter in Table 5.10 against each technique purported to fulfil the role of the most ideal production system. It would then become clear which technique is likely to become equivalent to the stirred tank reactor, of general utility to the rest of the fermentation industry. However, each proponent of a particular technology has used a cell line unique (often) to that proponent's laboratory, a medium formulated to a unique specification and a diversity of product assay systems which wholly precludes real comparisons between the performance of various techniques and laboratories (2). Yet it remains important to focus on this issue. For there will emerge a dominant technique, and those skilled in the art of that technique will have a competitive advantage over those who belatedly move in the direction of the dominant trend. The subsequent sections of this chapter will, therefore, review those techniques which are in competition for the achievement of the dominant position. The authors do not claim to be prescient; so the outcome of the present activities cannot be judged with certainty. There is, however, a superfluity of opportunity to which the authors hope to offer the reader a guide, along with an appreciation of the prospects and the problems. This should lead to the inspiration of those insights which will promote the achievement of better decision making.

5.6.1. *The scope of the problem*

The challenge to the decision makers is to choose a front runner from a wide-ranging and diverse plethora of alternative technologies. There are on offer systems of cells in suspension at operating concentrations from 5×10^6 cells/ml to 5×10^7 cells/ml: cells attached to surfaces under conditions of relatively low cell densities (in the reactor itself), 10^6 cells/ml to 10^7–10^8 cells/ml, or cells held, entrapped or immured at concentrations (in the cell-containing portion of the reactor) of up to and beyond 5×10^8 cells/ml.

5.6.1.1. *The units of measurement*

The yield of product from animal cells can be expressed in a number of ways; the reader should be clear about what he is being informed.

Yield of product per unit animal cell (or per unit weight or measure of biomass) tells readers about the physiology of the cells and the degree to which those cells are performing in relation to some 'animal cell biomass ultimate capability'; it

Table 5.10. *Properties of an idealised unit process for monoclonal antibody production from cells in culture*

(The process involves the conversion of raw materials to final products.)

Can be scaled up and down
  Operational range 0.01–10 000 l
Reliable and reproducible
  straightforward operating procedures: technician friendly
  sterilisable at 121 °C and with a maintainable asepticity
  ready availability of components
  available without legal requirements
Cost effective
  low capital and space requirements
  labour- and consumable-sparing
  high-yielding
    homogeneous: a sample represents the whole
    monitorable and controllable
Upstream process yields materials which render the downstream operations efficient
High quality, purity, activity and consistency of product
Flexible
  process intensity
  scale
  mode of operations
All cell substrates
  hybridomas (murine, human, bovine, ovine)
  immobilised cells
All product types
Regulatory agency clean bill of health

does not necessarily relate to economic or system performance.

Yield of product per unit of medium used expresses one of a number of important factors which may be relevant to the overall economics of the process but which may also relate to the physiology of the cell; when a recycle or make-up system is used, it may reflect a more materially efficient process. Clearly the factor of overall raw material cost to the process is contained within this parameter, as is some indication of the cost of the downstream process concentration and purification procedures.

Yield of product per unit volume of bioreactor per unit of time is a measure of the efficiency of one of the key elements in the production system; however, this factor can be misleading because in some bioreactors where the cells are held at high cell densities per unit volume (in excess of 10^8/ml) either a large or small volume of medium may be made to flow through the cell-containing part of the system. Under such circumstances it is more relevant to the determination of the space requirement of the bioreactor system to consider the volume of all the components which have been used to hold and feed the mass of animal cells in the system.

Cost of a unit weight of final product at a defined state of purity is perhaps a valuable determinant of the efficiency of a process, yet it is a parameter which is seldom determined and often difficult to acquire. It is also critically dependent on the performance of the cell and on medium utilisation efficiencies; however, it does represent an economic absolute which is of great relevance to a manufacturer when deciding on a system for the generation of a particular bioproduct using animal cells as the primary production agent.

5.6.2. *Cells in suspension*

Cells, unidisperse and homogeneously distributed throughout the volume of suspending culture medium, may be held to be cells in suspension. There are three major manifestations of this technology. The most common is based on the stirred tank reactor; the second is a modification of that type of reactor to enable medium perfusion or continuous culture with cell removal from the discharge stream and cell recycling back into the main bioreactor; and the third alternative is the use of air-lift reactors which are most often, but not always, characterised by the absence of a stirrer in the culture fluids.

5.6.2.1. *The basic stirred tank reactor*

There is little doubt that the basic stirred tank reactor is a highly versatile, reliable and cost-effective tool for the production of monoclonal antibodies from hybridoma cells. It works well over scales of operation from 0.01 l to 10 000 l (Figs 5.4–5.6) and over the whole of this range the stirrer can be impelled by a magnetic coupling which obviates the need for a shaft which penetrates the vessel wall and thereby constitutes a hazard to the ascepticity of the culture. These reactors score highly on most of the major points of Table 5.9 with the exception that they have limited scope for increasing the process intensity (defined in terms of cell concentration) nor are they particularly adaptable to operating in the perfused or continuous modes over long periods of time. Their prime advantage is that they scale up and down with facility and represent the

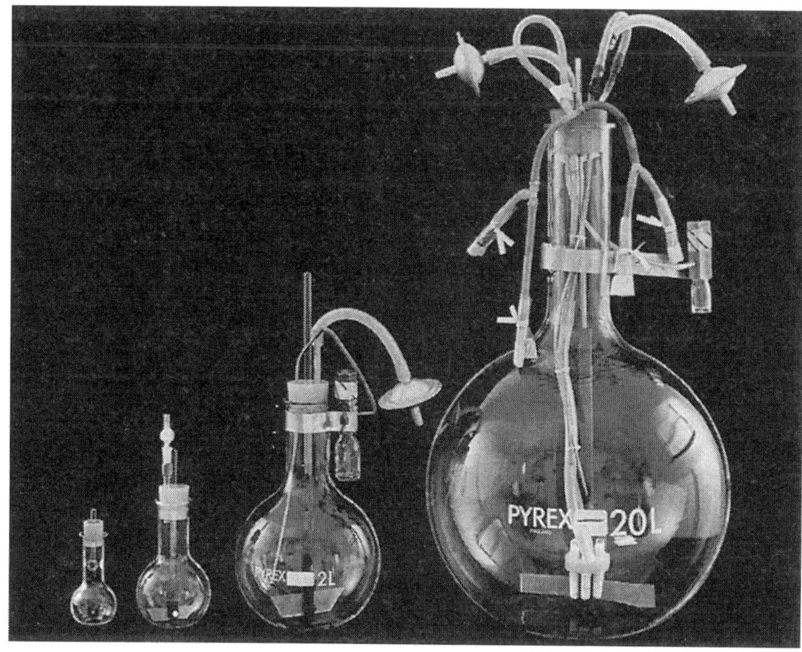

Fig. 5.4. Bottom-driven, magnetically coupled, simple stirred tank reactors for cultures of volume 0.1–10 l.

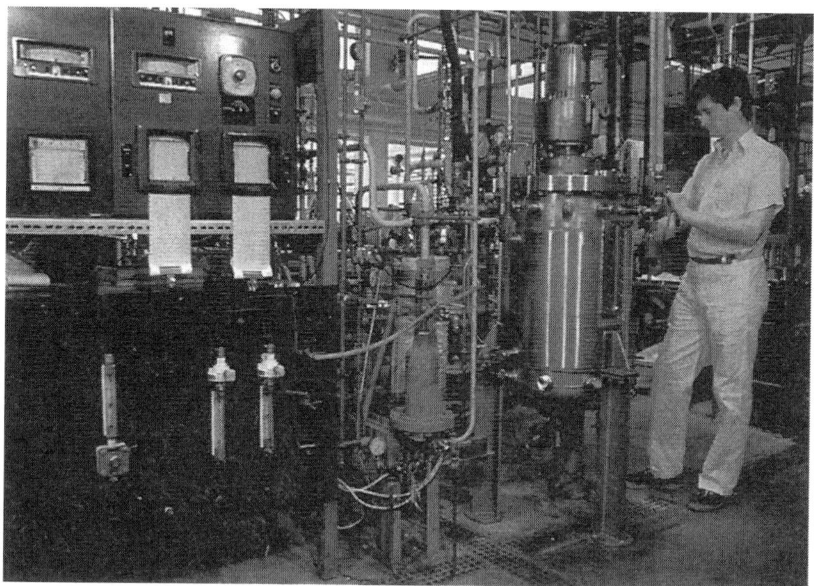

Fig. 5.5. A top-driven, magnetically coupled, stirred tank reactor at the 100 l culture volume scale.

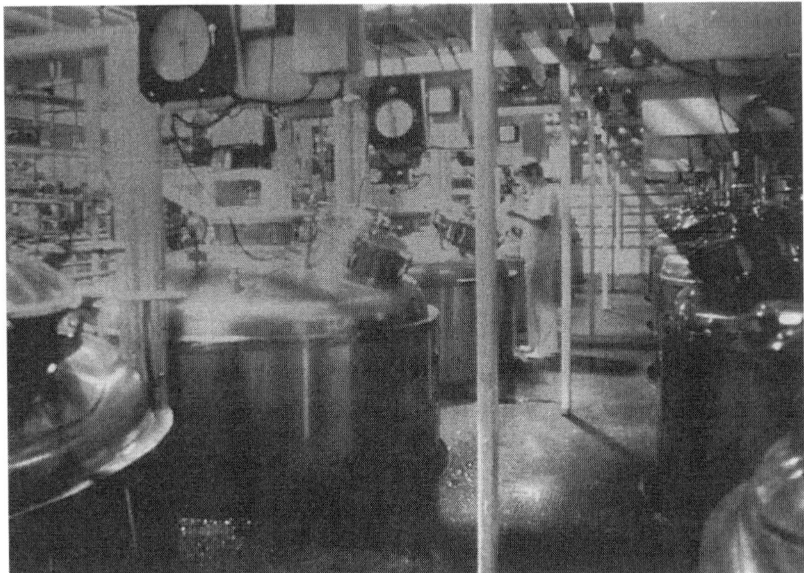

Fig. 5.6. Culture tanks at the 8000 1 scale, driven by a magnetically coupled stirrer (courtesy of Wellcome Biotechnology plc).

most simple and hence most straightforward and robust technology that enables a moderate level of cost and effective performance to be achieved with relative ease.

5.6.2.2. *The developed stirred tank reactor*

To overcome the limitations of the basic stirred tank reactor, investigators have operated the system in such a way that it (a) runs continuously, as opposed to a batch mode and (b) operates with cell recycle back to the main reactor. This latter option can be achieved either by preventing the cells from leaving the reactor with the discharging culture fluids or by allowing the cells and culture fluid to leave the reactor, then separating the cells from the discharged fluids and returning them to the reactor. The three modes of operation are depicted in Fig 5.7.

(i) The continuous culture option: This option does not attempt to concentrate the cells in the bioreactors. Thus it has an advantage over the basic stirred tank reactor in that

(i) it generates a constant environment in terms of nutrient concentrations of which one can be held to be growth limiting (a consequence of operating under a known and definable growth-limiting nutrient is that it presents the cells with a controllable stress

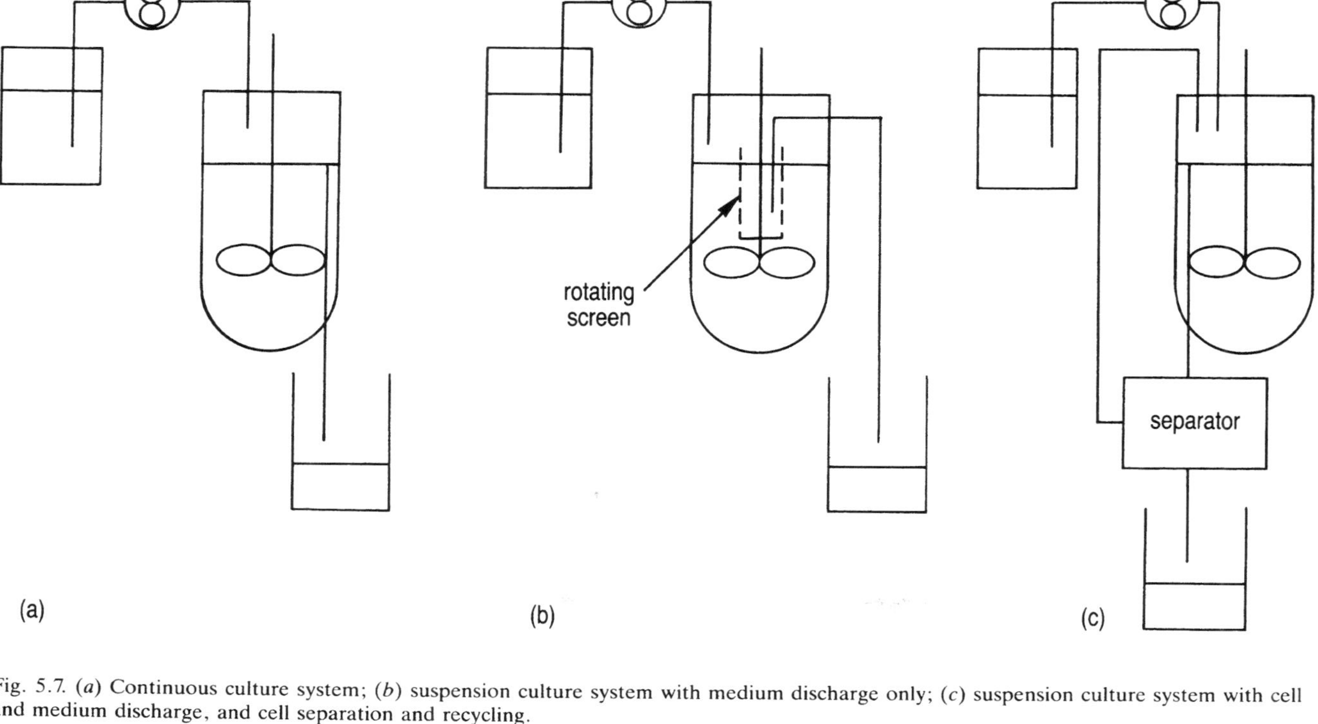

Fig. 5.7. (*a*) Continuous culture system; (*b*) suspension culture system with medium discharge only; (*c*) suspension culture system with cell and medium discharge, and cell separation and recycling.

of the type known to enhance the production of secondary metabolites in the antibiotic industry);

(ii) once set up the system is easy to operate and less labour-intensive than the batch system, and also uses fermenter capacity most efficiently;

(iii) it is possible to discover the effect of changes in the level of a single physical parameter on growth rate or productivity;

(iv) it is possible to run the system under computer control for self-optimisation (76).

In spite of such advantages cell concentrations rarely exceed 5×10^6 cells/ml and indeed tend to hover in the 1–3 $\times 10^6$ cells/ml area (1, 19, 62). Thus the potential gains in cost-effectiveness from process intensification have not been achieved in this type of system.

(ii) Continuous cultivation with cell concentration: The first such perfusion system was that of Himmelfarb *et al.* in 1969 (32). It was based on removing medium, but not cells, by using a spinning filter mounted on the vessel stirrer shaft. Van Wezel (63) and others (35, 68) have adapted this technology for monoclonal antibody-producing hybridoma cells. The system can be operated in four modes: (i) batch, (ii) continuous without filtration, (iii) continuous with filtration and (iv) continuous with filtration and with spent medium recycle at different flow rates and discard rates. With such a system, cell concentrations of about 3×10^7/ml (35, 63, 68) can be sustained and maintained for up to seven weeks of continuous operation (35). In such systems it is often observed that two to three times as many cells can be kept in the culture system for the expenditure of a given volume of medium, compared with normal continuous cultures. Such an observation would corroborate the data in Table 5.9, which show that cultures with static numbers of cells require ⅓–⅒ as much glucose as do cultures whose overall cell numbers are increasing.

The filters used in these systems have pores in the 1–10 μm range and are made of sintered metal (stainless steel) or porous ceramic. The essential problem in these systems is filter blockage. This becomes particularly acute when a high flow rate of medium is required to nurture the cells, particularly with oxygen, at the high cell concentrations generated in the main body of the reactor. It is possible to control the blinding of the filter to some degree by spinning it at 80 r.p.m. in a side chamber or by 'wiping' its face with a rotating cleaning device (35). However, such heroic techniques do not scale up or scale down well. Furthermore, as the cell concentration increases the blocking problems are disproportionately exacerbated. This feature is reflected in the maximum cell concentrations quoted for such systems: 3×10^7 cells/ml (35, 68). A futher disadvantage of such systems is that the time or extent of filter blockage cannot be predicted, so the process is less reliable than one in which the performance of all the component parts can be relied upon. In summary, this process suffers from limitations in process intensity, technological complexity, unreliability and lack of scaleability; although it offers a way of modifying an easy system (the basic or developed continuous suspension system) into a system operating at higher intensity it runs into complications that defeat the aim of the exercise.

(iii) Continuous cultivation with cell recycling: The logistics of cell recycle are depicted in Fig. 5.7. The difficulty is in the continuous separation of the cells from the cell–medium slurry which discharges from the vessel. There are several ways in which this can be achieved. One method is based on tangential filtration using a 0.22 pore size sterilisation membrane (51); this method has already been demonstrated as having the capability of separating animal cells from their culture fluid. An alternative is continuous flow centrifugation. Although such a method has been developed for use in single-cell protein production systems, the engineering difficulties inherent in using a steam-sterilisable centrifuge are not easy to overlook. The most significant problem is the maintenance of a sterile barrier around the drive shaft that rotates the separation chamber of the centrifuge. From a technical viewpoint this suffers from the same disadvantages as the previously described methods of adapting suspension cell culture to the intensive mode. It has some advantages over the spinning filter systems described above in that the turbulent flow of fluid over the membrane prevents the membrane from blocking, and also because such filtration systems can be bought 'off the shelf' and in diverse sizes, thus enabling some degree of experimentation at smaller as well as larger scales of operation.

5.6.2.3. *The air-lift reactor*

H. Katinger was the first proponent of the air-lift reactor as a bioreactor suitable for growing the allegedly 'shear-sensitive' animal cells (33). Indeed, the concept that animal cells are shear-sensitive has persisted without solid justification. Such views may well be misfounded, as was observed by R.C. Dean, Jr, who noted that the fragility of red blood cells was not brought about by turbulent hydrodynamics in pumps but by biochemical reactions induced by the blood vessel walls (77). Nevertheless, this concept, that air-lift reactors generate a benign hydrodynamic environment, was taken up by Smart for use in cultivating plant cells (78) although Fowler has now reverted to the use of a stirred tank reactor for those cells (79). (See also 20.)

The air-lift reactor was given prominence in two unrelated contexts. The one was a 10^6 l (working volume) air-lift reactor for single-cell protein (ICI, Billingham: numerous news items, 1983–85); the other was a 10^3 l reactor for hybridoma cells (1). The latter works at a cell concentration of 3–7 × 10^6 cells/ml and generally operates in the batch mode. The cells normally require serum (0.5–10%) and the product has to be concentrated prior to purification; this process must perforce also concentrate serum proteins, resulting in technically difficult purification processes downstream from the bioreactor. This system also requires the application of antifoam and probably makes use of polyols such as Pluronic F68 to reduce the damage induced by bubble disengagement (20).

In engineering terms, a reactor without an impeller must offer the advantages of simplicity and robustness with a bonus that cultures are not exposed to the contamination hazard of a discontinuous vessel exterior. On the other hand the unit is not flexible in that both mixing and aeration are achieved by one agent, the bubbles. There is little doubt that oxygen transfer rates in such systems are adequate or even energetically efficient. It is also possible to change the composition of the gas bubbles so as to control aeration rates without changing the hydrodynamic mixing conditions. Yet the span of conditions between those which cause adequate mixing and those which lead to blow-out is limited and although reasonable reactors can be built and operated down to the 1–2 l scale the more extensive flexibility of the 0.01 l reactor is denied by this technology. A further limitation is built into the operational flexibility where the pH is controlled by the gas composition.

A low-intensity process with limited flexibility yet simple and robust, easy to sterilise although requiring specialised buildings once the scale of operations exceeds 1000 l, the air-lift forms a useful introduction to cell cultivation, as does the basic stirred tank reactor, but in a highly competitive environment the need for efficient production militates against this low-intensity technology.

5.6.3. *Cells attached to surfaces*

Section 5.6.2.2. described some of the problems of cells which cannot easily be separated from the culture medium. Were cells attached to a surface, then the culture medium could be removed from the reactor and replaced by further medium at will. Although there are many techniques for growing, in unit process systems, large quantities of anchorage-dependent cells (reviewed by R.E.S. in 1980 and 1985 (48, 80) the process intensity is generally low. Typically, cells may be present in a part of a bioreactor at a concentration of 1.5 × 10^6 cells/ml. (This would apply to both glass sphere and microcarrier-based anchorage-dependent cell bioreactors.) However, surface-based cultures may be effected at cell densities in excess of this (Table 5.11). It is clear from the table that, in the part of the reactor containing the beads, cell densities from 4 × 10^7 to 1 × 10^9 cells/ml can be obtained, in theory.

Table 5.11. *Number of monolayer cells on beads of different sizes*

bead diam. (mm)	bead SA (mm^2)	beads/ ml	cells[1]/ bead	cells/ ml
3	28.6	37	278 407	10×10^6
1	3.14	1000	30 877	30×10^6
0.3	0.286	37 000	2784	100×10^6
0.1	0.0314	1 000 000	308	300×10^6

Note:
[1] As a monolayer of 12 μm diameter spheres made cuboid.

Thus it is possible, in a packed bed reactor of 3 mm glass spheres, to obtain a cell concentration in the bed of about 10^7 cells/ml of fluid in the bed (the fluid in a bed of randomly packed spheres occupies about half its volume). At the other extreme a bed of packed, hydrated microcarriers of 0.1–0.2 mm diameter could provide enough surface for about 10^9 cells, or manifest a cell concentration of twice that. Clearly, in the latter case there is insufficient space for the cells, so the system would operate at cell concentrations below this calculated value.

Most hybridoma cells do not stick readily to normal surfaces, although some do adhere to glass (25) and others may attach to microcarriers (35). People have attempted to grow hybridomas or microcarriers in the dynamic quasi-suspension cell mode without much success (work in the laboratory of R.E.S. and others) so the surface-dependent cultures which have been developed have been designed so that the medium is made to flow past the cells, which are held stationary on a stack of horizontal glass discs (25) or in a packed bed of microcarriers (35).

It is implicit in such systems that the primary problem is that of inhomogeneity. Medium flowing across or down a bed has nutrients removed and waste products added as it moves through the bed. The cells at the discharge end are exposed to a different set of nutritional conditions than those at the entry side. A second source of inhomogeneity is that caused by channelling. This results from the preferential flow of the irrigating medium through some parts of the bed, where the resistance to flow is less than in other parts of the bed where the cells may have grown so as to occlude spaces which would have been used by the circulating medium. Clearly, this problem is much accentuated when the bead sizes decrease to about 1 mm or below, yet problems can be observed in packed beds of 3 mm spheres which have been perfused continuously for many months. Two solutions to such problems are available. The first involves the periodic alternation of the direction of flow of the perfusing medium; the second requires the use of pumps capable of operating against a sizeable pressure head (10 lbf/in^2 or more). Such pumps could be magnetically coupled gear pumps, as opposed to the positive-displacement peristaltic pumps, which generate a reliability hazard resulting from the wearing away of the deformable pump tubing by the incessant friction of the driven rollers.

However, the attached-cell system does offer the opportunity for process intensification. For such a process to work the cell has to be such that it will attach to the surface made available. This reduces the availability of the systems to many of the existing hybridoma cells and to those cells which have been specifically designed or engineered to stick to commonly available surfaces. Modification of a glass or polystyrene substratum so that all kinds of cells will adhere (R.E.S, unpublished work, 1986) is an alternative but in the absence of proven materials this approach is not available at the time of writing. There is, however, the possibility of using open sponge-like matrices made of polyester (81).

By most of the other criteria of Table 5.10, however, the production of antibodies from cells immobilised in a static bed can be recognised as an advantageous method. The scale range of 0.1 l to about 400 l medium volume has already been demonstrated (82) (P. Brown (Bioresponse), personal communication, Jan. 1986). The equipment is simple, free of legal encumbrance (to the authors' present knowledge) and capable of operating under a wide variety of modes and control options. Its chief disadvantage is the lack of homogeneity and also the difficulty in obtaining a representative sample of the cellular materials (48). Nevertheless, such systems provide a useful introduction into high-intensity processes although their productivities may be difficult to maximise with regard to cost-efficiency.

5.6.4. *Cells entrapped*

Cells which are entrapped are those which are held within a restraining matrix where the boundaries of the matrix allow for some degree of escape from that matrix. This category of reactor includes some of the situations depicted in Figure 5.8. The ingenuity of the animal cell biotechnologists has led to the development and testing of three types of entrapped system and three types of immured system. These techniques will be described below.

5.6.4.1. *Inertial entrapment*

A development of the concept of trapping cells by virtue of their tendency to settle into a hole or pit and stay there while the fluid medium passes

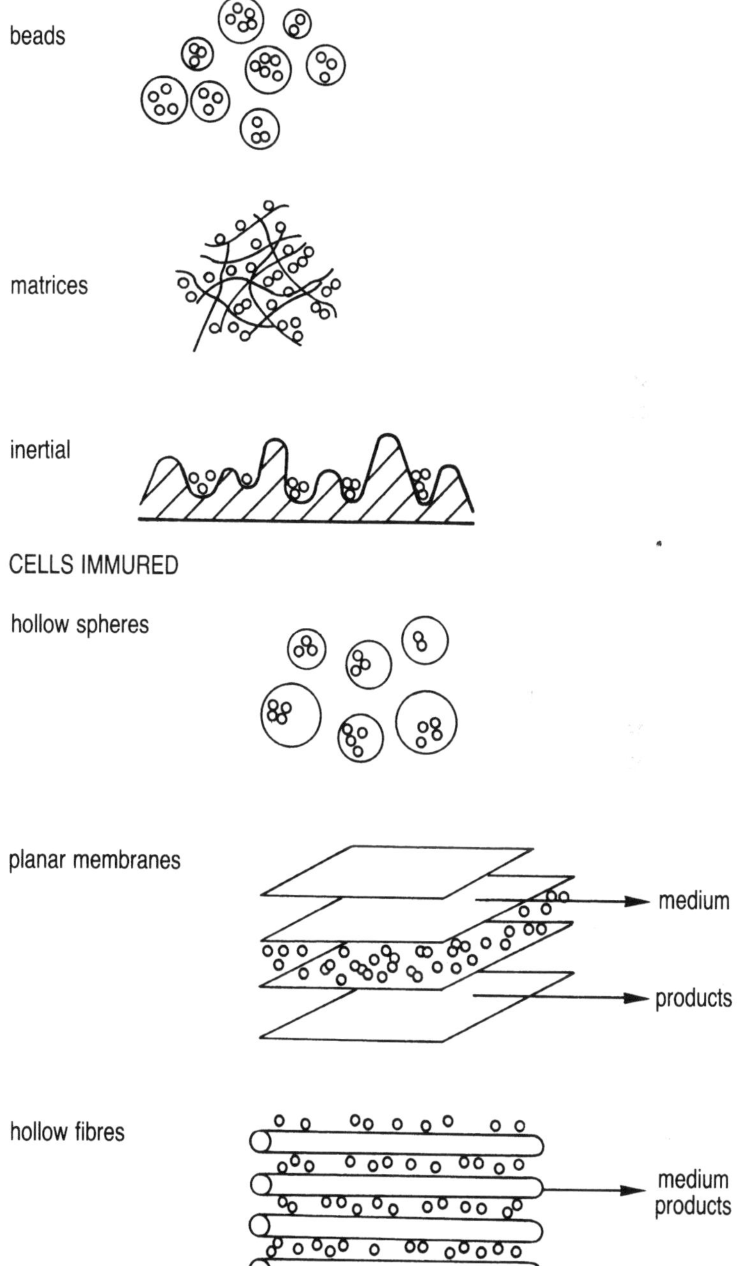

Fig. 5.8. Cells, entrapped and immured.

by is the construction of a tubular film reactor (83). This device may be likened to a roller bottle with partitions stationed down its length in a manner which divides the bottle into a number of cylindrical segments. The partitions are annular and extend about a quarter of a diameter from the bottle periphery towards the centre. When medium and cells are poured into the bottle the segments partially fill to the point when the liquid laps over from one segment to the next. The result is that, when the bottle is rotating at about 1 r.p.m., the unattached cells stay in their compartment in the fluid at the bottom of the bottle while a thin film of medium is carried round with the bottle and is aerated as in a normal roller-bottle culture. In this system, however, when medium is added at one end the overflow may be removed from the other while retaining the cells in the segmented section of the vessel. This system can be further developed by coating the material of the segments with polyester fibres so as to (a) allow some cell types to form an attached cell system (see above) or (b) to move more medium and cells into the gas phase for better gas transfer. This system is as yet untried; it serves to advance the technology in demonstrating the feasibility of holding cells which do not normally attach to surfaces in indentations or pits. While so entrapped the cells may be developed to the high cell densities required.

5.6.4.2. *Porous ceremic entrapment*

The adaptation of the normal ceramic matrix, to which hybridoma cells would not adhere, to a novel and more porous ceramic matrix in which hybridoma cells could become entrapped is a relatively recent development (84). The performance data available suggest that in the volume of the reactor, defined as the volume of the porous or textured ceramic cartridge of approximately 1500 ml, it is possible to produce and hold some 5×10^{10} cells; this gives a cell concentration of about 3×10^7 cells per millilitre of reactor volume. Assuming that the cartridge has to be kept full of fluid all the time (a fluid volume of about half the reactor volume) this would give a maximum cell concentration, in the fluid that has to be present, of 6×10^7 cells/ml. Although the feasibility of this system has been clearly demonstrated, certain questions remain in that it seems that such a system cannot be purchased without purchasing the peripheral control equipment. There is a difficulty in scale-up and scale-down. Although a smaller cartridge may be available the major route to scale-up is by ganging a number of the larger cartridges in a manifold. Although the system can achieve a moderate cell intensity, its lack of flexibility and relatively high capital cost would tend to weigh against its becoming a dominant technique for monoclonal antibody production.

5.6.4.3. *Gel entrapment systems*
The use of gel-entrapped animal cells for the production of monoclonal antibodies was first reported in 1983 (85). Since that time much work has been done (5) to demonstrate the feasibility of the system. Indeed little other than feasibility has, so far, resulted. The possibilities open to the plant biotechnologist of using calcium alginate gels is rendered more difficult for their animal cell counterparts as incubation temperatures are somewhat higher (+10 °C) which results in the beads becoming unstable in a relatively short time (a day or so). The alternative gel matrix, agarose, has also presented technical problems. An early problem came to light when it was reported that the quality of the paraffin oil has to be clearly specified (31). The method of bead formation is crucial: the beads should be formed without air pockets in them, neither should the bead contain droplets of the oil. This feat is relatively difficult to achieve with complete success. Indeed, it now seems clear that some of the early work quoted was done with that fraction of the beads which had separated themselves out from the 'contaminated' oil- and air-containing beads as a result of their higher density and tendency to sink to the bottom of the container in the bead-forming system (S. Musgrave, personal communication, 1986).

Subsequent discussion on this subject revealed that small (100 ml) quantities of beads can be made readily; difficulty was experienced, however, when this process was scaled up to the one or multi-litre scale (86).

A further problem of the bead system is that in a nutritive medium the cells grow and either grow out of the bead or cause the bead to break down (C. Morrison, unpublished undergraduate project, Surrey University, 1985). This requires that the cells be immobilised at the level at which they are to be maintained and held at that cell number by a judicious selection of a nutritive medium which enables the number of cells within the particle to remain stationary. This is an inherent disadvantage of the method, as the large numbers of cells needed for dense cell cultures would have to be made in a dilute cell system before entrapment. Also, individual workers have claimed that gases (in the form of bubbles) discharged from metabolising cells (carbon dioxide) could be responsible for bead breakdown (87). This contention requires careful examination as the possibility of gas entrapment during bead formation was not excluded.

Such beads can be held stationary in a packed bed reactor configuration (80, 82); they can also be fluidised. The motive force for the latter has generally been supplied by a rotary shaker, although other alternatives such as bubble or liquid medium flow-based fluidisation are possible. The overriding problem in such systems remains bead stability:

broken or compacted beads would cause blockage and channelling in static bed reactors, and in reactors where the beads are fluidised particle–particle attrition can result in a loss of homogeneity and problems of filter and column blockage in downstream processing operations. Nevertheless, it should be noted that yeast systems immobilised by calcium alginate gel have been used in multiples of the 4000 l scale static reactors for ethanol production at 30–32 °C (88).

There are clear alternatives to bead systems. Gel sheets have been used for plant cell systems (89, 6). Such sheets are built up about a sheet of coarse woven material which provides the sheet or slab with physical toughness and enables large gel sheets to be manipulated into and out of reactors. In the reactor the sheets are arranged in parallel format, rather like the plates in a heat exchanger or plate and frame filter press. The potential advantage of the sheet system or the bead has not been established for animal cell systems and indeed the inherent problems of such a system, such as casting the gel slab and then manipulating it into its position in the bioreactor, requires technologically complex processes and equipment.

Although gel entrapment offers an attractive method for immobilisation because of the wide range of options for the gel support, which, for animal cells can include gelatin and chitosan (90) as well as the carbohydrate gels referred to above, there are also many forms in which the system can be manipulated. Relatively few attempts have been made to exploit animal cells in such systems (91) so it is not possible to conclude that the systems are inappropriate, but rather that they have not been explored to a level which enables the inherent problems to be eliminated and where elegant, simple, robust and flexible techniques have been developed to capitalise on the entrapment properties of soft gels.

Fibroid systems: Gels offer a solvated fibrous matrix in which cells can be entrapped; it is also possible to use fibres which are solvated to form cell masses, balls or clumps (2, 92, 93). Such clumps are maintained in suspension either by a stirred agitator or by fluid or gas bubble mechanisms of fluidisation. Clearly, such systems are simple compared with the gel entrapment systems. The problems with them are that the clumps are not homogeneous; bits break away to the detriment of the downstream operations. The size of the particle, which forms by generating itself, is not easy to control, whereas using a pre-formed open mesh matrix of defined size enables some degree of control in this area. There are clear inhomogeneities within the morulae themselves. Gradients of nutrients and wastes will exist between the exterior and centre of the particle. At equilibrium the centre of the particle may be inhabited by dead cells which need not materially interfere with the production rate of the systems as a whole.

Data for such systems indicate that cell densities of 5×10^7/ml of the bioreactor are practicable, yet 10% of the cells remain in the supernatant. Even though the supernatant is far from devoid of particulates, recirculation rates of 10 l/min have been achieved. Downstream processing involves (i) cell and cell debris removal using a microporous filter, (ii) removal of all but 5% of the water by tangential flow ultrafiltration, (iii) a DEAE-derivatised column to remove proteins of lower molecular weight, (iv) HPLC final stage purification before (v) filter sterilisation and (vi) lyophilisation (2).

It is clear that such systems could be made to operate at both the 0.1 l and 10 000 l or more scales. Using sterilisable (at 121 °C) fibrous support materials, a simple, robust and reliable system can be built. Were such systems to move to higher cell intensities, improvements in cost effectiveness could be achieved. Overall, such systems offer many advantages and seem worthy of more intensive investigation and development.

5.6.4.4. *Cells immured*

Cells held within walls can be treated somewhat differently from cells entrapped within particles. Within the boundaries defined by the firm outer physical barrier to spatial movement, the cells are free to move or be moved. Under such circumstances the cell population may, if suitably manipulated, be (within itself) homogeneous. A further feature of such systems is that the nutrient medium provides the cell with sustenance only after it has crossed the boundary envelope while waste materials and products cross the boundary to return to the main body of the medium or are held within the boundary and are liberated when the boundary is dissolved for the purpose of product recovery. Three different systems conform to this description. The first is the microcapsule system (41); the second is a system where the cells, sandwiched between two porous planar membranes, are nurtured via one or both of those membranes (47); and the third manifestation involves the use of membranes in the form of hollow tubes or 'capillaries' (94).

(i) Microencapsulation: The basic method of producing microencapsulated cells consists of (i) forming a calcium alginate gel bead; (ii) coating the cell-containing, 500 μm diameter, gel sphere with a mixture of a number of long-chain polycations (poly-L-lysine, poly-L-arginine and poly-L-ornithine); and (iii) removing the original gel following its dissolution by the removal of the calcium ions by sodium citrate. Once the cell-containing capsule has been made, the cells are supplied with a nutrient medium which they obtain via the capsular wall. This enables them to grow to a concentration of 5×10^8 cells/ml of settled capsules and with a concentration in the bioreactor such that the capsules occupy

20–50% of the available space. However, the important parameter is the concentration of the product in the fluids prior to downstream processing, a feature which is determined by the mechanism of product release from the microcapsules (41). The need to add material to the settled capsules and process the resulting cell and cell debris results in a product concentration equivalent to that which would be made from having the settled capsules suspended in an equal volume of product-liberating solution. To convert this to terms by which the other systems have been discussed, it gives an effective cell concentration of 2.3×10^8 cells/ml.

Such microcapsule-immured cells can be nurtured in a more or less conventional stirred tank reactor. A feature of the market for monoclonal antibodies is that not only is there a need for large quantities of a single type of material, which could be many hundreds of kilograms, there is also a need to produce many batches of different antibodies, each of some tens of grams of material. This need is most appropriately met by fielding a suite of bioreactors. The majority would be small, 5–50 l volume units, while there would also be available units of scale of 1000–10 000 l in volume. The microencapsulated cell system just described lends itself to such developments.

A feature of this system is that the product is manufactured at a level of 20% of the non-cellular solid materials contained within the microcapsule. This facilitates the downstream processing. In one step, using an ion exchange column, material of 90% purity can be obtained. It is then relatively easy to upgrade this to 98%. The leading proponents of this field (Damon, Biotech, Inc.) hold that affinity purification is not without its problems. The difficulties may be listed as: (i) the antibody-capturing ligand may leak off the column, thus contaminating and deactivating, to an unknown extent, the resulting product; (ii) for each antibody produced a unique column has to be generated, a procedure which can make it difficult to obtain a standard and effective adsorbant; and (iii) processing monoclonal antibodies by affinity methods can decrease the biological activity of the antibody. Clearly, much remains to be achieved as many other manufacturers (Celltech UK for example) extol the virtues of affinity purification and even purifications based on the use of immobilised protein A (see also ref. 95 for review). It therefore can be concluded that each antibody–column system is, as yet, a unique entity and that the successes or failures of one laboratory do not necessarily carry over to the next laboratory, even when it tries to make this 'same material'. The trial and error approach is very much in evidence while the experiments needed to gain the understandings necessary to gain control of the technologies have yet to be commissioned.

To review: the microencapsulation technique excels in operating at high intensity with the ability to move easily into the downstream operations which are thereby, and as expected, simplified and cost-effective. The major drawback is the encapsulation process itself which represents a cost factor (for the polycations) and a technically sophisticated series of procedures to generate the microcapsules. A further problem is inherent in the use of a 500 μm diameter sphere which has been shown (see Appendices I–III) to be a size which curtails the oxygenation of the cells in the centre of the capsule. None the less, such systems do offer pointers to the art of the possible and hence the way ahead.

(ii) Parallel planar membrane reactors: Building on the concept of the plate and frame filter press and the plate heat exchanger, both well-tried and widely used process techniques in the chemical industry, a bioreactor which relied on holding cells in a series of membrane bounded compartments mounted in an array or stack can be perceived as having a potential for the growth and exploitation of animal cells. Such a reactor has been built (36) and a commercial version is available. The membranes used for the reactor can be based on the 0.2 μm medium sterilisation membranes, which can withstand sterilisation at 121 °C in flowing, wet steam. Clearly, other membranes which can both withstand the conditions of sterilisation and express different kinds of filtration properties can be used. This enables the cells to be provided with nutrient via one membrane while products and/or toxic wastes are separated from the cells by the second of the two bounding membranes.

The results reported to date (47) quote cell concentrations in the cell compartment of 6×10^7 cells/ml, a level approaching the level of process intensity which leads to cost-effectiveness. However, the investigators also report problems in sealing the edges of the membranes which, to retain the necessary spatial format, have to be kept apart by the use of stainless steel grids. This feature is carried through to the design of the massive header plates needed to generate the compressibilities required, without the bending in the centre, which would lead to poor sealings round the periphery. The system controls operate via an external reservoir and, as the medium compartment is an open and unblockable cavity, high pump-around rates can be achieved.

Although such systems can be scaled up, scale-down is not achieved without the involvement of all the peripheral systems. The system is not so robust and simple that it can be readily translocated from the development department to the production shop floor. It can, however, be operated aseptically for long periods and offers a high degree of versatility in terms of the ability to control process and product streams independently.

(iii) Tubular membrane reactors: For many years the American Vitafibre system with a 2 ml volume chamber was used to mimic conditions pre-

valent in living tissue (see (37) for review). Since about 1982–83, however, workers have made cartridges of 200 ml liquid capacity and have incorporated them into sophisticated computer-controlled environments, wherein they have demonstrated a capacity for sequestering and maintaining cells at high concentrations (*c*. 5 × 10^8 cells/ml) generally on the shell side of the tubular membranes, although it is also possible to grow the cells within the lumens of the tubes themselves (94, 55, 56). At present, the capillary tube units are purchased sterile as they have been X-ray decontaminated after manufacture. The scale-up of this system is dependent on using multiples of three 200 ml modules presently available. However, by the judicious use of the computer and its controlled hardware, it is possible to run each of a battery of modules as a separate reactor. In practice it is simpler to keep processes separate, and indeed were the products to be used as human injectibles it would be required that each cell line be kept in a separate area, let alone a module within a composite reactor.

The system is capable of providing for the mixing of the cells on the shell side of the reactor as the reactors can be rotated, shaken or rocked, or the fluids on the cell side can be pulsed or made to flow in alternate directions. Such attempts at mixing do bring rewards in terms of the achievement of longer times under conditions of continuous perfusion and higher yields per unit of cost expended (P. Brown, personal communication). Smaller (approximately 20 ml capacity) systems are available for test work so that although the cartridges do not have larger manifestations (2 l, 20 l) useful exploratory work can be effected on the small scale.

Systems can be based on cartridges presently used for kidney dialysis (55) or they may be units originally made for reverse osmosis systems. Unlike the planar membrane system, the user of the tubular membranes is constrained by those tubular membrane systems that are presently available from a commercial source. Inhomogeneities are expressed in terms of the lack of regularity in the spaces on the shell side of the tubular membrane reactor as well as in gradients set up between the tube membranes and those cells furthest away from such membranes. A further gradient is set up in the direction of nutrient flow. Such a gradient can be reversed by alternating the direction of flow of the nutrients, although the cells at the centre of the reactor will be disadvantaged vis-à-vis those at the ends of the cartridge.

A further development of the system would be the construction of cartridges in which two different kinds of tube were embedded. Arrangements at the end of the tube bundle could allow for nutrient flow in one set of tubes while the second set catered to the waste and/or product removal. Such a variant has not yet been described in operational circumstances.

The fully monitored, controlled and automated version of this system is a versatile and flexible operational package. It is more complex and less robust than other systems discussed and its capital cost is significant, although this latter feature could be lost were it amortised over the quantity of products generated. There is little doubt that as the process intensity is high the system offers some advantages; it has clearly and unequivocally demonstrated the feasibility of operating systems with cells held as dense masses for extended periods of time (months). Whether it can dominate this technique from this demonstrated feature remains to be seen, but it is a technique which is yet to be.

5.7. **Conclusions**

There have been many developments in the last few years, leading to hybridomas which excrete large quantities of antibody molecules, as well as to media low in (or free of) high-molecular mass proteinaceous materials. The technology to exploit such 'soft' process features has developed apace. This chapter has reviewed over twelve such techniques and some of their variants against a set of criteria which are used to establish the technique which will eventually dominate the field. That technique will be the most cost-effective when all factors have been fully taken into account. Such factors will include the way operators take to the system as well as the way the regulatory agencies view the quality of the resulting products. In addition, the ability of a system to be sparing of the expensive components of the nutritive medium will also weigh heavily in determining the outcome. The contesting techniques have, each in its unique way, demonstrated their prowess in generating and exploiting over long periods the antibody-generative potential of hybridoma cells in culture.

It would be premature to nominate the technique that is likely to dominate the field of dense cell cultures as the stirred tank reactor has dominated the field of suspension cell systems. From the various reactors described above and the delineation of the factors which affect their evaluation it may be possible to discern that type of technique likely to survive to the greatest extent. Whichever it is, it will open up a new era for the animal cell biotechnologist in that it will provide a capability to produce and exploit biomass, in media that will be almost as inexpensive as, and at scales of operation which will challenge, the most cost-effective processes which seek to make animal cell proteins in prokaryotes.

6 In conclusion: the diversity of application of monoclonal antibodies and hybridoma technology

The previous chapters dealt with the reasoning of how and why the mammalian immune system can be manipulated such that monoclonal, antibody-secreting hybridomas can be produced. The various biological, chemical and physical requirements for the production and culture of hybridomas were presented, as was a detailed description of the various assays used for detecting and characterising the hybridoma antibodies. The present chapter will be used to demonstrate, in conclusion, that monoclonal antibodies have found a wide range of uses, being applied in many different areas of the clinical and veterinary fields. The areas will be divided into research, diagnostics, preparative protein chemistry and immunochemistry, prophylaxis and therapeutics, and anti-idiotype antibodies. These categories will be discussed in this order, since this is the approximate chronological order of the development and application of monoclonal antibodies. Because the application of monoclonal antibodies in basic research has received most attention, particularly with respect to publication, this section will be subdivided into the different areas of microbiology, immunobiology and cell biology.

It is, however, impossible to cover all of these areas adequately in a single chapter, particularly a concluding chapter, nor can they be covered in a single volume. In the individual sections and subsections of this chapter, extensive reference will be made to recent reviews, monographs and books on each area of monoclonal antibody application, followed by selected examples to show how the MAb have been used and what the benefit of that application has been. An idea of how extensive this field is can be seen from the number of reviews already written (Table 6.1).

6.1. Research applications

The largest area in which MAb have been used is that of scientific research. This area can be divided, rather generally, under a number of heading: antigens and their structure; variation of the antigen under normal environmental conditions (especially under pressure of the immune system, for example, evasion by a pathogen of immune defences through alteration of the antigenic determinant repertoire by the microorganism); identification of subcompartments of the immune response,

Table 6.1. *Examples of the reviews concerning applications of monoclonal antibodies*

Subject	Reference
antigenic characterisation	1,2,3,4,5,6,7,8,9,10,11
antigenic variation	1,5,6,7,10,11
leukocyte differentiation	1,4,5,6,12,13,14,15
immunological function	4,6,11,12,13,14,15,16,17,18
cancer research	1,4,5,8,15,19
diagnosis	7,9,11,20,21
drug targetting	1,4,8,22,23,24,25
protection against disease	4,5,7,9,10,11,19,25
embryo development	15
receptor structure and function	8,26
cytoskeletal structure	8
plant sciences	9
neurology	1,4
enzymes	8

through analysis of the cell surface proteins on leucocytes, and the characterisation of regulatory pathways (helper and suppressor circuits); analysis of neoplasia; and other applications for MAb in research.

6.1.1. *Studies of antigens and epitopes*

The use of MAb in this area has produced a large amount of research material, culminating in a number of reviews, particularly in the fields of virology (1,2,3,5,6,7,9,10,11), immunology (1,5,6,9,11,12), cell biology (1,5,8,9), and biochemistry and genetics (1,5,8,9) (see Table 6.1 for a list of these and other reviews). The research in virology and immunology offers good examples of how MAb can be used to study the structure of antigens and epitopes. This section will concentrate on virological applications for MAb; whilst the work in the area of immunology will be discussed in §6.1.3.

Research into epitope expression on viral antigens began with influenza virus, and has continued since; it now covers representatives from each of the taxonomic groups of viruses. Table 6.2 gives examples, primarily of some of the first reports, of this work with different virus groups, in order to show how the research grew and expanded. The work

Table 6.2. *Examples of the research on epitope topology of viruses from each taxonomic group*

Virus group	Representative virus	References
herpesvirus	herpes simplex virus I	Howes *et al.* (27)
adenovirus	adenovirus 5	Russell *et al.* (28)
parvovirus	simian virus 40	Martinis & Croce (29)
	canine parvovirus	Burtonboy *et al.* (30)
hepadnavirus	hepatitis B virus	Cote *et al.* (31) Imai *et al.* (32)
rhinovirus	human rhinovirus 14	Sherry *et al.* (33)
aphthovirus	foot-and-mouth disease virus type O_1	McCullough & Butcher (34); McCullough *et al.* (35)
enterovirus	poliovirus	Ferguson *et al.* (36); Emini *et al.* (37); Minor *et al.* (38); Wiegers & Dernick (39)
	coxsackievirus	Cao *et al.* (40)
rotavirus	rotavirus	Greenberg *et al.* (41)
reovirus	reovirus	Burstin *et al.* (42)
orbivirus	bluetongue virus	Appleton & Letchworth (43)
myxovirus	influenza virus A	Gerhard *et al.* (44); Gerhard & Webster (45); Yewdell *et al.* (46); Laver *et al* (47); Webster & Laver (48)
paramyxovirus	Newcastle disease virus	Iorio & Bratt (49)
morbillivirus	measles virus	Norrby *et al.* (50); Sheshberdaran *et al.* (51); Sheshberdaran & Norrby (52)
	distemper virus	Orvell *et al.* (53)
	rinderpest virus peste des petits ruminants virus	McCullough *et al.* (54)
pneumovirus	respiratory syncytial virus	Gimenez *et al.* (55)
rhabdovirus	rabies virus	Wiktor & Koprowski (56); Lafon *et al.* (57)
	vesicular stomatitis virus	Volk *et al.* (58); Pal *et al.* (59)
alphavirus (togavirus)	sindbis virus	Chanas *et al.* (60); Schmaljohn *et al.* (61); Roehrig *et al.* (62)
	Venezuelan equine encephalomyelitis virus	Roehrig *et al.* (63)
flavivirus (togavirus)	tick-borne encephalitis virus	Heinz *et al.* (64)
bunyavirus	La Crosse virus	Gonzales-Scarano *et al.* (65)
retrovirus	mouse mammary tumour virus	Massey & Schochetman (66)
	murine leukaemia virus	Nowinski *et al.* (67); Lostrom *et al.* (68)
	bovine leukaemia virus	Bruck *et al.* (69)
	feline leukaemia virus	Grant *et al.* (70)

of Croce, Gerhard, Laver, Webster and co-workers with influenza virus, Nowinski, Lostrom and co-workers with murine retroviruses and Norrby, Sheshberadaran and co-workers with morbilliviruses are good examples of how certain types of antigenic determinant can be identified. They used viruses composed of an inner nucleoprotein core surrounded by a matrix protein, and a lipoprotein envelope through which glycoprotein 'spikes' protruded. The infectivity of the virus was associated with these glycoproteins, and the MAb showed that there was in fact more than one epitope on the glycoprotein spike related to virus infectivity. It was already known that certain viruses, indeed groups of viruses, carried more than one type of glycoprotein. This had been shown through differences in the functional activity of the glycoproteins. For example, influenza virus carries haemagglutinin and neuraminidase glycoproteins; measles virus carries haemagglutinin and haemolysin glycoproteins. The latter glycoprotein of measles virus has been related to fusion of adjacent infected cells; several viruses which do not have haemolytic activity have been shown to carry a fusion protein.

With the application of other more molecular analyses, the sites of the epitopes within the different glycoprotein molecules and the structure of those determinants were identified. The site of the epitopes was revealed from analyses of the amino acid sequence of glycoproteins from virus variants with which the MAb could or could not react. When a consistent difference between the sequences on MAb-resistant variants and the MAb-sensitive virus was noted, that was taken to be the region within which the MAb reacted, although amino acid changes outside the region could influence MAb reactivity through alterations of the tertiary and quaternary structure of the protein, glycoprotein, etc. X-ray crystallographic studies were able to put a three-dimensional structure on the glycoprotein, and as such a more accurate determination of both the site and structure of the epitopes. Consequently, it was demonstrated that some determinants relied on simple sequences of amino acids, whereas others were due to the conformational twisting of the protein. These types of epitope are termed, respectively, sequential or conformation-independent, and conformational or conformation-dependent epitopes. Such discrimination of epitopes was first described, using MAb, with the proteins of myoglobin and hen egg lysozyme. This description of epitopes has now been used for most antigens studied with MAb.

Viruses such as influenza virus, measles virus and the retroviruses, which are composed of a nucleoprotein core surrounded by an envelope through which glycoprotein 'spikes' protrude, are termed enveloped viruses. Much of the structural study on these viruses has concentrated on the glycoproteins, because these are the subunits most often associated with the infectivity of the virus and thus the protective immune response against infection by such viruses. There is a second group of viruses, the non-enveloped viruses, which are basically a nucleoprotein structure with no envelope. In contrast to the enveloped viruses, infectivity of the non-enveloped virus and the protective immune response against infection by such viruses is associated with the surface topography of the nucleoprotein. The major exception is the adenovirus group, the members of which carry 'spikes' – the penton fibres – with which the virus infectivity is associated.

Most non-enveloped viruses (where the infectivity is associated with the nucleoprotein unit) have been studied in a similar fashion to the influenza virus glycoprotein. Analyses with MAb have identified a number of sites of infectivity on the virion particle of foot-and-mouth disease virus (35), poliovirus (36–38) and rhinovirus (33), all members of the picornavirus group (the smallest known complete viruses). With the latter two, X-ray crystallographic studies have elaborated the findings with the MAb, identifying structures of sites and showing that more than one polypeptide in the nucleoprotein can be involved in the formation of an antigenic site (71). The latter results were important in the light of attempts to prepare polypeptide and synthetic peptide vaccines. An example of this is seen with foot-and-mouth disease virus, where MAb identified four sites involved in the protective immune response (72), only one of which was sequential and could therefore be synthesised simply from looking at the amino acid sequence of the virion polypeptides. Since foot-and-mouth disease virus has a high rate of antigenic variation, it may prove prudent to prepare vaccines which contain more than one of the infectivity-associated sites. Perhaps whole virus vaccines will always be more effective than peptide vaccines in the case of foot-and-mouth disease virus; only time will tell.

A natural extension to this work on epitope expression and variation was the application of MAb to the study and differentiation of variants of viral, bacterial and other parasitic pathogens. MAb have permitted an analysis of, for example, the antigenic determinants on streptococci, mycobacteria, *Neisseria, Plasmodium* spp., schistosomes, trypanosomes and other members of the family Trypanosomatidae, especially *Leishmania* spp. (1,4,8,9). Much of this research has led to applications in the study of the life-cycle of parasites and the more rapid, sensitive (accurate) or early diagnosis of infection. Although antigenic and immunogenic determinants have been identified, and have resulted in the possibility of producing and isolating new 'subunit' vaccines, it is the area of diagnosis where the MAb against such pathogens have had greatest impact. Because MAb can be used to diagnose, more accurately than antisera, the particular pathogen associated with a particular disease in a particular individual, a more efficient analysis of the epidemiology, pathogen variation, and perhaps also control of certain diseases may be made possible. The application of MAb to the diagnosis and epidemiology of diseases will be dealt with in §6.2; the following section will look at the application of MAb to study antigenic variation.

6.1.2. *Studies on antigenic variation and epidemiology*

As with epitope mapping, studies on antigenic variation with MAb found considerable applications in the field of virology. Here, again, much of the pioneering work was done with influenza virus (2,7,10,45,46,47,73,74). Before the application of MAb to the study of antigenic variation, considerable work had been done with influenza virus. Using antisera, it had been shown that the virus could, in the natural environment, undergo considerable variation quite frequently. This resulted in virus variants which were antigenically related but not identical. The term given to this variation was 'antigenic drift'. If an individual had strong immunity against a certain influenza virus variant, he could resist infection from those variants which subsequently arose through antigenic drift. This did not mean that he would be totally immune to infection, although that may be the case, but that if there was an infection, there would be no obvious signs of illness. Variants could arise, however, which would produce classical influenza; these had a greater degree of antigenic drift. Such variants are said to have arisen through 'antigenic shift'.

There were a number of questions as to how drift and shift could occur, which remained unanswered from the work with antisera. One of the advantages of using MAb was that virus variants could be selected, which had changed at only a single epitope. In this way, the antigenic changes that occured in the virus when under pressure to escape the antibody population in nature (in human sera) could be studied at the epitope level. For example, from the work with MAb on the identification and mapping of epitopes (§6.1.1) four independent infectivity-associated sites had been identified on the influenza virus haemagglutinin glycoprotein by using MAb. Antigenic variants were selected from a population of an H3N2 type influenza A virus (A/Texas/77 virus) by applying excess MAb. These variants failed to react with human antisera which reacted with the parental A/Texas/77 virus (75), suggesting that a change in all four infectivity-associated epitopes was not a prerequisite for the selection of epidemiologically significant variants. What appears to happen in nature is that certain humans have a limited range of effective (with respect to protection) anti-influenza virus antibody, often restricted to one or two of the four infectivity-associated epitopes. Such restrictions were seen most often with children's sera, compared to adult sera, which may explain the means of epidemiological spread of influenza virus.

MAb have also shown, more accurately than antisera, where antigenic changes are occurring in drift and shift. It was known from work with antisera that both of the glycoproteins – the haemagglutinin (H) and neuraminidase (N) – were involved (hence the nomenclature for the virus variants of H1N1, H2N2, H1N2, H3N2). MAb could be used to both select virus variants, and to analyse the protein changes which occurred during the selection (see Laver (74)). The sites of change were mapped, and the amino acid alterations (often only a single replacement in any one variant) identified. From this, 'hot-spots' of variation were found: that is, areas on the glycoprotein molecules where variation most often occurred. Although the H protein showed the largest number of variations which were of relevance to neutralisation of virus infectivity and the protective immune response, significant variation was also found in the neuraminidase protein.

Similar variation was found with the glycoproteins of measles virus (where these glycoproteins have either haemagglutinating or haemolytic–fusion properties) and of rabies virus. However, with these viruses greater differentiation of virus variants (that is, more antigenic variation) could be seen when MAb were used with specificities for other virion proteins, in addition to those specific for the glycoproteins.

With measles virus, and the other viruses of the morbillivirus group (canine distemper, rinderpest and peste des petits ruminants viruses), the H glycoprotein showed the highest degree of antigenic variation, whereas the F glycoprotein was the most stable between variants of measles virus and between the different members of the morbillivirus group (51,54,76). In addition to those variations seen with the glycoproteins, the internal nucleoproteins and matrix protein were also shown to display epitopic differences between isolates. Variation was also seen in the internal proteins of influenza virus virions (74).

This work with the nucleoprotein antigen highlights the potential of MAb to identify antigenic variation not previously recognised. Only very low levels of variation had been seen with influenza virus nucleoproteins before MAb were used. Measles virus, rinderpest virus and rabies virus had been considered stable with respect to antigenic variation in their nucleocapsids. In fact, this had also been considered the case for the glycoproteins of these three viruses. With the MAb, it has been possible to 'fingerprint' almost every isolate of these viruses. The application of such 'antigenic fingerprinting' to virus isolates has been of considerable value in the work with rabies virus, where it has permitted both the identification of isolates and the separation of street or wild-type rabies from the vaccine (56,77,78). Similarly, the separation of wild-type from vaccine virus using MAb has proved useful with poliovirus (38,79,80).

MAb have also been used to identify previously unseen antigenic variation in coxsackievirus and foot-and-mouth disease virus (FMDV). With coxsackievirus B4, conventional serology had been unable to differentiate virus isolates. MAb were able to show that antigenic variation did occur, and to a frequency as high as 10^{-4} (81). The FMDV serotype O_1 had been considered relatively antigenically stable between isolates. Again, however, MAb were used to 'fingerprint' each isolate (82). Examples of such increased differentiation of virus isolates has been reported for other viruses (see reviews, 1,2,4,5,7,10,11,20,21).This topic of the

Table 6.3. *Advances in parasitology made possible through the use of monoclonal antibodies*

Parasite	Advance due to MAb
Plasmodium	Identification of protective epitopes; MAb adoptive transfer of resistance; purification of immunogenic antigens; potentially effective and well-defined vaccines.
Schistosoma	Identification of protective epitopes; MAb adoptive transfer of protection; isolation of surface antigens.
Leishmania	Serodiagnosis and differentiation.
Trypanosoma	Antigen isolation; diagnosis; preparation of vaccines.

identification of virus isolates will be dealt with further in §6.2, which will consider the application of MAb to diagnosis.

So far this section has concentrated on the applications of MAb in the study of virus variation. They have also been applied to both bacteriological (83,84) and parasitological analyses of variations (85–87). The reason for the concentration on viruses is that studies on virus variation has had a more substantial application, especially with respect to diagnosis where reliable assays were not always available before the use of MAb. This is particularly relevant in the case of vaccine–wild-type virus differentiation. It is most important to know the antigenic characteristics of a virus isolate, since this will determine whether or not a vaccination will have induced the correct population of antibodies with respect to protection of the host against a particular isolate or variant. In virology, there are few, and then not necessarily reliable, chemotherapeutic measures, and control of virus infections relies on vaccinations and the efficient induction of protective immune responses. With bacteria and other parasites, there are many fewer effective vaccines available. More frequently, the control of bacterial and protozoal infections relies on chemotherapy. Thus, differentiation and antigenic analyses of bacterial and protozoal isolates is of less importance than the analysis of sensitivity to the chemotherapeutic agent.

However, MAb have enabled the identification of important epitopes on bacteria and parasites, and how these can vary during infection. This is important with certain protozoa which can vary rapidly in order to evade the protective immune response. MAb have been used in epidemiological analyses, in studies of vaccine preparation, and the interaction between the host and the parasite (Table 6.3). However, with the exception of the few successful bacterial vaccines such as those against tuberculosis and whooping cough, and those using the toxoid for protection against diphtheria and tetanus toxins, further applications of MAb in the bacteriology and parasitology fields must await the generation of better vaccines. The usefulness of MAb in this context can be seen from the advances made towards vaccines against certain parasites (Table 6.3). Nevertheless, for vaccines and MAb to have greater applicability, there must be a need for antigenic analysis and a production of factors (such as vaccines) which are both more effective and cheaper to make than currently available systems (for example chemotherapeutic measures).

6.1.3. *Leukocyte markers*

MAb have been used to separate populations and sub-populations of murine, human, bovine, ovine and porcine leukocytes (1,4,5,6,12,13,14, 15,88,89,90). They have also given considerable insight into the structure and function of molecules of the major histocompatibility complex (12,91,92). From this, it is clearer how self-recognition (the body's immune system recognition of its own cells), and cell surface communication during antigen-presentation and T lymphocyte cytotoxicity take place.

The analysis of the surface antigens on leukocytes has resulted in the capacity to identify, more accurately, the roles which different cells play in particular immune responses. Many functional subsets of murine leukocytes, such as helper, cytotoxic, suppressor and DTH T lymphocytes, had been identified by using allo-antisera and rosetting techniques. The MAb confirmed and extended these observations, but also identified in greater detail the existence of such sub-populations in humans, cattle, pigs and sheep. Furthermore, maturation and differentiation pathways for lymphocytes, monocytes–macrophages and granulocytes were elucidated. MAb can, of course, separate these major populations, but they can also separate T and B lymphocytes in different stages of differentiation; bone marrow cells from thymocytes from peripheral blood cells; and different stages of leukocyte development and maturation in the primary and secondary lymphoid organs (in the latter, also after stimulation with antigen).

An additional advantage of this enhanced differentiation of leukocyte sub-sets is in the analysis of disease conditions, particularly leukaemia. Since the leukaemic cells have de-differentiated, or differentiated such as to have cell surface markers typical of a particular phase in the development of leukocyte sub-populations, these leukaemic cells can be used to target the detection system, thus permitting an earlier and more rapid identification and diagnosis of the malignancy. This targetting also permits the MAb to focus any anti-tumour drug, which may be linked to the MAb, on to the tumour cell; the subject of drug targetting will be dealt with in §6.4.

MAb against leukocyte markers have been used to study two other aspects of leukocyte differentiation. The first is ontogeny: following the differentiation of a particular leukocyte type in order to determine the organs in which different phases of differentiation occur, and which environmental factors influence this development. The second is the study of effector cell development: how and where the mature leukocytes differentiate into effectors after stimulation from an infection or from leukokines produced by leukocytes which have themselves responded to the same or another stimulation. In this latter area, the analysis of macrophage sub-populations provides a good example.

Monocytes are the mature precursors of the phagocytic and antigen-presenting mononuclear cells of the body. MAb have identified the cell surface changes which occur during differentiation into macrophages. Four antigens were originally found on macrophages: MAC-1, MAC-2, MAC-3 and MAC-4 (93). MAC-1 is found on resident and induced peritoneal macrophages, and these cells express 8–10 times as much MAC-1 as do the MAC-1 positive cells found in the spleen and bone marrow. The peritoneal macrophages carry considerably more MAC-1 than do blood monocytes and granulocytes. During maturation of monocytes to macrophages, there is a concomitant increase of MAC-1 and decrease of another marker: M1/69 heat-stable antigen. An antigenically similar MAC-1 is found on human monocytes and granulocytes, and appears to be a marker for NK and ADCC activity. MAC-2,3 and 4 antigens are on all thioglycollate-induced peritoneal macrophages, but, in contrast to MAC-1, they are not expressed on bone marrow cells.

It would appear that MAC-1 is on the common precursor of monocytes and granulocytes, and continues to be expressed on both granulocyte precursors and promonocytes, although increases in MAC-1 expression apparently occur under environmental influences such as those found in the peritoneal cavity and, to a lesser degree, the spleen and bone marrow. In contrast, MAC-2,3 and 4 appear to be expressed only on the monocytic line of differentiation, some time after the divergence from the granulocytic line. Furthermore, the MAC-2,3 and 4 antigens may be a late differentiation or maturation marker. Not only are they absent from bone marrow cells, they are found on less than 10% of spleen cells and less than 2% of resident peritoneal monocytes. The antigens may identify a particular subpopulation of macrophages; over 90% of thioglycollate-induced macrophages carry MAC-2,3,4, but only 10–20% of peptone-induced cells and less than 2% of *Listeria*-, lipopolysaccharide- or concanavalin A-induced macrophages express these antigens.

Another example of how MAb have been used with respect to the identification of leukocyte populations is where they have shown variations in functional activity of subpopulations of cells. MAb against the surface antigens of macrophages were able to separate these cells into functionally different subpopulations: cytotoxic macrophages which were dependent upon lymphokines for activation; macrophages involved in ADCC reactions against tumour targets; macrophages with natural killer cell-like activity; and antigen-presenting monocytes (94). These MAb were not directed against Ia (MHC class II) antigens, MHC class I antigens or F_c receptors, as so many of the MAb used in the study of leukocyte surface markers have been. Instead, they fall into the same group as the MAC-1,2,3,4 antigens mentioned above (93).

Nevertheless, many of the studies with MAb, in particular the early studies, concentrated on characterising the structure, role and genetic control and variation of the Ia antigens and the class I MHC antigens (1,4,5,6,12–15,88–92). This work was extended to identify the roles of some of these antigens in disease, but the MAb have also been used to attribute particular immunological function to cells bearing class I or class II MHC antigen. Furthermore, the topography of the surface molecules has also been identified using MAb. For example, MAb against MHC class I antigens H-2K, or H-2D were able to inhibit the function of cytotoxic T lymphocytes (95). On the basis of their results, the authors proposed that the MHC molecules must be located either within or very close to the T cell receptor complex which the T lymphocytes use for binding to their target cells.

The studies on leukocyte antigens using MAb have covered a wide variety: epitope topology, membrane topology, receptor function, leukocyte differentiation, leukocyte maturation, leukocyte function, and the subdivision of leukocytes into different sub-populations. Thus, it forms one of the largest areas of application of MAb, alongside epitope topology on antigens. One aspect of the work which requires further mention is that dealing with the identification of T lymphocyte activities with respect to co-operation with the rest of the immune system; that is, the studies on helper and suppressor T lymphocytes (T_h and T_s), and the factors which they produce.

6.1.4. *Lymphocyte helper and suppressor factors*

It had been known for several years before the application of MAb to immunological studies that there were sub-populations of lymphocytes which produced 'helper' or 'suppressor' factors acting on immune response pathways. These sub-populations could be differentiated by using allo-antisera, but the MAb enabled a more detailed division and analysis of both the cells and their products (16,14,96,97). MAb could also be used to identify such sub-populations in animal species which were not inbred, and for whom allo-antisera preparations could not achieve the same result as in the inbred animals. Through the use of MAb, the roles of T_h and T_s lymphocytes could be studied in many animal species including man (reviewed by Reinherz *et al.* (98)). The studies demonstrated that the T_h and T_s populations are very heterogeneous and that inter-sub-population communication (idiotype network) was present. These T_h cells would also communicate directly with other T lymphocytes (T_h,T_s,T_c,T_d), B lymphocytes, antigen-presenting monocytes and both macrophages and their monocytic precursors. Much of this communication was through the production of the so-called 'helper' and 'suppressor' factors.

Analysis of these factors was also possible with MAb, but a further expansion of this work was made by applying hybridoma technology, in place of simply the MAb, to the subject. This resulted in the T cell hybridomas (6,17) from which a large variety of monoclonal factors were identified. Through the analyses of the factors, by their production from T cell hybridomas or with the use of MAb, the soluble mediators of 'helper' and 'suppressor' function were studied in considerable detail. These analyses demonstrated that T lymphocytes could produce a wide range of lymphokines which stimulated or enhanced the proliferation (activation) of other cells: other T lymphocytes, B lymphocytes, monocytes, macrophages, granulocytes, and fibroblasts (99). These lymphokines included IFN-γ, TCGF (IL-2), BCGFs and BCDFs (the BSF family), MIF and MAF. In addition, there are the so-called T_hF (helper factors) and T_sF (suppressor factors), which could be subdivided into idiotypic, anti-idiotypic and anti-anti-idiotypic factors (T_hF_1, T_hF_2, T_hF_3, T_sF_1, T_sF_2, T_sF_3) (see Chapter 1).

Therefore, both MAb and hybridoma technology have identified the relationships between cells of the immune system, both at the membrane level and at the sub-population level. Furthermore, the factors which leukocytes produce in order to facilitate the various methods of immunological control – help or induction, and regulation or suppression – have also been more accurately defined and characterised, both epitopically and functionally.

6.1.5. *Cancer research*

Monoclonal antibodies have many applications in the field of cancer: therapy, diagnosis, analysis of tumour antigens. The review by Boss *et al.* (100) demonstrates the number and variety of these applications. One of the earlier reports by Goodfellow *et al.* (101) showed that the use of monoclonal antibodies permitted the isolation and characterisation of a teratocarcinoma-specific surface antigen, which was distinct from a second antigen (also characterised with a monoclonal antibody) common to all normal cells.

The definition and characterisation of tumour antigens by monoclonal antibodies has found use with many different solid tumours (3,102–105). Table 6.4 shows the variety of solid tumours, the antigens of which have been characterised by using monoclonal antibodies. Berthold (105) and Kennett *et al.* (104) give considerable detail of the specificity and the number of monoclonal antibodies used to characterise tumour-associated antigen. From this, the potential which monoclonal antibodies have for the accurate diagnosis and 'typing' of solid tumours can be seen.

Strand *et al.* (106) and Haskell *et al.* (107) have summarised the work on the application of monoclonal antibodies to the screening of human carcinomas by radioimaging; Taylor-Papadimitriou *et al.* (108) have used antibodies to study the antigenic composition of human mammary carcinomas and applied these antibodies to the diagnosis, differentiation and detection of the tumours.

In addition to the direct detection of solid tumours, monoclonal antibodies have also been used to characterise and study tumour-related factors present in serum. A good example of this is the α-fetoprotein, which has been studied in both mice (109) and humans (110,111). Furthermore, monoclonal antibodies have been used to study the other class of tumours, the leukaemias (112). There are a large number of groups working on the applications for monoclonal antibodies to the study, diagnosis and characterisation of leukaemias. One of the areas of study comes directly from the diagnostic potential of monoclonal antibodies, and has been applied also to the studies on solid tumours. This area is the application of monoclonal antibodies to the therapy and treatment of solid tumours and leukaemias (100).

Monoclonal antibodies have been shown to have a therapeutic potential in the control of lymphocytic leukaemia and cutaneous lymphoma (113), which probably acts through the antibody binding to the tumour cell and thus enhancing the destruction of the tumour by the antibody-dependent cytotoxic immune defences (lymphocyte, macrophage and granulocyte) of the host. In addition, monoclonal antibody therapy can result in a direct interference with the biological function of tumour cells. For example, Trowbridge (114) has shown that one of several monoclonal antibodies against the transferrin receptor was able to interfere with the growth of a mouse T cell leukaemia *in vivo*. The author suggested that such treatments may have applications in humans, and in this context he proposed that the efficiency of such treatment was due to the presence of much higher levels of transferrin receptor on certain tumours than on normal cells. Furthermore, there may be other receptors against which monoclonal antibodies may have a potential with respect to the interference with tumour cell growth or function. Again, the reasoning

Table 6.4. *Monoclonal antibodies to solid tumour-associated antigens*

colon carcinoma
germ cell tumours and teratocarcinomas
glioblastoma
Hodgkin disease
leiomyosarcoma
lung cancer
mammary carcinoma
melanoma
neuroblastoma
osteosarcoma
ovarian carcinoma
prostatic cancer
tumour markers:
CEA
α-fetoprotein
acid phosphatase

Source: From Bechtol (in reference 8).

is that certain tumours express elevated levels of these receptors, in particular those for epidermal growth factor, insulin and interleukin 2 (TAC). It has also been argued that monoclonal antibodies against the factors themselves may have a therapeutic effect with respect to the *in vivo* inhibition of metastatic tumour cells.

These are only a small number of reports on the current work which is attempting to find therapeutic applications for monoclonal antibodies in cancer. One area of such applications which has received a great deal of attention is that of the immunotoxin or 'magic bullet'. The immunotoxin consists of a monoclonal antibody specific for a tumour surface antigen, attached to a cytotoxic drug such as ricin, vinblastine or methotrexate. In other words, the monoclonal antibody is being used to target the drug onto the tumour cells. This area of drug targetting will be dealt with in more detail in §6.4, since drug targetting may find applications in areas other than those concerned with cancer.

Suffice it to say that monoclonal antibodies have proven as useful to cancer research as they have been in other areas of cell biology, immunology and microbiology. As a tool for the diagnosis and early detection of tumours they are invaluable, but they have also given us insight into the antigenic nature of tumour cell antigens. For example, monoclonal antibodies have identified that the carbohydrate moieties of membrane glycoproteins and glycolipids can form onco-developmental antigens (115), and that certain structures such as lacto-*N*-fucopentose are common to the antigenic sites of several tumours (116). In addition, monoclonal antibodies are finding potential applications in cancer therapy.

However, we must await further research in this area, in order to appreciate more fully the extent to which monoclonal antibody therapeutic reagents will have a place in clinical medicine.

6.1.6. *Other fields*

Monoclonal antibodies have been used in several other areas of research, although not with the same degree of application as seen with the above areas. Similar to the work in immunology and tumour research, cell biologists have studied differentiation antigens in cells of the nervous system (117,118), neurotransmitters (119), and the structure and characteristics of membrane receptors (8,120). In this last area, research in certain areas of neurology and endocrinology, in particular the studies on acetylcholine receptors (121,122) and the receptors involved in growth promotion or anabolic signals (123–126), has provided information on the function of the receptors, as well as their structure. Some of the antibodies have been used to induce autoimmune disorders, such as experimental autoimmune myasthenia gravis. From such work, a clearer appreciation of the interaction between the immune system and the physiological processes of the body has been forthcoming. Monoclonal antibodies have also shown that certain reovirus infections will induce autoimmune antibodies that react with endocrine tissues (127).

Endocrinological studies using monoclonal antibodies have not been restricted to hormone receptors. There are numerous reports in which antibodies have been raised against peptide hormones such as growth hormone (128), insulin and adrenocorticotrophic hormone (129). Such antibodies have made it possible to study in greater detail the antigenic make-up of hormones, and the influence of their presence or absence on physiological functions.

Enzymes have also received considerable attention with respect to the application of monoclonal antibodies (130). Table 6.5 lists examples of several of the enzymes studied. Further information can be found in the review by Harris (130).

The structure and function of cytoskeletal proteins and carbohydrate structures on cell surfaces (see 8) have also been studied with monoclonal antibodies. Allergic reactions have been analysed using monoclonal IgE antibodies, and monoclonal antibodies against antibody isotypes have proved very sensitive and most useful reagents in the quantitation of immunoglobulin isotypes formed during immune responses.

However, two major areas in which monoclonal antibodies have proved invaluable are the analysis of antigen–antibody affinities, and the study of plant sciences. There are a large number of reports studying antibody affinity for an epitope, but only a few examples can be given here. Frankel & Gerhard (131) applied monoclonal antibodies to a rapid

Table 6.5. *Monoclonal antibodies to enzymes*

Enzyme	Species	Tissue source
phenylalanine hydroxylase	monkey	liver
phosphofructokinase	human	red blood cells
tyrosine hydroxylase	rat	caudate nucleus and substantia nigra
glucose-6-phosphate dehydrogenase	human,	red cells
	rat	liver
acetylcholinesterase	human	red cells
choline acetyltransferase	bovine	caudate nucleus
	Drosophila melanogaster	—
catalase T	yeast (*Saccharomyces cerevisiae*)	—
xanthine oxidase	bovine	milk
5-aminolevulinate dehydrogenase	spinach	—
guanylate cyclase	rat	lung
	rat	brain
ß-D-galactosidase	*E. coli*	—
Acid α-glucosidase	human	placenta
RNA polymerase II	*D. melanogaster*	—
	calf	thymus
S-adenosylhomocysteine hydrolase	human	placenta
γ-cystathionase	human	liver
monoamine oxidase B	human	platelets
5′-nucleotidase	rat	liver
ATPase	barley	protoplast
cytochrome P-450, (phenobarbitol induced)	rabbit	liver
3-hydroxy-3-methylglutaryl-CoA-reductase	rat	liver
lysozyme c	chicken	egg white
urokinase	human	kidney
alkaline phosphatase	human	placenta
	human	cultured cells
	human	liver

Source: From Harris (130).

determination of binding constants. From this, the relative affinity of particular monoclonal antibodies for different influenza virus isolates and variants was easily determined. Lew (132) used monoclonal antibodies to analyse the relationships between epitope density and antibody affinity, and to identify the influences which these have on the performance of an ELISA. Finally, Jacobsen & Steensgaard (133) analysed the binding properties of antibody during immune complex formation. They were able to show that, when monoclonal (homogeneous) antibody systems were used, genuine antibody–antigen complex formation did not obey the expected linearity of commonly used binding equations. Furthermore, the methods used gave a variation in the end result, but overall the most important factor controlling antigen–antibody association (the binding pattern) was the antibody concentration. It is probable that this is due to the fact that monoclonal antibodies are relatively homogeneous in their binding properties for a particular antigen, whereas most antigens are an arrangement of a number of antigenic sites containing unique and/or overlapping epitopes. Of course, if monoclonal antibodies were to be assayed against different, but closely related antigens, homogeneity in binding characteristics would be lost.

The application of MAb to the study of plant sciences has made considerable advances. This can be seen from the review of the meeting on the application of MAb in agricultural research (9, pp. 231–252) and the concentrated effort in plant sciences by the AFRC Monoclonal Antibody Centre at Babraham in England. The AFRC Centre have been using MAb to analyse phytochrome function in *Chlamydomonas* cells; the Ministry of Agriculture, Food and Fisheries Plant Pathology Laboratory have developed ELISA kits based on MAb, for the diagnosis of certain plant viruses such as potato virus Y.

Although monoclonal antibodies have been, and are being, applied to the analysis of antigenic sites and antigenic variation in plant sciences, they are also having considerable impact on the diagnosis of plant disease. This area is, of course, not confined to plant diseases. Animal disease – infections, tumorigenic, autoimmune, congenital – are also studied in great detail using MAb, with respect to the more rapid, efficient and accurate diagnosis. It is this area of diagnosis which the next section will now consider.

6.2. **Diagnostic applications of MAb**

This area is quite extensive. However, the basis of its success lies in the capacity of MAb to accurately identify epitopes and epitopic changes (both intra- and interepitopic). From this, variations in antigens and in the antigenic 'make-up' of pathogens, hitherto unrecognised, were identified. The obvious extension of this work was to apply MAb to identify and diagnose the pathogens associated with particular diseases, or the antigenic changes occurring during neoplasia and autoimmune or physiological disorders. From these applications, the MAb were not only able to identify the pathogens, tumours or antigenic changes, but also to identify them more accurately and more rapidly than with assays that used polyclonal antibody preparations. This increase in efficiency of diagnosis could lead to a more effective basis for treatment. Some of the best examples as to how MAb have been applied in these areas can be seen with the diagnosis of pathogen infections.

The study of antigenic drift in influenza viruses led to the application of MAb to the identification of the changes in the virus proteins which occurred during the spread of the virus through a susceptible, and, subsequently, partly immune population (see §§6.1.1 and 6.1.2) (2,21,45,47,48,73,74,75). This typifies the potential which MAb have in the area of diagnosis. Other good examples can be seen with viruses which are not recorded as demonstrating much antigenic change between isolates. The morbilliviruses – measles, distemper, rinderpest and peste de petits ruminants viruses – did not show a high level of antigenic variation. However, MAb were able to identify several antigenic differences between isolates (51,53,54,76). Based upon this work, 'antigenic fingerprinting' of morbillivirus isolates was possible, permitting an accurate epidemiological analysis to be made from the diagnostic applications of the MAb. In fact, the MAb provided, for the first time, the possibility of differentiating rinderpest virus isolates from peste de petits ruminants virus isolates by ELISA, instead of the more laborious, much less rapid, and sometimes variable virus neutralisation assay.

'Antigenic fingerprinting' has also proved most useful with respect to the diagnosis of foot-and-mouth disease virus (82). Although subtype variation of the seven serotypes of this virus has been satisfactorily studied using polyclonal antisera, it was the application of the MAb which made clearer the degree of variation which exists with this virus. For example, a number of isolates of the O_1 subtype of the virus which were indistinguishable antigenically using polyclonal antisera were all shown to be quite distinct using MAb. This 'antigenic fingerprinting' of foot-and-mouth disease virus was put to good use during the recent epizootic (1984–86) in Italy, where it was able to show that the virus present in the animal population was antigenically similar to the vaccine virus, and thus would be susceptible to control by vaccination. Another good example of MAb application to accurate diagnosis came with an outbreak of foot-and-mouth disease in Denmark in 1983. The MAb showed that this O_1 subtype virus was indistinguishable from the virus which had recently been isolated in the German Democratic Republic. None of the other O_1 subtype viruses which had been isolated in Europe at that time, or for several years previously (including one responsible for an earlier Danish outbreak in 1982) were antigenically identical to this 1983 virus. Polyclonal antisera were totally ineffective in identifying any of these antigenic similarities and differences.

MAb have also been put to good use in the diagnosis of bacteria (83,84,134) and other parasites (85,86,87,135). Although the differentiation of such parasites uses, very successfully, diagnostic methods other than MAb (selective media, microscopy), the application of MAb has provided a new dimension. The successful diagnosis of many bacterial and other parasitic infections requires the culturing of the pathogen, or its isolation in large enough numbers. This type of diagnosis is not ideal for a patient who will often require treatment as soon as possible. MAb offer, as they have also done with viral infections, a more rapid, and therefore more efficient, diagnostic procedure. Furthermore, they can often be used to type very accurately, for example, a particular *Streptococcus* infection. It is not surprising to find that MAb are commercially available for exactly this purpose.

Also akin to the work with viruses, MAb are identifying more accurately antigenic variations in certain parasites such as *Theileria* and *Leishmania* species (85,87), *Trypanosoma* species (87,135) and *Plasmodium, Schistosoma, Onchocerca* and *Toxoplasma* species (86,87), and thus are demonstrating their epidemiological potential. Such MAb have been used to identify both species-specific and life cycle stage-specific antigens, which has potential for therapy and new vaccine production, as well as diagnosis. Despite the relatively large size of some of these parasites, their diagnosis (often by microscopic, and even macroscopic techniques) has not *always* been straightforward. For example, MAb have resulted in the improvement of a diagnostic test for *Echinococcus granulosis* in sheep; the MAb were able to distinguish this parasite from those which had given cross-reactions and thus confusion in conventional diagnostic assays (85). Other examples of this particular applicability of MAb in the diagnosis of parasites can be found for *Taenia*, *Schistosoma* and *Toxoplasma* species in the review by Mitchell (85).

Monoclonal antibodies have been, and are being, applied to the diagnosis and analysis of plant diseases, with the same efficiency as has been found with animal diseases (9). Viruses such as *Prunus* necrotic ringspot, apple mosaic, tobacco streak and alfalfa mosaic viruses have been studied by using MAb (136). Various epitopes have been defined, from which the identification of groups and subgroups of antigenic relationships has resulted in a diagnostic application for the MAb. With these antibody-based serological tests, the investigator does not have to rely solely on physical examination of diseased plants. Furthermore, diagnosis can be extended to analyse plants which are, as yet, not showing disease symptoms. Serological analyses, with MAb in particular, have allowed an analysis of seed stocks for contaminating virus infections which could only be achieved, otherwise, after germination of the seeds and analysis of the resultant progeny. This is of great potential in the field of seed health.

In the field of cancer diagnosis, MAb are having considerable impact. This was dealt with in §6.1.5 due to the way in which such work followed the identification and characterisation of tumour-associated antigens. The MAb bring into reality an earlier and much more accurate diagnosis of a particular cancer, which would not have been otherwise possible. A particular bonus with MAb is that the same MAb can be used to diagnose and treat a cancer; this latter application is the topic of the immunotoxin, which will be dealt with in §6.4.

Monoclonal antibodies have one great advantage over polyclonal antisera with respect to diagnosis, and that is their homogeneity. In other words, the reactions of the MAb are not complicated by other antibody specificities, as in antisera; the investigator can be more confident in his diagnosis. The problem is compounded by the fact that many pathogens, in particular several plant viruses, are currently impossible to purify. Often, the attempts to generate antisera against the virus result in an excess of antibodies against host proteins: the last thing required when attempting to generate diagnostic tools. With their homogeneity, MAb do not suffer from this problem. Although the investigator may have to generate a large number of hybridomas against such 'cell-associated' pathogens before obtaining the pathogen-specific MAb, the diagnostic tool is obtainable. A good example of this is actually found with bluetongue virus (137). This virus is difficult to diagnose in areas where vaccinations have been performed with BHK cell-grown vaccines. The reason is that the bluetongue virus is grown in BHK cells, and it is often impossible to distinguish between anti-viral reactions and anti-cellular reactions. It is not only BHK cell proteins which present this problem, since the virus can be grown in several other cell lines with the same result. A monoclonal antibody was isolated which would react with all known bluetongue virus serotypes, but not, of course, with cellular antigen. Using this antibody in a competition assay, it was possible to identify with great accuracy those animals which carried anti-bluetongue virus antibody, even in the presence of very high titres of anti-cellular antibody. The MAb had the additional advantage in being able to discriminate all bluetongue viruses from the group of bluetongue-related viruses which often produced the problem for diagnostics as to whether one was finding a bluetongue virus infection, or an infection due to one of the bluetongue-related viruses.

This topic of MAb application to bluetongue virus diagnosis brings to light the importance of the test involved. Many of the assays described in §4.1 have been used in the diagnostic applications of MAb. Nevertheless, the ELISA, RIA and immunofluorescence assays have been used most frequently, of which the most sensitive form of the assay is the competition assay.

The major problems with diagnostic techniques are the production of pathogen antigen of reasonable purity, and the detection of specific antibody against that pathogen. Both these problems are brought about by contaminating host proteins (present from the method of propagation and culturing of the antigen) and/or antibodies in test antisera which will react with non-pathogen material present in the antigen preparation. In order to obviate these problems, one can use two MAb in a sandwich ELISA. If the antigen is large, the two MAb can have the same specificity; otherwise it is better to use MAb of different specificities. The first MAb will be bound to the solid phase (the ELISA plate). This will trap or capture the antigen (no high degree of purification of the antigen is necessary, because the 'capture' MAb will perform all of the 'purification' required). The trapped antigen is detected by using the second MAb, which is conjugated with an enzyme such as peroxidase or phosphatase, or with biotin. For use in diagnosis, one can analyse sera for the presence of antigen-specific antibodies by adding dilutions of the test material into the ELISA reaction at the same time as the conjugated MAb. If antibodies of the same specificity as the MAb are present in the sera, they will compete with the conjugated MAb, resulting in a reduction in colour obtained on development of the ELISA. Similarly, antigen can be detected in samples, where the 'sample' antigen competes for the binding of the conjugated MAb to the trapped antigen. Such assays have proved particularly useful in diagnosis, and good examples of these are to be found with foot-and-mouth disease virus (82,138), morbilliviruses (54), and bluetongue virus (137).

Although the competition assay would appear to be the most effective diagnostic serological assay, the question still has to be put as to what is being asked of the diagnostic assay. Different characteristics of MAb reactivities can be obtained with different ELISA methods (139). For strain differentiation, the indirect or trapping (capture or sandwich) ELISA are probably best; but for a diagnosis which can be related to protection against disease, the liquid-phase ELISA (140) is the obvious choice. Once the assay has been chosen, the MAb must be selected to best answer the questions being asked. With respect to MAb for the diagnosis of protective immunity, a good example is the work with foot-and-mouth disease virus (72). MAb were selected on the basis of their capacity to protect animals from infection. When used in a competition ELISA, they would identify those animal sera which contained antibody of similar specificity (138). Armed with the assay and MAb of choice, the desired and defined diagnosis of the presence of a pathogen or anti-pathogen antibody is often easily achieved.

6.3. Preparative uses of MAb

The homogeneity of a monoclonal antibody preparation, in terms of both affinity of reaction and specificity for a particular epitope, can be put to use in the preparation and purification of antigens. There are two methods most favoured in this respect: immunoadsorbent columns, and pansorbin precipitation.

With immunoadsorbence, the MAb is attached to Sephadex G25, Sepharose CL-4B or Ultragel AcA40, to mention a few of the solid supports which can be used. A column is prepared with the support to which the MAb is irreversibly attached. After pH and molar equilibration, the crude antigen preparation is applied. Since the MAb will recognise only the antigen, this will bind to the MAb on the column, with the contaminating material eluting through. The bound antigen can then be removed by altering the strength of the MAb–epitope bonds through the use of ionic and pH changes brought about by the application of eluting buffer such as 4 M urea, 0.1 M citric acid (pH 2), 0.2 M glycine–HCl (pH 2), or 0.5 M acetic acid. The eluted antigen is collected into tubes containing an appropriate buffer to neutralise the pH of the eluting buffer.

Instead of using an immunoadsorbent column, pansorbin can be used to precipitate complexes formed by incubating MAb with the antigen. However, since the protein A in the pansorbin preparation has a much higher affinity for rabbit immunoglobulins than mouse antibodies, the method often uses pansorbin primed with rabbit anti-mouse immunoglobulins to precipitate the MAb–antigen complexes. These methods of immunoprecipitation are described in §4.1.19. Elution of antigen can be achieved as for the immunosorbent columns (or as described in §4.1.19, if the method is used to analyse the MAb–antigen reaction or isolate polypeptides of the antigen, and not to prepare complete antigen).

A combination of the two methods uses MAb attached to a solid support matrix, such as Sepharose, for an immunoprecipitation. Instead of preparing a column, the MAb–Sepharose is reacted with the crude antigen preparation in suspension. Antigen which has reacted with the MAb can be precipitated as with the pansorbin-based immunoprecipitation method. Elution of the antigen is achieved by using the same buffers as for immunoadsorption columns, centrifuging to remove the MAb–Sepharose, and transferring the supernatants containing the eluted antigen to fresh tubes containing an appropriate buffer to neutralise the eluting buffer.

These methods for the affinity purification of antigens using MAb have found a large number of applications. One of the earliest and most publicised of these was the purification of human leukocyte interferon

(141). This example reflects one major use of MAb affinity columns: the ability to purify antigens which could not otherwise be purified from crude preparations. Such was the situation with purification of interferons. The antigen could not be purified to the degree required to produce polyclonal antibody which would have the specificity for use in affinity chromatography. MAb had to be generated, where the 'specificity' was assured through the methodology of hybridoma technology. However, interferons can now be prepared by recombinant biotechnology, and the usefulness of MAb-based affinity purification is not so great.

Nevertheless, such affinity chromatography can be applied to the purification of the engineered protein being produced by the bacteria, yeast or mammalian cells in recombinant biotechnology. In addition, it has been found that some biologically active molecules, in particular certain leukokines such as interferon-ß, require glycosylation, which cannot be achieved when using bacterial cloning systems. Thus, affinity chromatography using MAb can still have a very significant role to play, both with and in place of recombinant biotechnology.

As with the early affinity purification of interferon, MAb-based affinity purification is most useful with those antigens which cannot otherwise be purified, or are in very low concentrations during their production. The homogeneity of the MAb has meant that the complications found with polyclonal antibody preparations binding more than one antigen in an immunosorbent column do not arise. Furthermore, the single affinity of reaction of the MAb is also of tremendous use. An affinity of reaction can be chosen which will permit the most effective adsorption and subsequent elution of antigen during the immunoadsorption procedure; effective in the sense that only the antigen being sought will be bound, and that the elution can be performed under conditions which do not alter the structure, and in particular the antigenicity and/or biological activity, of the antigen. With polyclonal antibodies, the combination of affinities can result in a situation where elution is a gradual procedure, with complete elution requiring, at times, elution buffers which are not the most desirable (such as the very low pH glycine–HCl and acetic acid buffers). A MAb-based immunoaffinity column can bind the antigen of choice under conditions in which that antigen will be eluted with relatively mild buffers. This was the situation found with the affinity purification of α-fetoprotein (142). Binding of the antigen by the MAb cannot reach those highest avidities found when more than one antibody specificity and/or affinity are involved. The elution can use milder reagents, such as 2 M urea, and a gradation of elution is not seen.

Thus, monoclonal antibodies have significant applicability to the purification of antigens which will remain both antigenically and biologically active. The homogeneity in specificity and affinity of reaction of the MAb results in a more efficient and effective affinity purification procedure. Monoclonal antibodies can be chosen to give the most desirable result; selectivity (specificity) and ease of purification (affinity). Even with material derived from recombinant biotechnology, MAb-based affinity chromatography is of use with respect to the rapid isolation of the material in a pure and active form.

6.4. **Drug targetting using MAb**

The control of a large number of diseases in both human and veterinary fields is achieved through the application of drugs, which will interfere with the metabolism of the host or, in the case of infectious diseases, the invading pathogen. In the latter case, there may be relatively high tolerance of the drug by the host. A good example of this is the tolerance of the majority of the population to certain anti-bacterial antibiotics such as the penicillins, erythromycins and gentamycin. Unfortunately, this is not always the case. One major problem is found with the response of the liver and kidneys to the presence of the drug. Because the application is often systemic, high concentrations of drug have to be injected in order that enough will reach the target in the body. Sometimes, this concentration is above or too close to the tolerability level for the host, and toxic side-effects may be seen.

One method of circumventing such problems would be to deliver the drug in much lower concentrations to the site of action. In a few situations, this can be achieved physically; with the majority of diseases, however, this is not possible. Monoclonal antibodies have provided a solution, in that they can be used to target the drug. If the MAb has a specificity for an antigenic determinant which is unique to, or in a much higher density in, the site of action for the drug, and the drug is attached to or associated with the MAb, then the MAb can act as a targetting agent for the drug.

Much of the work in this area of drug targetting has concentrated on cancer therapy (100,143,144,145,146), although there is also an interest in controlling allergic reactions and immunologically mediated disease. MAb also have the potential to deliver anti-parasite drugs to the individual parasitic cell, if the MAb has a specificity for an antigenic determinant on the surface of the parasite.

With respect to cancer therapy, the MAb acts as a carrier for a cytotoxic drug. The drugs are often derived from naturally occurring poisons, usually of plant origin (145). These immunotoxins, as they are called, are formed by linking the drug, or the active part or side-chain of the drug, with an antibody specific for the target cell (145,146). Although it had been known for some time that cytotoxic agents covalently bound to tumour-specific antibodies could have therapeutic applications (see 147), it was not until the early 1980s that the monoclonal antibody-based immunotoxin was shown to have promise. Blythman *et al.* (148) used an immunotoxin carrying the A-piece of ricin to selectively kill T cell leukaemic cells in mice. This type of work has been extended to cover other types of tumours, and to use other cytotoxic drugs such as daunomycin, vindesine, methotrexate and adriamycin (100,146).

Although the potential for the immunotoxin 'magic bullet' is apparently high, its application has not met with overwhelming success. There are a number of reasons for this. Firstly, the MAb must have a specificity and affinity which will allow it to react with tumour cells, but not normal cells, and remain in contact with the cell long enough to allow an irreversible interaction between the cell and the toxin. However, not all MAb have these properties, and the characteristics of the reaction with the cell membrane may differ between different tumours and even between the same class and type of tumour. Furthermore, many of the determinants on cancer cells are merely an increased expression of those found on normal cells. If the dose of immunotoxin is too high, it may react with normal cells. Following from this comes the second group of problems: those associated with the clearance rate of the immunotoxin. The idea of the MAb is to target the drug such that the concentrations which would have to be used with the drug alone (owing to the relatively rapid rate at which the body may clear the drug) may be reduced considerably. Since the MAb is also, in most instances, a foreign protein, the body will attempt to clear this, as it would any foreign material. If MAb were used which were more closely related to the recipient (e.g. human MAb instead of murine, when attempting to treat human cancer patients), this would not necessarily relieve the problem. Attaching the drug to the MAb would render some degree of foreignness to the antibody. Thirdly, when an antibody reacts on the surface of a cell, there is an induction of membrane activity brought about by the antibody–antigen interaction. This often results in internalisation of the antigens, and is called antigen modulation. If such modulation occurs before the drug on the immunotoxin can become active, or before the minimum quantity of drug to be irreversibly cytotoxic has become associated with the cell, then the efficacy of the immunotoxin will be greatly reduced or abrogated.

Attempts have been made to circumvent some of these problems and to create more effective immunotoxins (100). The A-chain of ricin has been used in place of the complete molecule. Immunotoxins with whole molecule ricin require high galactose or lactose levels to be effective and to reduce their binding (by the ricin B-chain) to normal cells. However, the cytotoxic efficacy of A-chain immunotoxins, which have a greatly reduced binding for non-target cells, is highly variable. Thorpe *et al.* (149) used a 'blocked' ricin molecule in their immunotoxins. These did not require the high galactose or lactose concentrations found with intact ricin immunotoxins, but did have greater non-specific cytotoxicity than the A-chain immunotoxins. Nevertheless, they were more potent and consistent in their cytotoxicity than those immunotoxins carrying only the A-chain, but the half-life of activity was short; within five hours of infection, the toxin was no longer associated with the drug.

One possible means of increasing immunotoxin efficacy is to have the antibody or toxin associated via a liposome. This may prove to be a much more effective 'drug', and it is certainly the method currently favoured with respect to MAb–immunomodulator conjugates. Although interferons, tumour necrosis factors and interleukin-2 have been conjugated to MAb which will target these leukokines on to cancer cells (or cells of the immune system, if that is required, as in attempts to control infectious diseases) the current evidence would suggest that liposomes with the modulator inside and the MAb on the surface may be more effective (150). This type of conjugate appears to function by stimulating (or enhancing stimulation) and targetting the tumoricidal response by macrophages to the tumour with which the MAb has reacted. Toxicity for normal cells would be greatly reduced, since a large influx of monocytes is already present in a neoplastic site, and much higher levels of immunoconjugate would be required to activate any response against normal tissues. Furthermore, because the 'toxin' part is actually a naturally occurring leukokine, this will be self-regulating in two senses. The duration of time in which the immunoconjugate must remain on the tumour cell surface will not necessarily be as long as is required of the immunotoxin. This is because the action of the leukokine is not a direct effect on the tumour cell but an effect on the immune system resulting in a cascade of events which will continue and be self-amplifying in the subsequent absence of the leukokine. In addition, the immune system can then self-regulate its response such that an over-production, or over-application, of toxic material is not required. This, of course, is all dependent upon both a successful stimulation of the immune system, and, thereafter, a successful destruction of the neoplasm. Neither of these events can be absolutely guaranteed at the present stage of research and development.

The other problem which continually confronts researchers attempting to apply immunotoxins or immunoconjugates is the antigenic modulations which can occur at all cell surfaces after a bivalent antibody has reacted with antigenic determinants on the cell membrane. Research has now demonstrated that certain univalent monoclonal antibodies can perform the functions originally demanded of bivalent antibodies.

Glennie & Stevenson (151) produced a univalent monoclonal antibody against guinea pig lymphocytic leukaemia through controlled papain digestion of the bivalent antibody. The monovalent MAb had enhanced cell killing, both *in vitro* and *in vivo*, against lymphocytic leukaemia cells, and the authors related this to an absence of antigenic modulation when using the monovalent (univalent) MAb.

Cobbold & Waldmann (152) took the manufacture of monovalent antibodies one step further. They generated immune splenocytes against certain human cell-surface antigens in DA rats which they fused with the LOU rat myeloma cell line Y3/Ag 1.2.3. From the hybridomas produced, the bivalent molecules would be characterised as having two k1b light chains, whereas monovalent hybridoma antibodies would have one k1b chain (from the DA rat cells) and one k1a light chain (from the Y3 myeloma cells). These monovalent antibodies could be separated for characterisation using the MRC OX12 mouse monoclonal antibody, which binds preferentially to the k1a allotype. This 'natural' production of the univalent antibody avoids structural alteration of the antibody such as that which can occur with enzyme treatment (11).

Although these reports on the production of univalent antibodies were not considering drug targetting, it can be seen that the attachment of a drug, or a liposome carrying a drug, to a univalent antibody would have the advantage over the bivalent antibody system of not inducing antigenic modulation. Thus, the univalent antibody-based immunotoxin could direct a drug to a cell surface where it would remain in contact for longer, or would be phagocytosed rather than shed (as with certain types of antigenic modulation); in such instances, the drug would have considerably increased cytotoxic potential.

Of course, if the targetting antibody had one combining site (paratope) specific for the target, and the other paratope specific for the drug, this could have certain advantages: the risk of altering the antibody structure by the chemical binding of the drug would be averted. Unfortunately, many drugs are so small that an antibody reaction can interfere with their function. Nevertheless, hybrid antibodies (carrying two different paratopes, both of which are put to use) have been produced, and do show considerable promise for the future. However, this promise will probably be most fruitful in the field of prophylaxis or therapy, and not drug targetting. It is also possible that the univalent or monovalent MAb will have considerable prophylactic and/or therapeutic impact; this area of passive immunisation with monoclonal antibodies is the subject of the next section. It is probable that the future will see MAb being used both for a direct attack upon a pathogen or tumour cell, and for a targetting of drugs and immunomodulators, probably encapsulated in liposomes carrying the MAb on their surface.

6.5. Prophylactic and therapeutic uses of MAb

For the same reasons that MAb specific for a particular pathogen or tumour cell have been used to target drugs to that pathogen or tumour cell (see §6.4), the MAb can also be used to produce a direct attack. That is, they can be used for passive immunisation and therapy (1,4,7,8,9,10,11).

There are now several examples of the potential of MAb for the passive immunisation against viruses, bacteria and other parasites (see 11). Some very good examples are found in the field of virology. It is also worth noting that several of the reports use antibodies which, under the conditions used, would not neutralise the capacity of the viruses to infect susceptible cells *in vitro*. This highlights the lack of correlation between virus neutralisation *in vitro* and protection *in vivo*. In fact, the ideal antibodies with respect to passive immunisation are not those which neutralise pathogen infectivity *in vitro*, but those which efficiently opsonise the pathogen and enhance the phagocytosis and killing of that parasite.

Schmaljohn *et al.* (153) used non-neutralising monoclonal antibodies to protect mice against a fatal paralytic encephalitis due to Sindbis virus. Although the authors related this to the ability of the MAb to enhance complement-dependent lysis of virus-infected cells *in vitro*, it is equally possible that the protective mechanism was due to an opsonisation-enhancement of phagocytosis of the virus or macrophage killing of infected cells (with or without the additional enhancing effects of complement for these two reactions). Rector *et al.* (154) did demonstrate that non-neutralising antibodies probably could protect *in vivo* through enhancement of macrophage killing of virus-infected cells. They also described other antibodies which could protect animals through events which were concluded by McCullough (11) as reflecting the presence of opsonisation-enhanced phagocytosis, or the three activities of neutralising virus infectivity, opsonising and activating complement-mediated lysis.

The kinetics of antigen–antibody reactions would suggest that not all potentially infectious virus could be removed from the circulation by simple antigen–antibody complexing, even if this did interfere with virus adsorption to susceptible cells (neutralisation of infectivity). Work with foot-and-mouth disease virus (FMDV) has shown under the electron microscope that MAb can alter the structure of a virus, with complete loss of the virus genome and subsequent dissolution of the capsid form (155). Such events would probably occur when enough antibody was present. At lower concentrations of antibody, passive protection of mice was still noted, even when virus infectivity could not be neutralised, as estimated *in vitro* (72). This passive protection by the MAb was related to an opsonisation-enhanced phagocytosis of virus–antibody complexes (156). Reference to other examples of passive protection by MAb in mice can be found in the reviews by McCullough (11) and Carter & ter Meulen (7).

Passive immunisation using MAb has also been successfully achieved in animals other than mice. For example, Letchworth & Appleton protected sheep against bluetongue virus with a murine MAb (157). Passive immunisation with MAb has also been used in the therapy of cancer. As described in §6.4, MAb can be generated such that antigenic modulation of the cancer cell surface through the reaction of a bivalent antibody can be avoided. Such monovalent antibodies can be generated easily by selecting the appropriate myeloma cell line for the fusions. The basis of this was to use the splenocyte for the production of the heavy chains and one of the light chains, and the myeloma cell for the other light chain. Thus, the progeny antibody would have two different paratopes; that is, it would be monovalent for the antigenic determinant recognised by each paratope. The obvious progression on this idea was to fuse two hybridomas and select for those hybrid hybridomas secreting antibody which carried the paratope of each of the parent cells.

Consider the situation with two hybridoma cell lines. One secretes antibody specific for an antigenic determinant on the surface of a cancer cell, a virus-infected cell, a bacterium, or another parasite. The other secretes antibody specific for a leukocyte involved in the immune defence against the particular tumour or pathogen (for example, the T lymphocyte). After fusing these two hybridomas, certain hybrid cell lines could be selected which secreted antibody bearing the two specificities; that is, antibody which could react, for example, with both the cancer cell and T lymphocytes. Because the antibody (hybrid MAb as it is called) would be monovalent for each antigenic determinant, there would be little possibility of antigenic modulation. This hybrid MAb could react with, in this example, T lymphocytes and target them onto the cancer cell, or react with the cancer cell and trap T lymphocytes on to the tumour cell surface.

Staerz *et al.* (158) showed the potential of this idea by chemically linking two MAb. Their 'hybrid' molecules could react with the T cell receptor complex of cytotoxic and helper T lymphocytes (reaction of a MAb with this receptor mimics the reaction by antigen) and a surface antigen on S.AKR lymphoma cells (this was Thy1.1, so the cytotoxic T cells had to be Thy1.2†). The 'hybrid' molecule efficiently targetted the cytotoxic cells, and probably also enhanced their lytic potential, since antibody reaction with the T cell receptor would stimulate resting T cells.

The subsequent development of this work by Staerz and co-workers was to produce the hybrid hybridoma secreting the hybrid MAb (159).

This hybrid MAb was selected and partly purified, and shown to target S.AKR hybridoma cells for lysis by cytotoxic T cells, in much the same manner as with the chemically-produced 'hybrid' molecule.

The therapeutic potential for MAb has been recognised for several years (100,105,160–162). Some of this potential has already been discussed in §6.1.5, particularly with respect to those MAb which recognise certain tumour cell antigens and/or interfere with tumour cell function. The first six chapters of the review by Boss *et al.* (100) are devoted to this topic of MAb therapy of leukaemias (the next five chapters deal with immunotoxins). One of the major problems facing the therapeutic use of MAb is the fact that they are often mouse proteins. Although little toxicity has been observed in human patients given murine MAb therapeutically (probably due to the purity and the specificity of the material inoculated), their clinical benefits have not always been great; sometimes little or no effect upon the course of the cancer has been observed. Much of this lack of potency has been related to antigenic modulation, and the rapid production of anti-mouse antibodies. The former problem can be avoided using monovalent antibodies. The second problem is more difficult to resolve. If the hybrid antibody could not only increase the efficiency at targetting the immune system to destroy the tumour cells, but also reduce the risk of removal of the MAb by anti-mouse antibody this would be of considerable advantage. Indeed the potential for MAb in all fields of passive immunisation, whether prophylactic or therapeutic, could be augmented if the induction of anti-mouse antibodies were avoided. The answer to this problem would be to produce antibodies of the same species as the target species for treatment.

Both human and bovine monoclonal antibodies have been produced by using the heterohybridoma system: mouse myeloma cells fused with human (1,8,100,163–167) or bovine (168,169) immune lymphocytes. The procedure has been taken one step further, after the isolation or production of suitable human lymphoblastoid cell lines (167,170–173). These can be used in place of the mouse myeloma cells in the fusion procedure, in order to produce human × human homohybridomas. Such homohybridomas were apparently more stable, with respect to the production, assembly and secretion of human monoclonal antibody, than the human × mouse heterohybridomas. Human monoclonal antibodies have now been produced against several antigens: viral, bacterial and, in particular,

† Thy1.1 and Thy1.2 are two forms of the alloantigen carried by all murine T lymphocytes (both intra- and extrathymic); there are equivalent alloantigens in other species. The expression of these antigens is controlled by a single genetic locus (Thy-1), of which there are two alleles, Thy-1^a and Thy-1^b, coding for the Thy1.1 and Thy1.2 antigens respectively.

tumour (1,8,18,100,167). Their prophylactic and therapeutic potential has been assayed in a number of cases, but the results are often variable or inconclusive. It is probable that human monoclonal antibodies suffer from the same problem as found with murine MAb, that is antigenic modulation. Perhaps the generation of monovalent antibodies would increase the efficiency of human MAb, as has been found with their rodent counterparts.

Thus, the prophylactic and/or therapeutic potential of MAb is apparently high. The two major problems encountered with this application are (i) antigenic modulation of the target, and (ii) an immune response by the host against the injected MAb. With respect to the first problem, the answer appears to lie with the use of monovalent MAb; the second problem may be resolved by using species of MAb which are less xenogeneic for the host (e.g. human MAb for human patients). Probably the greatest potential application for MAb in prophylaxis and therapy is the use of the hybrid antibody: the MAb which has two paratopes, one of which reacts with the target, and the second of which binds with effector cells of the immune system and thereby targets (focuses) immune defences on to the target 'infection'.

There is one other area of prophylaxis and therapy where MAb have proved most useful. In this, the antibody acts as a vaccine. MAb could be given in a complex with antigen in an attempt to generate memory immune responses; however, the 'vaccine' application of MAb which is showing the greatest potential is the anti-idiotype. With anti-idiotypic MAb which mimic the antigenic determinant against which an immune response is desired (the 'internal image' MAb or 'surrogate antigen'), the possibility exists of focusing the immune response against a relevant epitope without having to use the complete antigen. This is of great advantage when the antigen cannot be purified enough to have a good vaccine, or when the antigen is a potent or dangerous pathogen. The theory, production and potential application of anti-idiotype antibodies is a large subject, and requires a section of its own.

6.6. **Idiotopes and idiotypes**

The idiotypic network and the theory of the surrogate antigen 'internal image' antibody has been described in Chapter 1. However, it is pertinent to reiterate some of this here, for ease of explanation.

When an antigen is recognised as foreign, the recipient animal's immune system responds against areas on the surfaces of the antigen: the antigenic determinants or epitopes. Similarly, an antibody molecule carries determinants which will be recognised as foreign by the immune system of an appropriate recipient animal. These antibody determinants are grouped into:

(i) those which differ between different animal species (xenotypic determinants);
(ii) those which differ between related animal species and/or between inbred strains of a single species (allotypic determinants);
(iii) those which are unique to particular antibody molecules within an individual animal or inbred strain (idiotypic determinants).

A rabbit can respond against xenotypic, allotypic and idiotypic determinants on Balb/c mouse antibody. C57/Bl6 mice can respond against allotypic and idiotypic determinants on Balb/c mouse antibody, but a Balb/c mouse antibody can only respond against the idiotypic determinants of syngeneic (from other Balb/c mice) or autologous (from the same Balb/c mouse) antibody. This response against idiotypic determinants (the anti-idiotype response) forms the basis of the network theory of immune regulation proposed by Jerne (174).

The term idiotope is used to describe that determinant on a single clone of antibody which confers 'selfness' on that antibody. Idiotypes are families of closely related idiotopes, or idiotopes which are common to a limited number of antibody clones (they often have closely related antigenic specificity). For ease of description, such determinants will be collectively referred to as Id.

6.6.1. *Induction of anti-idiotype antibody*

When mice are passively immunised with an anti-parasite antibody or monoclonal antibody, the animals may be protected against challenge with the parasite against which the MAb reacted. Another consequence of this passive transfer may be the induction of the regulatory anti-Id networks. Stimulation of an immune response against an Id can only occur when that Id reaches immunogenic levels, that is, when the antibody carrying it is produced in large quantities such as during an active immune response or after inoculation of immunogenic doses (usually 100 μg for small animals). Since the 'private' Id is relatively unique to a particular clone of antibody (and the 'cross-reactive' Id to a family of closely related antibodies), the Id can be recognised as foreign by the autologous immune system and anti-Id antibody produced. This idiotype–anti-idiotype network of immune regulation is effected through the idiotopy of lymphocyte receptors. All Id identified to date, and, thus, anti-Id specificities, are associated with F_v region of antibody, that is the V_H and V_L domains (175). They can be divided, generally, into Id associated with the antigen-binding crevice or paratope (Id_p), Id outside the paratope, and Id formed by combination of determinants on the antibody and antigen during antibody–antigen interaction (175,176,177).

6.6.2. *Internal image anti-idiotope*

When the Id associated with the antigen-binding crevice or paratope (Id_p) reaches immunogenic levels, anti-Id_p-bearing B cells can be stimulated. These lymphocytes, in the presence of antigen-presenting cells (APC) and the appropriate T helper (T_h) lymphocytes, differentiate and produce anti-Id_p antibody. This anti-Id_p antibody is a mirror image of the inducing paratope. Hence, the paratope of the anti-Id_p bearing antibody should be similar conformationally to the epitope with which the Id_p-bearing antibody combines; it is therefore called an 'internal image' of the epitope. This internal image antibody is central to the theory of the 'surrogate antigen', which is proposed to function as an 'immunogen' stimulating Id_p-bearing B cells to differentiate and produce Id_p-bearing antibody again.

The second route by which the Id_p-bearing B lymphocytes can be stimulated requires the inducing Id_p to be presented (by APC) to anti-Id_p-bearing T_h lymphocytes. These T_h cells can in turn trigger the differentiation of Id_p-bearing B cells through Id–anti-Id reaction. This route does not utilise an internal image antibody or surrogate antigen, but will be referred to subsequently.

6.6.3. *Surrogate antigen*

The evidence for idiotype–anti-idiotype networks in a protective immune response against pathogens has been reviewed by McCullough & Langley (177). Sacks *et al.* (178) protected mice by using anti-Id antisera raised against neutralising (by passive protection) monoclonal anti-trypanosome antibody. Reagan *et al.* (179) have used rabbit anti-Id antibody (anti-rabies virus glycoprotein MAb) to induce virus-neutralising antibody, while Kennedy & Dreesman (180) used anti-Id antibody to induce or enhance the production of anti-hepatitis B antibody which expressed an Id common with convalescent anti-hepatitis B antiserum. Forstrom *et al.* (181) used what may be such a reagent to induce delayed-type hypersensitivity against the mouse sarcoma MCA-1490. This raises the question as to whether a single anti-Id antibody, several different (or related) anti-Id antibodies, combinations of anti-Id with anti-allotype antibodies (some allotypes and idiotypes are genetically linked), or other combinations are required for an effective surrogate antigen preparation.

There is also the concentration-dependency of the immunostimulatory capacity of anti-Id antibody to be considered. Anti-Id antibody at 10–100 ng enhanced the expression of Id-bearing antibody, whereas 10 μg suppressed the response and 1 μg had no observable effect (182,183). Anti-idiotypic antibodies have also been used to study the functioning of, and communication within, the immune systems (see 11,175,177). In addition, these reagents have proved most useful in the analysis of epitope structure, and as probes for receptor structure and function (184).

However, there are reports of anti-Id inducing the converse to protective immunity. Kennedy *et al.* (185) produced an increase in the pathogenesis of herpes simplex virus type 2 after inoculating mice with a *particular* anti-Id antibody. Furthermore, not all apparently potential anti-Id 'internal image' antibodies will function as efficient surrogate image vaccines and protect animals. An example of this comes from the work of Uytdehaag & Osterhaus (186) with poliovirus. These authors used an anti-Id which would induce neutralising antibody against the virus in mice. However, no protection against virus challenge was found (this relates to the area of passive immunisation with MAb where the important fact has been shown, with MAb against foot-and-mouth disease virus, that protection is related to opsonisation-enhanced phagocytosis and not neutralisation of virus infectivity for tissue culture cells (72,156)).

In contrast to this lack of success, Ertl & Finberg (187) were able to protect mice using an anti-idiotype MAb against Sendai virus-specific T_h lymphocyte clone. This anti-Id antibody induced both a B and T lymphocyte response against the virus. Perhaps there are only certain anti-Id antibodies which can induce both B and T cell immunity. This would depend on which idiotypes are present on the B and T lymphocytes. Nevertheless, protective immunity will require the participation of both B and T cells (see Chapter 1), and the stimulation of both by an anti-idiotype antibody is absolutely necessary. The anti-Id antibody need not stimulate both B and T lymphocytes directly, and it is possible that this is the situation with those anti-Id MAb which have induced a protective response.

An additional factor has come to light concerning the induction of idiotypic networks (188). Monoclonal antibodies, which were passively protective against foot-and-mouth disease virus (FMDV), were used to immunise syngeneic mice in order to generate, subsequently, anti-idiotype antibody-secreting hybridomas. When these hybridoma antibodies were analysed, a number were identified as anti-idiotype. In addition, a large group of antibodies were found which reacted directly with the antigen; that is, they were Id-bearing antibody and not anti-Id. These antibodies were produced by hybridomas derived from the splenocytes of the mice immunised with the anti-FMDV MAb. These mice had no detectable antibody titres against the FMDV before the immunisation with the MAb. It is probable, therefore, that the splenocytes which gave rise to the Id-bearing antibody-secreting hybridomas were induced by the MAb immunisation. In order to achieve this, the MAb must have induced anti-idiotypic networks which, in turn, induced the production of Id-bearing cells and antibody.

The consequence of this work would be that passive immunisation with appropriate concentrations of the relevant MAb would offer, in the short term, passive protection, and, in the long term, the generation of a memory immune response and lymphocytes which could secrete antibody of similar specificity to the original immunising MAb. It is possible that the immunising MAb may have to be syngeneic or allogeneic for the animal species to be treated. Thus, the production of human, bovine, ovine and porcine MAb could have an additional significance.

6.7. Summary

The application of MAb has many facets, covering most areas of biology, from the analysis of the structure of antigens and receptors to the prophylactic and therapeutic treatment of diseases and disorders. It is now the accepted procedure to use MAb in most serological assays. A look at the catalogues of the many companies now selling and marketing antibodies will show the position which MAb have attained in research and diagnostics. The fact that MAb have not found greater applications in prophylaxis and therapy rests with the problems mentioned in §6.5. With the constant adaptation of technologies, it is probable that *in vivo* applications of MAb will soon be as common as the research applications. The identification of the potential of hybrid antibodies in therapy and prophylaxis, and the success at generating human and bovine MAb, will probably provide the sound base required for the successful launch of MAb into many *in vivo* applications. With anti-idiotype surrogate antigens, the future is not so certain. Hybrid antibodies, allogeneic to the recipient, will probably be the best method of applying anti-idiotype specificities, although some murine anti-Id MAb may prove most effective vaccines when no appropriate alternative vaccine is available. The question of the necessity to use anti-Id antibodies has now been posed. It is possible that future uses of the idiotypic network may be through a passive immunisation with a MAb which will generate, directly, the short-term protection, and, through stimulation of idiotypic networks, the long-term protection of the memory response.

Most of these prophylactic and therapeutic applications require further research. There is no doubt that MAb are here to stay, now being such well-established tools (often the first tools of choice) for research and diagnostic purposes. For the future, that is the prophylactic and therapeutic applications, we may well see the rise of the new age of monoclonal antibody and hybridoma technology: the production of the hybrid hybridoma. The secreted 'hybrid' MAb (with its two distinct paratopes) will have a multitude of uses, either alone, or linked to a drug- or leukokine-carrying vehicle such as the liposome. There is no doubt about it; monoclonal antibodies and hybridomas have been the greatest success story in biology over the past 10 years, and the next 10 years will probably see new heights reached, both in the technology of their manufacture, and in the variety and ingenuity of their application.

References

Chapter 1

1 HOOD, L. E., WEISMANN, I. L., WOOD, W.B. & WILSON, J. H. (1984). *Immunology* (second edition). The Benjamin Cummings Publishing Co., California, Massachusetts, London.

2 HUMPHREY, J. H. & WHITE, R. G. (1971). *Immunology for students of medicine*. Blackwell Scientific Publications, Oxford.

3 EDELMAN, G. M. & POULIK, M. D. (1961). In G.M. Edelman (1973) Antibody structure and molecular immunology. *Science* **180**, 830.

4 McCONNELL, I., MUNRO, A. & WALDMANN, H. (1981). *The immune systems. A course on the molecular and cellular basis of immunity*. Blackwell, Oxford, London.

5 LANCET, D., ISENMAN, D., SJÖDAHL, J., SJÖQUIST, J. & PECHT, I. (1978). Interaction between staphylococcal protein A and immunoglobulin domains. *Biochem. Biophys. Res. Commun.* **85**, 608–614.

6 OI, V. T., VUONG, M., HARDY, R., DANGL, J., REIDLER, J., STRYER, L. & HERZENBERG, L. A. (1982). Segmented flexibility and effector function of immunoglobulin isotope containing identical antidansyl variable regions. *Fed. Proc.* **41**, 289.

7 MIMS, C. A. & WHITE, D. D. (1984). *Viral pathogenesis and immunology*. Blackwell Scientific Publications, Oxford.

8 UNANUE, E. R. (1981). The regulatory role of macrophages in antigenic stimulations. Part two: symbiotic relationship between lymphocytes and macrophages. *Adv. Immunol.* **31**, 1–136.

9 KLAUS, G. G. B. (1978). The generation of memory cells. II. Generation of B memory cells with preformed antigen–antibody complexes. *Immunology* **34**, 643–652.

10 NISONOFF, A., REICHLIN, M. & MARGOLIASH, E. (1970). Immunological activity of cytochrome C. II. Localization of a major antigenic determinant of human cytochrome C. *J. Biol. Chem.* **245**, 940–948.

11 SMITH-GILL, S. J., WILSON, A. C., POTTER, M., PRAGER, E. M., FELDMANN, R. J. & MAINHART, C. R. (1982). Mapping the antigenic epitope for a monoclonal antibody against lysozyme. *J. Immunol.* **128**, 314.

12 SHESHBERADARAN, H. & NORRBY, E. (1984). Three monoclonal antibodies against measles virus F protein cross-react with cellular stress proteins. *J. Virol.* **52**, 955–999.

13 MÖLLER, G. (ed.) (1980). Accessory cells in the immune response. *Immunol. Rev.*, vol. 53. Munksgaard, Copenhagen.

14 UNANUE, E. R. (1984). Antigen-presenting function of the macrophage. *Ann. Rev. Immunol.* **2**, 395–428.

15 STEINMAN, R. M. & NUSSENZWEIG, M. C. (1980). Dendritic cells: features and functions. *Immunol. Rev.* (Ed G. Möller), vol. 53, pp. 127–148. Munksgaard, Copenhagen.
16 BELLER, D. I. & HO, K. (1982). Regulations of macrophage populations. V. Evaluation of the control of macrophage Ia expression *in vitro*. *J. Immunol.* **129**, 971.
17 THOMAS, D. W. & SHEVACH, E. M. (1976). Nature of the antigenic complex recognised by T lymphocytes. I. Analysis with an *in vitro* primary response to soluble protein antigens. *J. Exp. Med.* **144**, 1263–1273.
18 ERB, P. & FELDMANN, M. (1975). Role of macrophages in *in vitro* induction of T-helper cells. *Nature (London)* **254**, 352–353.
19 SMITH, K. A. & RUSCETTI, F. W. (1981). T-cell growth factor and the culture of cloned functional T cells. *Adv. Immunol.* **31**, 137–175.
20 HOWARD, M. & PAUL, W. E. (1983). Regulations of B-cell growth and differentiation by soluble factors. *Ann. Rev. Immunol.* **1**, 307–333.
21 GREEN, D. R., FLOOD, P. M. & GERSHON, R. K. (1983). Immunoregulatory T-cell pathways. *Ann. Rev. Immunol.* **1**, 439–463.
22 MOLLER, G. (ed) (1984). B cell growth and differentiation factors. *Immunol. Rev.*, vol. 78. Munksgaard, Copenhagen.
23 KISHIMOTO, T. (1985). Factors affecting B-cell growth and differentiation. *Ann. Rev. Immunol.* **3**, 133–157.
24 MOLLER, G. (ed.) (1983). T cell hybrids. *Immunol. Rev.*, vol. 76. Munksgaard, Copenhagen.
25 ALTMAN, A., SCHREIBER, R. D. & KATZ, D. H. (1983). Functional T cell hybridomas producing non-specific immunoregulatory factors. In *Monoclonal antibodies and T cell products* (ed. D. H. Katz), pp. 133–170. CRC Press, Florida.
26 ESHHAR, Z. (1983). Functional T cell hybridomas producing antigen-specific immunoregulatory factors. In *Monoclonal antibodies and T cell products* (ed. D. H. Katz), pp. 133–170. CRC Press, Florida.
27 JERNE, N. K. (1974). Towards a network theory of the immune system. *Ann. Immunol. (Paris)* **125**, 373.
28 GREENE, M. I., NELLES, M. J., SY, M.-S. & NISONOFF, A. (1982). Regulation of immunity to azobenzenearsonate hapten. *Adv. Immunol.* **32**, 253–300.
29 BONA, C. A. (1981). *Idiotypes and lymphocytes*. Academic Press, New York and London.
30 BONA, C. & CAZENAVE, P.-A. (eds) (1981). *Lymphocyte regulation by antibodies*. John Wiley and Sons, New York.
31 URBAIN, J., CAZENAVE, P.-A., WIKLER, M., FRANSSEN, J. A., MARIAME, B. & LEO, D. (1981). Idiotopic induction and immune networks. In *Immunology 80: Progress in Immunology IV.* (ed. M. Fougereau & J. Dausset), pp. 81–93. Academic Press, New York, London.
32 KELSOE, G., RETH, M. & RAJEWSKY, K. (1980). Control of idiotope expression by monoclonal anti-idiotope antibodies. *Immunol. Rev.* **52**, 75.
33 McCULLOUGH, K. C. & LANGLEY, D. (1985). Anti-idiotope vaccines: can they work? *Vaccine* **3**, 59–64.
34 KLAUS, G. G. B. & HUMPHREYS, J. H. (1977). The generation of memory cells. I. The role of C3 in the generation of B memory cells. *Immunology* **33**, 31–40.

35 LILET-LECLERCQ, C., RADOUX, D., HEINEN, E., KINET-DENOËL, C., DEFRAIGNE, J.-O., HOUBEN-DEFRESNE, M.-P. & SIMAR, L. J. (1984). Isolation of follicular dendritic cells from human tonsils and adenoids. I. Procedure and morphological characterization. *J. Immunol. Methods* **66**, 235–244.

36 SCHNIZLEIN, C. T., KOSCO, M. H., SZAKAL, A. K. & TEW, J. G, (1985). Follicular dendritic cells in suspension: identification, enrichment and initial characterization indicating immune complex trapping and lack of adherence and phagocyte activity. *J. Immunol.* **134**, 1360–1368.

37 MILLER, G. W. & NUSSENZWEIG, V. (1975). A new complement function: solubilisation of antigen–antibody aggregates. *Proc. Natl. Acad. Sci., U.S.A.* **72**, 418–422.

38 MILSTEIN, C. (1983). Monoclonal antibodies from hybrid myelomas: theoretical aspects and some general comments. In *Monoclonal antibodies in clinical medicine* (ed. A. J. McMichael & J. W. Fabre), pp. 3–16. Academic Press, London, New York.

39 McCULLOUGH, K. C. (1986). Monoclonal antibodies: implications for virology. *Arch. Virol.* **87**, 1–36.

40 MANDEL, B. (1979). Interaction of viruses with neutralizing antibodies. In *Comprehensive virology* (ed. H. Fraenkel-Conrat & R. R. Wagner), vol. 15, pp. 37–121. Plenum Press, New York, London.

41 OSAKI, Y. (1968). Neutralization kinetics of poliovirus by specific antiserum during the course of immunisation of rabbits. *Arch. Ges. Virusforsch.* **25**, 137–147.

42 ICENOGLE, J., SHIWEN, H., DUKE, G., GILBERT, S., RUECKERT, R. & ANDEREGG, J. (1983). Neutralisation of poliovirus by monoclonal antibody: kinetics and stoichiometry. *Virology* **127**, 412–425.

43 HORNICK, C. L. & KARUSH, F. (1972). Antibody affinity. III. The role of multivalence. *Immunochemistry,* **9**, 325.

44 HERZENBERG, L. A., BLACK, S. J., TOKUHISA, T. & HERZENBERG, L. A. (1980). Memory B cells at successive stages of differentiation. Affinity maturation and the role of IgD receptors. *J. Exp. Med.* **151**, 1071.

45 VITETTA, E. S., FORMAN, J. & KETTMAN, J. R. (1976). Cell surface immunoglobulin. XVIII. Functional differences of B lymphocytes bearing different surface immunoglobulin isotope. *J. Exp. Med.* **143**, 1055.

46 UNANUE, E. R., PERKINS, W. D., & KARNOVSKY, M. V. (1972). Ligand-induced movement of lymphocyte membrane macromolecules. I. Analysis by immunofluorescence and ultrastructural radioautography. *J. Exp. Med.* **136**, 885.

47 MACKENZIE, I. F. C. & POTTER, T. (1979). Murine lymphocyte surface antigens. *Adv. Immunol.* **27**, 179–338.

48 STÄHLI, G., STAEHELIN, T., MIGGIANO, V., SCHMIDT, J. & HARING, P. (1980). High frequencies of antigen-specific hybridomas: dependence on immunisation parameters and prediction by spleen cell analysis. *J. Immunol. Methods* **32**, 297–304.

49 KOHLER, G. & SHULMAN, M. J. (1978), Cellular and molecular restrictions of the lymphocyte fusion. *Curr. Top. Microbiol. Immunol.* **81**, 143–148.

50 SISSONS, J. G. P. & OLDSTONE, M. B. A. (1980). Antibody-mediated destruction of virus-infected cells. *Adv. Immunol.* **29**, 209–260.

51 COOPER, N. R. (1979). Humoral immunity to viruses. In *Comprehensive virology* (ed. H. Fraenkel-Conrat & R. R. Wagner), vol. 15, pp. 123–170. Plenum Press, New York, London.

52 LEVINE, B. B. & VAZ, N. M. (1970). Effect of combinations of inbred strain, antigen and antigen dose on immune responsiveness and reagin production in the mouse. *Int. Arch. Allergy* **39**, 156.

53 LESLIE, R. G. Q. (1985). Complex aggregations: a critical event in macrophage handling of soluble immune complexes. *Immunol. Today* **6**, 183–186.

54 McCULLOUGH, K. C., CROWTHER, J. R. & BUTCHER, R. N. (1985). Alteration in antibody rectivity with foot-and-mouth disease virus (FMDV) 146 S antigen before and after binding to a solid phase or complexing with specific antibody. *J. Immunol. Methods* **82**, 91–100.

55 CLICK, R. E., BENCK, L. & ALTER, B. J. (1972). Immune responses *in vitro*. I. Culturing conditions for antibody synthesis. *Cell. Immunol.* **3**, 264–276.

56 CLICK, R. E., BENCK, L. & ALTER, B. J. (1972). Enhancement of antibody synthesis *in vitro* by mercaptoethanol. *Cell. Immunol.* **3**, 155–160.

57 KIRKLAND, T. N., SIECKMANN, D. G., LONGO, D. L. & MOSIER, D. E. (1980). Cellular requirements for antigen presentation in the induction of a thymus-independent antibody response *in vitro*. *J. Immunol.* **124**, 1721–1726.

58 BOSWELL, H. S., SHARROW, S. O. & SINGER, A. (1980). Role of accessory cells in B cell activation. I. Macrophage presentation of TNP-Ficoll: Evidence for macrophage–B cell interaction. *J. Immunol.* **124**, 989–996.

59 MOND, J. J., MONGINI, P. K. A., SIECKMANN, D. G. & PAUL, W. E. (1980). Role of T lymphocytes in the response to TNP-AECM-Ficoll. *J. Immunol.* **125**, 1066–1070.

60 LETVIN, N. L., BENACERRAF, B. & GERMAIN, R. N. (1981). B-lymphocyte responses to trinitrophenyl-conjugated Ficoll: requirement for T lymphocytes and Ia-bearing adherent cells. *Proc. Natl. Acad. Sci., U.S.A.* **78**, 5113–5117.

61 ENDRES, R. O., KUSHNIR, E., KAPPLER, J. W., MARRACK, P. & KINSKY, S. C. (1983). A requirement for non-specific T cell factors in antibody responses to 'T cell independent' antigens. *J. Immunol.* **130**, 781–784.

62 DEKRUYFF, R. H., CLAYBERGER, C. & CANTOR, H. (1985). Monoclonal helper T cells induce B cell responses to T-independent antigens: antigen specific T cells are directly stimulated by activated B cells in the absence of antigen. *J. Immunol.* **134**, 89–90.

63 MOSIER, D. E., ZITRON, I. M., MOND, J. J., AHMED, A., SCHER, I. & PAUL, W. E. (1977), Surface immunoglobulin D as a functional receptor for a subclass of B lymphocytes. *Immunol. Rev,* **37**, 89.

64 MOND, J. J., CAPORALE, L.A. & THORBECKE, G. J. (1974). Kinetics of B cell memory: development during a thymus independent immune response. *Cell. Immunol.* **10**, 105.

65 SHARON, R. P., McMASTER, R. B., KASK, A. M., OWENS, J. D. & PAUL, W. E. (1975). DNP-Lys-Ficoll: a T independent antigen which elicits both IgM and IgG anti-DNP antibody secretory cells. *J. Immunol.* **8**, 459.

66 CAPRA, J. D. & KEHOE, J. M. (1975). Hypervariable regions, idiotopy, and the antibody-combining site. *Adv. Immunol.* **20**, 1–40.
67 DAVIES, D. R. PADLAN, E. A. & SEGAL, D. M. (1975). Immunoglobulin structure at high resolution. *Contemp. Top. Molec. Immunol.* **4**, 127–155.
68 DAVIS, D. R. & METZGER, H. (1983). Structural basis of antibody function. *Ann. Rev. Immunol.* **1**, 87–117.
69 HUDSON, L. & HAY, F. C. (1980). *Practical Immunology.* Blackwell, Oxford.

Chapter 2

1 KOHLER, G. & MILSTEIN, C. (1975). Continuous culture of fused cells secreting antibody of predefined specificity. *Nature (London)* **256**, 495–497.
2 McMASTER, W. R. & WILLIAMS. A. F. (1979). Identification of Ia glycoproteins in rat thymus and purification from rat spleen. *Eur. J. Immunol.* **9**, 426–433.
3 CROCE, C. M., LINNENBACH, A., HALL. W., STEPLEWSKI, Z. & KOPROWSKI, H. (1980). Production of human hybridomas secreting antibodies to measles virus. *Nature (London)* **288**, 488–489.
4 SCHWABER, J. (1977). Human lymphocyte–mouse myeloma somatic cell hybrids selective hybrid formations. *Somatic Cell Genetics* **3**, 295–302.
5 YARMUSH, M. L., GATES, F. T., WEISFOGEL. D. R. & KINDT, T. J. (1980). Identification and characterization of rabbit-mouse hybridomas secreting rabbit immunoglobulin chains. *Proc. Natl. Acad. Sci., U.S.A.* **77**, 2899–2903.
6 SRIKUMARAN, S., GUIDRY, A. J. & GOLDSBY, R. A. (1983). Production and characterization of monoclonal bovine immunoglobulins G_1, G_2 and M from bovine × murine hybridomas. *Vet. Immunol. Immunopathol.* **5**, 323–342.
7 CLICK, R. E. BENCK, L. & ALTER, B. J. (1972). Immune responses *in vitro*. I. Culturing conditions for antibody synthesis. *Cell. Immunol.* **3**, 264–276.
8 HERBERT, W. J. & WILKINSON, P. C. (1971). *A dictionary of immunology.* Blackwell Scientific Publications, Oxford.
9 POTTER, M. (1972). Immunoglobulin-producing tumours and myeloma proteins of mice. *Physiol. Rev.* **52**, 631–719.
10 STÄHLI, G., STAEHELIN, T., MIGGIANO, V., SCHMIDT, J. & HARING, P. (1980). High frequencies of antigen-specific hybridomas: dependence on immunisation parameters and prediction by spleen cell analysis. *J. Immunol. Methods* **32**, 297–304.
11 GALFRE, G., MILSTEIN, C. & WRIGHT, B. (1979). Rat × rat hybrid-myelomas and monoclonal anti-Fd portion of mouse IgG. *Nature (London)* **277**, 131–133.
12 MANDEL, B. (1979). Interaction of viruses with neutralising antibodies. In *Comprehensive virology* (ed. H. Fraenkel-Conrat & R. R. Wagner), vol. 15, pp. 37–121. Plenum Press, New York, London.
13 McCULLOUGH, K. C. (1986). Monoclonal antibodies: implications for virology. *Arch Virol.* **87**, 1–36.
14 McCULLOUGH, K. C., BUTCHER, R. N. & PARKINSON, D. (1983). Hybridoma cell lines secreting monoclonal antibodies against foot-and-

mouth disease virus. I. Cell culturing requirements. *J. Biol. Stand.* **11**, 171–181.

15 FAZEKAS de ST. GROTH, S. & SCHEIDEGGER, D. (1980). Production of monoclonal antibodies: strategy and tactics. *J. Immunol. Methods* **35**, 1–21.

16 MILSTEIN, C. (1982). Monoclonal antibodies from hybrid myelomas: theoretical aspects and some general comments. In *Monoclonal antibodies in clinical medicine* (ed. A. J. McMichael & J.W. Fabre), chapter 1, pp. 3–16. Academic Press, London, New York.

17 HUMPHREY, J. H. & WHITE, R. G. *Immunology for students of medicine*, pp. 292–295. Blackwell, Oxford.

18 MISHEL, B. B. & SHIIGI, S. M. (1980). *Selected methods in cellular immunology*, pp. 24–25. W. H. Freeman & Co., San Francisco.

19 KENNETT, R. H., DENIS, K. A., TUNG, A. S. & KLINMAN, N. R. (1978). Hybrid plasmacytoma production: fusions with adult spleen cells, monoclonal spleen fragments, neonatal spleen cells and human cells. *Curr. Top. Microbiol. Immunol.* **81**, 77–91.

20 BUTTIN, G., LeGUERN, G., PHALENTE, L., LIN, E. C. C., MEDRANO, L. & CAZENAVE, P. A. (1978). Production of hybrid lines secreting monoclonal anti-idiotypic antibodies by cell fusion on membrane filters. *Curr. Top. Microbiol. Immunol.* **81**, 27–36.

21 WESTERWOUDT, R. J. (1985). Improved fusion methods. IV. Technical aspects. *J. Immunol. Methods* **77**, 181–196.

22 HUDSON, L. & HAY, F. C. (1980). *Practical immunology.* Blackwell, Oxford.

23 LAEMMLI, U. K. (1970). Cleavage of structural proteins during the assembly of the head of bacteriophage T4.1. *Nature (London)* **227**, 680–682.

24 SPITZ, M., SPITZ, L., THORPE, R. & EUGUI, E. (1984). Intrasplenic primary immunization for the production of monoclonal antibodies. *J. Immunol. Methods* **70**, 39–43.

25 ADAM, A. (1985). *Synthetic adjuvants*. John Wiley and Sons, New York.

26 BRODEUR, B. R., TSANG, P. & LAROSE, Y. (1984). Parameters affecting ascites tumour formation in mice and monoclonal antibody production. *J. Immunol. Methods* **71**, 265–272.

Chapter 3

1 STÄHLI, G., STAEHELIN, T., MIGGIANO, V., SCHMIDT, J. & HARING, P. (1980). High frequencies of antigen-specific hybridomas: dependence on immunisation parameters and prediction by spleen cell analysis. *J. Immunol. Methods* **32**, 297–304.

2 RUSSELL, W. C., PATEL, G., PRECIOUS, B., SHARP, I. & GARDNER, P. S. (1981). Monoclonal antibodies against adenovirus type 5: preparation and preliminary characterization. *J. Gen. Virol.* **56**, 393–408.

3 UNANUE, E. R. (1982). The regulatory role of macrophages in antigenic stimulation. Part two: symbiotic relationship between lymphocytes and macrophages. *Adv. Immunol.* **31**, 1–136.

4 McCULLOUGH, K. C., BUTCHER, R. N. & PARKINSON, D. (1983). Hybridoma cell lines secreting monoclonal antibodies against foot-and-mouth disease virus. II. Cloning conditions. *J. Biol. Stand.* **11**, 183–194.

5 MILSTEIN, C. (1982). Monoclonal antibodies from hybrid myelomas: theoretical aspects and some general comments. In *Monoclonal antibodies in clinical medicine* (ed. A. J. McMichael & J. W. Fabre), chapter 1, pp. 3–16. Academic Press, London, New York.

6 FAZEKAS de ST. GROTH, S. & SCHEIDEGGER, D. (1980). Production of monoclonal antibodies: strategy and tactics. *J. Immunol. Methods* **35**, 1–21.

7 NABHOLZ, M. (1979). Production and maintenance of antibody-secreting hybridoma. In *Hybridoma technology with special reference to parasitic diseases*, (ed. V. Houba, T. J. Linna, F. Michal & D. S. Rowe) chapter 3, pp. 23–32. WHO, Geneva.

8 DAVIS, J. M., PENNINGTON, J. E., KUBLER, A. M. & CONSCIENCE, J. F. (1982). A simple single step technique for selecting and cloning hybridomas for the production of monoclonal antibodies. *J. Immunol. Methods* **50**, 161–171.

9 WOLOSCHAK, G. E. & SENITZER, D. (1983). Effect of mitogenic stimulation of murine splenocytes on PEG-induced cell fusion. *Hybridoma* **2**, 341–349.

10 ISCOVE, N. N. & MELCHERS, F. (1978). Complete replacement of serum by albumin, transferrin and soybean lipid in cultures of lipopolysaccharide-reactive B lymphocytes. *J. Exp. Med.* **147**, 923–933.

11 DULBECCO, R. (1970). Topoinhibition and serum requirements of transformed and untransformed cells. *Nature (London)* **227**, 802–806.

12 CHANG, T. H., STEPLEWSKI, Z. & KOPROWSKI, H. (1980). Production of monoclonal antibodies in serum-free medium. *J. Immunol. Methods* **39**, 369–375.

13 CLICK, R. E., BENCK, L. & ALTER, B. J. (1972). Enhancement of antibody systems *in vitro* by mercaptoethanol. *Cell. Immunol.* **3**, 155–160.

14 CLICK, R. E., BENCK, L. & ALTER, B.J. (1972). Immune responses *in vitro*. I. Culturing conditions for antibody synthesis. *Cell. Immunol.* **3**, 264–276.

15 DULBECCO, R. & ELKINGTON, J. (1973). Conditions limiting multiplication of fibroblastic and epithelium cells in dense cultures. *Nature (London)* **246**, 197–199.

16 STOKER, M. G. P. (1973). Role of diffusion boundary layer in contact inhibition of growth. *Nature (London)* **246**, 200–203.

17 RUBIN, H. & REIN, A. (1967). In *Growth regulatory substances for cells in culture*, (Wistar Institute symposium monograph 7) (ed. V. Defeni & M. Stoker), p. 51. Wistar Institute Press, Philadelphia, U.S.A.

18 ASTALDI, G. C. B., JANSSEN, M. C., LANSDORP. P., WILLEMS, C., ZEIJLEMAKER, W. P. & OOSTERHOF, F. (1980). Human endothelial culture supernatant (HECS): A growth factor for hybridomas. *J. Immunol.* **125**, 1411–1414.

19 PINTUS, C., RANSOM, J. H. & EVANS, C. H. (1983). Endothelial cell growth supplement: a cell cloning factor that promotes the growth of monoclonal antibody producing hybridoma cells. *J. Immunol. Methods* **61**, 195–200.

20 BUTCHER, R. N., McCULLOUGH, K. C., JARRY, C. & BRYANT, J. (1988). Mitomycin C-treated 3T3/A31 cell feeder layers in hybridoma technology. *J. Immunol. Methods.* **107**, 245–251.

21 McCULLOUGH, K. C., BUTCHER, R. N. & PARKINSON, D. (1983). Hybridoma cell lines secreting monoclonal antibodies against foot-and-mouth disease virus. I. Cell culturing requirements. *J. Biol. Stand.* **11**, 171–181.

Chapter 4

1 ENGVALL, E. & PERLMAN, P. (1971). Enzyme-linked immunosorbent assay (ELISA). Quantitative assay of immunoglobulin G. *Immunochemistry* **8**, 871–874.

2 VOLLER, A., BIDWELL, D.E. & BARTLETT, A. (1976). Enzyme immunoassay in diagnostic medicine: theory and practice. *Bulletin WHO* **53**, 55–65.

3 McCULLOUGH, K. C. & PARKINSON, D. (1984*a*). The standardisation of a 'spot-test' ELISA for the rapid screening of sera and hybridoma cell products. I. The determination of the optimum buffering system. *J. Biol. Stand.* **12**, 67–74.

4 McCULLOUGH, K. C. & PARKINSON, D. (1984*b*). The standardisation of a 'spot-test' ELISA for the rapid screening of sera and hybridoma cell products. II. The determination of binding capacity, binding ratio and coefficient of variation of different ELISA plates in sandwich and indirect ELISA. *J. Biol. Stand.* **12**, 75–86.

5 EPSTEIN, S. L. & LUNNEY, J. K. (1985). A cell surface ELISA in the mouse using only poly-L-lysine as cell fixative. *J. Immunol. Methods* **76**, 63–72.

6 BUTLER, J. E., McGIVERN, P. L. & SWANSON, P. (1978). Amplification of the enzyme-linked immunosorbent assay (ELISA) in the detection of class-specific antibodies. *J. Immunol. Methods* **20**, 365–383.

7 McCULLOUGH, K. C., CROWTHER, J. R. & BUTCHER, R. N. (1985). A liquid-phase ELISA and its use in the identification of epitopes on foot-and-mouth disease virus antigens. *J. Virol. Methods* **11**, 329–338.

8 HAEGERT, D. G., HURD, C. & COOMBS, R. R. A. (1978). Comparison of the direct antiglobulin rosetting with direct immunofluorescence in the detection of surface membrane immunoglobulin on human peripheral blood lymphocytes. *Immunology* **34**, 533.

9 BINNS, R. M., LICENCE, S. T., SYMONS, D. B. A., GURNER, B. W., COOMBS, R. R. A. & WALTERS, D. E. (1979). Comparison of direct anti-globulin rosetting reaction (DARR) and direct immunofluorescence (DIF) for demonstration of sIg-bearing lymphocytes in pigs, sheep and cattle. *Immunology* **36**, 549.

10 COOMBS, R. R. A. (1981). Assays utilizing red cells as markers. In *Immunoassays for the '80's* (ed. A. Voller), p. 17. M.T.P. Press.

11 BINNS, R. M. LICENCE, S. T., GURNER, B. W. & COOMBS, R. R. A. (1982). Factors which govern the sensitivity of direct and indirect rosetting reactions and reverse passive haemagglutination in the identification of cell surface and free macromolecules. *Immunology* **47**, 717.

12 BINNS, R. M., LICENCE, S. T., GURNER, B. W. & COOMBS, R. R. A. (1983). The demonstration of sIg, MHC and T cell antigens and Fc receptors on the lymphocyte surface by anti-globulin rosetting reactions: some technical considerations. *J. Immunol. Methods* **63**, 69–80.

13 HUDSON, L. & HAY, F. C. (1980). *Practical immunology.* Blackwell Scientific Publications, Oxford.
14 RODRICK, M. L. (1980). Preparation of protein-conjugated red blood cells with bis-diazotized benzidine. In *Selected methods in cellular immunology* (ed. B. B. Mishel & S. M. Shiigi), pp. 105–108. W. H. Freeman & Co., San Francisco.
15 LING, N. R. (1961). The coupling of protein antigens to erythrocytes with difluorodinitrobenzene. *Immunology* **4**, 49.
16 KIPP, D. & MILLER, A. (1980). Preparation of protein-conjugated red blood cells with ECDI (modification). In *Selected methods in cellular immunology* (ed. B. B. Mishel & S. M. Shiigi), pp. 103–105. W. H. Freeman & Co., San Francisco.
17 JANDL, J. H. & SIMMONS, R. L. (1957). The agglutination and sensitisation of red cells by metallic cations: Interactions between multivalent metals and the red cell membrane, *Brit. J. Haematol.* **3**, 19.
18 WEIR, D. M. (1986). *Handbook of experimental immunology,* vols 1 and 2. Blackwell Scientific Publications, Oxford.
19 CRANAGE, M. P., GURNER, B. W. & COOMBS, R. R. A. (1983). Glutaraldehyde stabilisation of antibody-linked erythrocytes for use in reverse passive and related haemagglutination assays. *J. Immunol. Methods* **64**, 7–16.
20 OUCHTERLONY, O. (1958). Diffusion in gel methods for immunological analysis. In *Progress in allergy* (ed. P. Kallos), vol. 5, pp. 1–78. Karger Press, Basle and New York.
21 WILLIAMS, C. A. & CHASE, M. W. *Methods in immunology and immunochemistry,* vol. 3, pp. 234–94. Academic Press, New York and London.
22 LAURELL, C. B. (1965). Antigen–antibody crossed electrophoresis. *Anal. Biochem.* **10**, 358.
23 LAEMMLI, U.K. (1970). Cleavage of structural proteins during the assembly of the head of bacteriophage T4.1. *Nature (London)* **227**, 680.
24 LAURELL, C. B. (1966). Quantitative estimation of proteins by electrophoresis in agarose gel containing antibodies. *Anal. Biochem.* **15**, 45.
25 MISHEL, B. B. & SHIIGI, S. M. (eds) (1980). *Selected methods in cellular immunology.* W. H. Freeman & Co., San Francisco.
26 JERNE, N. K. & NORDIN, A. A. (1963). Plaque formation in agar by single antibody producing cells. *Science* **140**, 405.
27 MISHELL, R. I. & DUTTON, R. W. (1966). Immunization of normal mouse spleen cell suspensions *in vitro*. *Science* **153**, 1004–1006.
28 SHARON, J., MORRISON, S. L. & KABAT, E. A. (1979). Detection of specific hybridoma clones by replica immunoadsorption of their secreted antibodies. *Proc. Natl. Acad. Sci., U.S.A.* **76**, 1420–1424.
29 McCULLOUGH, K. C. (1986). Monoclonal antibodies: implications for virology. *Arch. Virol.* **87**, 1–36.
30 KENNETT, R. H., McKEARN, T. J. & BECHTOL, K. B. (eds) (1980). *Monoclonal antibodies, hybridomas: a new dimension in biological analyses,* pp. 171–274; pp. 376–378. Plenum Press, New York and London.
31 COLLEN, T., McCULLOUGH, K. C. & DOEL, T. R. (1984). Induction of antibody to foot-and-mouth disease virus in presensitized mouse spleen cell cultures. *J. Virol.* **52**, 650–655.

32 HOUBA, V., LINNA, T. J., MICHAL, F. & ROWE, D. S. (eds) (1979). *Hybridoma technology with special reference to parasitic diseases*. WHO, Geneva.

33 KOHLER, G. (1979). SDS-polyacrylamide gel electrophoresis. In *Hybridoma technology with special reference to parasitic diseases* (ed. V. Houba *et al.*), pp. 75–78. WHO, Geneva.

34 KOHLER, G. (1979). Isoelectric focusing. In *Hybridoma technology with special reference to parasitic diseases* (ed. V. Houba *et al.*), pp. 79–84. WHO, Geneva.

35 TRINCHIERI, G. (1979). Competition assay on cells. In *Hybridoma technology with special reference to parasitic diseases* (ed. V. Houba *et al.*), pp. 85–86. WHO, Geneva.

36 McCULLOUGH, K. C., BUTCHER, R. N. & PARKINSON, D. (1983). Hybridoma cell lines secreting monoclonal antibodies against foot-and-mouth disease virus (FMDV). II. Cloning conditions. *J. Biol. Stand.* **11**, 183–194.

37 FAZEKAS de ST. GROTH, S. (1982). The evaluation of limiting dilution assays. *J. Immunol. Methods* **49**, R11–23.

38 DAVIS, J. M., PENNINGTON, J. E. KUBLER, A. M. & CONSCIENCE, J. F. (1982). A simple single step technique for selecting and cloning hybridomas for the production of monoclonal antibodies. *J. Immunol. Methods* **50**, 161–171.

39 BUTCHER, R. N., McCULLOUGH, K. C., JARRY, C. & BRYANT, J. (1988). Mitomycin C-treated 3T3/A31 cell feeder layers in hybridoma technology. *J. Immunol. Methods* **107**, 245–251.

40 BUTCHER, R. N., OBI, T. U. & McCULLOUGH, K. C. (1989). Rapid isolation of monoclonal hybridoma cultures by a 'fusion-cloning' method: the requirement of aminopterin. *J. Biol. Stand.* (submitted).

41 McCULLOUGH, K. C., CROWTHER, J. R. & BUTCHER, R. N. (1985). Alteration in antibody reactivity with foot-and-mouth disease virus (FMDV) 146 S antigen before and after binding to a solid phase or complexing with specific antibody. *J. Immunol. Methods* **82**, 91–100.

Chapter 5

1 BIRCH, J. R., THOMPSON, P. W., LAMBERT, K. & BORASTON, R. (1985). The large-scale cultivation of hybridoma cells producing monoclonal antibodies. In *Large-scale mammalian cell culture* (ed. J. Feder & W. R. Tolbert), pp. 1–16. Academic Press, London.

2 KARKARE, S. B., PHILLIPS, P. G., BURKE, D. H. & DEAN, R. C. Jr (1985). Continuous production of monoclonal antibodies by chemostatic and immobilised hybridoma culture. In *Large-scale mammalian cell culture* (ed. J. Feder & W. R. Tolbert), pp. 127–149. Academic Press, London.

3 RANDERSON, D. (1984). Hybridoma technology and the process engineer. *The Chemical Engineer, Dec 1984*, pp. 12–15.

4 PHILLIPS, A. W., BALL, G. D., FANTES, K. H., FINTER, N. B. & JOHNSON, M. D. (1985). Experience in the cultivation of mammalian cells on the 8,000 1 scale. In *Large-scale mammalian cell culture* (ed. J. Feder & W. R. Tolbert), pp. 87–93. Academic Press, London.

5 DAVIS, J. M., PENNINGTON, J. E., BAKER, A. M. & CONSCIENCE, J. F. (1982). A simple, single-step technique for selecting and cloning hybridomas for the production of monoclonal antibodies. *J. Immunol. Methods* **50**, 161–171.

6 VAN WEZEL, A. J. (1984). Figures quoted at a meeting on hybridoma scale-up held under the aegis of the Institution of Chemical Engineers Biochemical Engineering Sub-Group at Unilever, Colworth House, 26 November 1984.

7 MERTEN, O. W., REITER, S., HIMMLER, G., SCHEIRER, W. & KATINGER, H. (1984). Production kinetics of monoclonal antibodies. *Dev. Biol. Standard.* **60**, 219–227.

8 NABHOLZ, M. (1979). Production and maintenance of antibody-secreting myeloma hybrids. In *Hybridoma technology with special reference to parasitic diseases* (ed. V. Houba *et al.*), part II *(Hybridoma technology)*, pp. 23–31. WHO, Geneva.

9 CLARKE, J. B. & SPIER, R. E. (1980). Variation in the susceptibility of BHK populations and cloned cell lines in three strains of foot-and-mouth disease virus. *Arch. Virol.* **63**, 1–9.

10 FEDER, J. (1985). Discussion. In *Large-scale mammalian cell culture* (ed. J. Feder & W. R. Tolbert), pp. 153–154. Academic Press, London.

11 RUKER, F., REITERS, S., JUNGBAUER, A., LIEGL, W., HIMMLER, G., STEINKELLNER, H., WENISCH, E., STEINDE, F., WAGNER, K. & KATINGER, H. (1987). Self-hybridisation of hybridomas leads to stabilisation of clones and increased yield of monoclonal antibodies. *Dev. Biol. Standard.* **66**, 71–74.

12 WOOD, C. R., BOSS, M. A., KENTEN, J. H., CALVERT, J. E., ROBERTS, N. A. & EMTAGE, J. S. (1985). The synthesis and *in vivo* assembly of functional antibodies in yeast. *Nature (London)* **314**, 446–449.

13 WAYMOUTH, C. (1972). Construction of tissue culture media. In *Growth, nutrition and metabolism of cells in culture*, vol. 1 (ed G. H. Rothblat and V. C. Cristofalo), ch. 2, pp. 11–47. Academic Press, London.

14 LAMBERT, K. J. & BIRCH, J. R. (1985). Cell growth media. In *Animal cell biotechnology* (ed. R. E. Spier & J. B. Griffiths), ch. 4, pp. 85–122. Academic Press, London.

15 MORANDI, M., STANGHELLINI, L. & VALERI, A. (1985). Problems involved in the large-scale production of biological products, such as beta-interferon, using diploid fibroblast as substrate. *Dev. Biol. Standard.* **60**, 405–412.

16 FLEISHAKER, R. J. & SINSKEY, A. J. (1981). Oxygen demand and supply in cell culture. *Eur. J. Appl. Microbiol. Biotechnol.* **12**, 193–197.

17 MILTENBURGER, H. G. & DAVID, P. (1980). Mass production of insect cells in suspension. *Dev. Biol. Standard.* **46**, 183–186.

18 SPIER, R. E. & GRIFFITHS, B. (1984). An examination of the data and concepts germane to the oxygenation of cultured animal cells. *Dev. Biol. Standard.* **55**, 81–92.

19 LEHMANN, J., PIEHL, G. W. & SCHULZ, R. (1987). Bubble-free cell culture aeration with porous moving membranes. *Dev. Biol. Standard.* **66**, 227–240.

20 HANDA, A., EMERY, N. & SPIER, R. E. (1987). On the evaluation of gas-liquid interface effects on hybridoma viability in bubble column bioreactors. *Dev. Biol. Standard.* **66**, 241–254.

21 BOEDEKER, B. G. D., BERG, G. J., HEWLETT, G. & SCHLUMBERGER, H. D. (1985). A screening method to develop serum-free culture media for adherent cell lines. *Dev. Biol. Standard.* **60**, 93–100.

22 CLEVELAND, W. L., WOOD, I. & ERLANGER, P. F. (1983). Routine large-scale production of monoclonal antibodies in a protein-free culture medium. *J. Immunol. Methods* **56**, 221–234.

23 BAKER, P., KNOBLOCK, K., NOLL, L., WYATT, D. & LYDERSEN, B. (1985). A serum-independent medium effective in all aspects of hybridoma technology and immunological applications. *Dev. Biol. Standard.* **60**, 63–72.

24 MALDONEDO, R. L. & FULBRIGHT, J. G. (1984). Processed serum: a consistent growth support for hybridomas. *Int. Biotechnol. Lab., March–April 1984*, pp. 34–36.

25 PANKRATOV, V. P., MANTZYGIN, Y. A., MORENKOV, O. S. & SWYATUKHINA, N. (1985). Continuous cultivation of hybridoma cells in a cell reactor. *Biotechnol. Lett.* **7**, 141–146.

26 REUVENY, S., VELEZ, D., RISKE, F., MACMILLAN, J. D. & MILLER, L. (1985). Production of monoclonal antibodies in culture. *Dev. Biol. Standard.* **60**, 185–197.

27 HIMMLER, G., PALFI, G., FUKER, R., KATINGER, H. & SCHEIRER, W. (1985). A laboratory fermenter for agarose immobilised hybridomas to produce monoclonal antibodies. *Dev. Biol. Standard.* **60**, 291–296.

28 RADLETT, P., PAY, T. W. F. & GARLAND, A J. M. (1985). The use of BHK suspension cells for the commercial production of foot-and-mouth disease vaccines over a twenty year period. *Dev. Biol. Standard.* **60**, 163–170.

29 MONTAGNON, B., VINCENT-FALQUET, J. C. & FANGET, B. (1984). Thousand litre scale microcarrier culture of vero cells for killed polio virus vaccine: promising results. *Dev. Biol. Standard.* **55**, 37–42.

30 McALEER, W. (1986). Operational unit process system for Marek's vaccine at the 70 1 scale. (Personal communication to R.E.S.).

31 GRIFFITHS, J. B. (1985). Discussion (following paper by G. Himmler). *Dev. Biol. Standard.* **60**, 296.

32 HIMMELFARB, P., THAYER, P. S. & MARTIN, H. E. (1969). Spin filter culture: the propagation of mammalian cells in suspension. *Science* **164**, 555–557.

33 KATINGER, H. W. D., SCHEIRER, W. & KRAMER, E. (1979). Bubble column reactors for mass propagation of animal cells in suspension culture. *German Chem. Eng.* (English translation) **2**, 31–38.

34 BIRCH, J. (1985). Tape recording of presentation to Nature New Technology, London, 27 June 1985.

35 TOLBERT, W. R., LEWIS, C., WHITE, P. J. & FEDER, J. (1985). Perfusion culture systems for production of mammalian cell biomolecules. In *Large-scale mammalian cell cultures* (ed. J. Feder & W. R. Tolbert), pp. 97–119. Academic Press, London.

36 KLEMENT, G., SCHEIRER, W. & KATINGER, H. W. F. (1987). Construction of a large-scale membrane reactor system with different compartments for cells, medium and product. *Dev. Biol. Standard.* **66**, 221–226.

37 HOPKINSON, J. (1985). Hollow fibre cell culture systems for economical cell-product manufacturing. *Biotechnology* **3**, 225–230.

38 SEFTON, M. V. (1982). Encapsulation of live animal cells. U.S. Patent no. 4 353 88.
39 LIM, F. (1983). Reversible microencapsulation of a core material. U.S. Patent no. 4 407 957.
40 LIM, F. (1983). Preparation of substances with encapsulated cells. U.S. Patent no. 4 409 331.
41 RUPP, R. G. (1985). Use of cellular microencapsulation in large-scale production of monoclonal antibodies. In *Large-scale mammalian cell culture* (ed. J. Feder & W. R. Tolbert), pp. 19–36. Academic Press, London.
42 KROGH, G. (1919). *J. Physiol.* 52, 409, 457.
43 BELL, G. H., DAVIDSON, J. N. & SCARBOROUGH, H. (1956). *Textbook of physiology and biochemistry* (3rd edn.).
44 TANNOCK, I. F. (1968). The relation between cell proliferation and the vascular system in a transplanted mouse mammary tumour. *Brit. J. Cancer* **22**, 258–273.
45 HOPKINSON, J. (1983). Hollow fibre cell culture: applications in industry. In *Immobilised cells and organelles.* vol. 1 (ed. B. Mattiasson), pp. 90–99. CRC Press, Boca Raton, Florida.
46 GREENE, H. S. H. (1941). Heterologous transplantation of mammalian tumours. I. Transfer of rabbit tumours to other species. *J. Exp. Med.* **73**, 462–474.
47 MURDIN, A. D., KIRKBY, N. F., WILSON, R. & SPIER, R. E. (1977). Immobolised hybridomas: oxygen diffusion. In *Animal cell biotechnology* (ed. R. E. Spier & J. B. Griffiths), vol. 3, pp. 56–75. Academic Press, London.
48 SPIER, R. E. (1980). Recent developments in the large-scale cultivation of animal cells in monolayers. *Adv. Biochem Eng.* **14**, 119–162.
49 BELL, G. D. (1985). Clarification and sterilisation. In *Animal cell biotechnology* (ed. R. E. Spier & J. B. Griffiths), vol. 3, pp. 87–127. Academic Press, London.
50 Cell removal filtration system. Derwent Patent Abstracts, December 1985.
51 RADLETT, P. J. (1972). The concentration of mammalian cells in a tangential flow filtration unit. *J. App. Chem. Biotechnol.* **22**, 495–496.
52 MORROW, A. W. (1972). Concentration of the virus of foot-and-mouth disease in a tangential flow ultrafiltration unit. *J. Appl. Chem. Biotechnol.* **22**, 501–505.
53 CARTWRIGHT, J. & DUCHESNE, M. (1985). Purification of products from cultivated animal cells. In *Animal cell biotechnology* (ed. R. E. Spier & J. B. Griffiths), vol. 2, pp. 151–184. Academic Press, London.
54 REIN, A. & RUBIN, H. (1968). Effects of local cell concentrations upon the growth of chick embryo cells in tissue culture. *Exp. Cell. Res.* **49**, 666–678.
55 SCHONHERR, O. T., VAN GELDER, P. T. J. A., VAN HEES, P. J., VAN OS, A. J. V. & ROELOFS, H. W. M. (1987). A hollow fibre dialysis system for the *in vitro* production of monoclonal antibodies replacing *in vivo* production in mice. *Dev. Biol. Standard.* **66**, 211–220.
56 ENDOTRONICS (1985). AcuSyst-P production system brochure. Endotronics, 8500 Evergreen Blvd, Coon Rapids, MN55433, U.S.A.
57 REUVENY, S., VELEZ, D., RISKE, F., MACMILLAN, J. D. & MILLER, L. (1985). Production of monoclonal antibodies in culture. *Dev. Biol. Standard.* **60**, 185–197.

58 MONSANTO CO. (1978). Culture reactor and method. Brit. Patent no. 1 514 906.

59 THRELFALL, G. & GARLAND, S. G. (1985). Equipment sterilisation. In *Animal cell biotechnology* (ed. R. E. Spier & J. B. Griffiths), vol. 1, pp. 123–140. Academic Press, London.

60 STRATHMANN, H. (1985). Membranes and membrane processes in biotechnology. *Trends Biotechnol.* **3** (5), 112–118.

61 LAVERY, M., KEARNS, M. J., PRICE, D. G., EMERY, A. N., JEFFERIES, R. & NEINOW, V. A. W. (1985). Physical conditions during batch cultures of hybridomas in laboratory scale stirred tank reactor. *Dev. Biol. Standard.* **60**, 198–205.

62 FAZEKAS de ST. GROTH, S. (1983). Automated production of monoclonal antibodies in a cytostat. *J. Immunol. Methods* **57**, 121–136.

63 VAN WEZEL, A. J. (1984). Marine impellor operating at 150 rpm. (Paper presented at a meeting on hybridoma scale-up held under the aegis of the Institution of Chemical Engineers Biochemical Engineering Sub-Group at Unilever, Colworth House, 26 November 1984.)

64 LITWIN, J. (1985). Discussion following ref. 61.

65 WANG, R. J. (1976). Effect of room fluorescent light on the determination of tissue culture medium. *In Vitro* **12**, 19–22.

66 HU, W.-S., DODGE, T. C., FRAME, K. K. & HIMES, V. B. (1987). Effect of glucose on the cultivation of mammalian cells. *Dev. Biol. Standard.* **66**, 279–290.

67 BORASTON, R. THOMPSON, P. W., GARLAND, S. & BIRCH, J. R. (1984). Growth and oxygen requirements of antibody-producing mouse hybridoma cells in suspension culture. *Dev. Biol. Standard.* **55**, 103–111.

68 REUVENY, S., VELEZ, D., MACMILLAN, J. D. & MILLER, L. (1987). Factors affecting monoclonal antibody production in culture. *Dev. Biol. Standard.* **66**, 169–176.

69 IMAURA, T., CRESPI, C. L., THILLY, W. G. & BRUNENGRABER, H. (1982). Fructose as a carbohydrate source yields stable pH and redox parameters in microcarrier cell culture. *Analyt. Biochem.* **124**, 353–358.

70 BAUGH, C. L., LECHER, R. W. & TYTELL, A. A. (1967). The effect of pH on the propagation of the diploid cell W138 in galactose medium. *J. Cell Physiol.* **70**, 225–228.

71 ZIELKE, H. R., AIELKE, C. L. & OZAND, P. T. (1984). Glutamine: a major energy source for cultivated mammalian cells. *Fed. Proc.* **43**, 121–125.

72 ZIELKE, H. R., OZAND, P. T., TILDON, J. T., SEVDALIAN, D. A. & CORNBLATH, M. (1978). Reciprocal regulation of glucose and glutamine utilisation by cultured human diploid fibroblasts. *J. Cell Physiol.* **95**, 41–48.

73 TELLING, R. C. & RADLETT, P. J. (1970). Large-scale cultivation of mammalian cells. *Adv. Appl. Microbiol.* **13**, 91–119.

74 ARMS, K. & CAMPS, P. S. (1982). In *Biology*, p. 17. Saunders College Publishing, Philadelphia.

75 BUTLER, M. & SPIER, R. E. (1984). The effects of glutamine utilisation and ammonia production on the growth of BHK cells in microcarrier cultures. *J. Biotechnol.* **1**, 187–196.

76 SPIER, R. E. (1980). Advantages of a microprocessor-monitored and controlled continuous culture of BHK suspension cells. *Dev. Biol. Standard.* **46**, 159–165.

77 DEAN, R.C. Jr (1985). Discussion. In *Large-scale mammalian cell culture* (ed. J. Feder & W. R. Tolbert), p. 154. Academic Press, London.
78 SMART, N. J. (1984). *Lab Practice*, July 1984.
79 FOWLER, M. (1985). Presentation given at Biotechnica '85, Hannover, F.R.G., October 1985.
80 SPIER, R. E. (1985). Monolayer growth systems: heterogeneous unit processes. In *Animal cell biotechnology* (ed. R. E. Spier & J. B. Griffiths), vol. 1, pp. 243–265. Academic Press, London.
81 MURDIN, A. D., THORPE, J. S., KIRKBY, N., GROVES, D. J. & SPIER, R. E. (1987). Immobilisation and growth of hybridomas in packed beds. In *Proceedings of the international conference on bioreactors and biotransformations, Gleneagles, Scotland*. Elsevier Applied Science Publishers, Amsterdam.
82 WHITESIDE, J. P. & SPIER, R. E. (1981). The scale-up from 0.1 to 100 litres of a unit-process system based on 3 mm diameter glass spheres for the production of four strains of FMDV from BHK monolayer cells. *Biotech. Bioeng.* **23**, 551–565.
83 KATINGER, H. (1987). Principles of animal cell fermentation. *Dev. Biol. Standard.* **66**, 195–210.
84 LYDERSEN, B. J., PUTNAM, J. BOGNAR, E., PATTERSON, M., PUGH, G. G. & NOTT, L. A. (1985). The use of a ceramic matrix in a large-scale cell culture system. In *Large-scale mammalian cell culture* (ed. J. Feder & W. R. Tolbert), pp. 39–58. Academic Press, London.
85 NILLSON, K., SCHEIRER, W., MERTEN, O.-W., OSTBERG, L., LIEHL, L., KATINGER, H. & MOSBACH, K. (1983). Entrapment of animal cells for the production of monoclonal antibodies and other biomolecules. *Nature (London)* **302**, 629–630.
86 NILLSON, K. & MOSBACH, K. (1987). Immobilised animal cells. *Dev. Biol. Standard.* **66**, 183–194.
87 EMERY, N. & MITCHELL, D. A. (1986). Operational considerations in the use of immobilised cells. In *Process engineering aspects of immobilised cell systems* (ed. C. Webb, G. M. Black & F. Mavituna). Institution of Chemical Engineers, Rugby.
88 ODA, G., SAMEJIMA, H. & YAMEDA, T. (1983). Continuous alcohol fermentation technologies using immobilised yeast cells. In *Biotech '83*. pp. 597–611. Online Publications, Northwood, U.K.
89 ROSEVEAR, A. & LAMBE, C. A. (1983). Immobilised plant and animal cells. In *Topics in enzymes and fermentation biotechnology*, vol. 7 (ed. A. Wiseman), ch. 2, pp. 13–37. Ellis Horwood, Chichester.
90 NILLSON, K. & MOSBACH, K. (1980). Preparation of immobilised animal cells. *FEBS Lett.* **118**, 145–150.
91 KLEIN, J. & VARLOP, K.-D. (1985). Immobilisation techniques – cells. In *Comprehension biotechnology* (ed. Murray Moo-Young), vol. 2, pp. 203–224. Pergamon Press, Oxford.
92 LITWIN, J. (1985). The growth of human diploid fibroblasts: aggregates with cellulose fibres in suspension. *Dev. Biol. Standard.* **60**, 237–242.
93 REUVENY, S., BINO, T., ROSENBERG, H. & MIZRAHI, V. A. (1987). A new cellulose-based microcarrier culturing system. *Dev. Biol. Standard.* **46**, 137–145.
94 BROWN, P. C., COSTELLO, M. A. C., OAKLEY, R. & LEWIS, J. L. (1985). Applications of the mass culturing technique (MCT) in the large

scale growth of mammalian cells. In *Large-scale mammalian cell culture* (ed. J. Feder & W. R. Tolbert), pp. 59–71. Academic Press, London.
95 HILL, S. A. & HIRTENSTEIN, M. D. (1983). Affinity chromatography: its application to industrial scale processes. *Adv. Biotechnol. Process.* **1**, 31–66.
96 DIEM, K. & LENTER, C. (1970). *Documenta Geigy* (scientific tables). (7th edn.)
97 GRIFFITHS, J. B. & RILEY, P. A. (1985. Cell biology: basic concepts. In *Animal cell biotechnology,* vol. 1 (ed. R. E. Spier & J. B. Griffiths), pp. 17–48. Academic Press, London.
98 DIEM, K. & LENTER, C. (1970). *Documenta Geigy* (scientific tables). (7th edn.).
99 DAVIS, D. V. & COUPLAND, R. E. (eds) (1967). *Gray's Anatomy* (34th edn.), p. 740.
100 ARATHOON, W. R. & TELLING, R. C. (1982). Uptake of amino acids and glucose by BHK 21 Clone 13 suspension cells during cell growth. *Dev. Biol. Standard.* **50**, 145–154.

Chapter 6

1 KENNETT, R. H., McKEARN, T. J. & BECHTOL, K. B. (eds) (1980). *Monoclonal antibodies, hybridomas: a new dimension in biological analyses*. Plenum Press, New York and London.
2 YEWDELL, J. W. & GERHARD, W. (1981). Antigenic characterisation of viruses by monoclonal antibodies. *Ann. Rev. Microbiol.* **35**, 185–206.
3 YELTON, D. E. & SCHARFF, M. D. (1981). Monoclonal antibodies: a powerful new tool in biology and medicine. *Ann. Rev. Biochem.* **50**, 657–680.
4 McMICHAEL, A. J. & FABRE, J. W. (eds) (1982). *Monoclonal antibodies in clinical medicine*. Academic Press, London.
5 HURRELL, J. G. R. (ed.) (1982). *Monoclonal hybridoma antibodies: techniques and applications*. CRC Press, Florida.
6 KATZ, D. H. (1982). *Monoclonal antibodies and T cell products*. CRC Press, Florida.
7 CARTER, M. J. & ter MEULEN, V. (1984). The application of monoclonal antibodies in the study of viruses. *Adv. Virus. Res.* **29**, 95–130.
8 KENNETT, R. H., BECHTOL, K. B. & McKEARN, T. J. (eds) (1984). *Monoclonal antibodies and functional cell lines*. Plenum Press, New York.
9 STERN, N. J. & GAMBLE, H. R. (eds) (1984). *Hybridoma technology in agricultural and veterinary research*. Rowman and Allanheld, New Jersey.
10 POLLOCK, R. R., TEILLAUD, J.-L. & SCHARFF, M. D. (1984). Monoclonal antibodies: a powerful tool for selecting and analyzing mutations in antigens and antibodies. *Ann. Rev. Microbiol.* **38**, 389–417.
11 McCULLOUGH, K. C. (1986). Monoclonal antibodies: implications for virology. *Arch. Virol.* **87**, 1–36.
12 MÖLLER, G. (ed.) (1979). Hybrid myeloma monoclonal antibodies against MHC products. *Immunol. Rev.*, vol. 47. Munksgaard, Copenhagen.
13 MÖLLER, G. (ed.) (1983). B cell differentiation antigens. *Immunol. Rev.*, vol. 69. Munksgaard, Copenhagen.
14 MÖLLER, G. (ed.). (1983). Functional T cell subsets defined by monoclonal antibodies. *Immunol. Rev.*, vol. 74. Munksgaard, Copenhagen.

15 MELCHERS, F., POTTER, M. & WARNER, N.L. (eds) (1978). Lymphocyte hybridomas. *Curr. Top. Microbiol. Immunol.*, vol. 81. Springer-Verlag, Berlin.
16 MÖLLER, G. (ed.) (1982). Effects of anti-membrane antibodies on killer T cells. *Immunol. Rev.*, vol. 68. Munksgaard, Copenhagen.
17 MÖLLER, G. (ed.) (1983). T cell hybrids. *Immunol. Rev.*, vol. 76. Munksgaard, Copenhagen.
18 TOM, B. H. & ALLISON, J.P. (1983). *Hybridomas and cellular immortality.* Plenum Press, New York.
19 BOSS, B. D., LANGMAN, R., TROWBRIDGE, I. & DULBECCO, R. (eds) (1983). *Monoclonal antibodies and cancer.* Academic Press, New York.
20 YOLKEN, R. H. (1983). Use of monoclonal antibodies for viral diagnosis. *Curr. Top. Microbiol. Immunol.* **104**, 177–195.
21 OXFORD, J. (1982). The use of monoclonal antibodies in virology. *J. Hyg. Camb.* **88**, 361–368.
22 MÖLLER, G. (ed.) (1982). Antibody carriers of drugs and toxins in tumor therapy. *Immunol. Rev.*, vol. 62. Munksgaard, Copenhagen.
23 VITETTA, E. S. & UHR, J. W. (1985). Immunotoxins: Redirecting nature's poisons. *Cell* **41**, 653–654.
24 HAHN, G. S. (1986). Immunoglobulin-derived drugs. *Nature (London)* **324**, 283–284.
25 KLAUSNER, A. (1986). Taking aim at cancer with monoclonal antibodies. *Biotechnology* **4**, 185–194.
26 GREAVES, M. F. (ed.) (1985). *Monoclonal antibodies to receptors*. Chapman and Hall, London.
27 HOWES, E. L., CLARK, E. A., SMITH, E. & MITCHISON, N. A. (1979). Mouse hybrid cell lines produce antibodies to herpes simplex virus type 1. *J. Gen. Virol.* **44**, 81–87.
28 RUSSELL, W. C., PATEL, G., PRECIOUS, B., SHARP, I. & GARDNER, P. S. (1981). Monoclonal antibodies against adenovirus type 5: preparation and preliminary characterisation. *J. Gen. Virol.* **56**, 393–408.
29 MARTINIS, J. & CROCE, C. M. (1978). Somatic cell hybrids producing antibodies specific for the tumour antigen of simian virus 40. *Proc. Natl. Acad. Sci., U.S.A.* **75**, 2320–2323.
30 BURTONBOY, G., BAZIN, H. & DELFERRIERE, N. (1982). Rat hybridoma antibodies against canine parvovirus. *Arch. Virol.* **71**, 291–302.
31 COTE, P.J. Jr, DAPOLITO, G. M., SHIH, J. W. & GERIN, J. L. (1982). Surface antigenic determinants of mammalian 'Hepadnaviruses' defined by group and class specific monoclonal antibodies. *J. Virol.* **42**, 135–142.
32 IMAI, M., NOMURA, M., GOTANDA, T., SANO, T., TACHIBANA, K., MIYAMOTO, H., TAKAHASHI, K., TOYAMA, S., MIYAKAWA, Y. & MAYUMI, M. (1982). Demonstration of two distinct antigenic determinants on hepatitis Be antigen by monoclonal antibodies. *J. Immunol.* **128**, 69–72.
33 SHERRY, B., MOSSER, A. G., COLONNO, R. J. & RUECKERT, R. R. (1986). Use of monoclonal antibodies to identify four neutralization immunogens on a common cold picornavirus, human rhinovirus 14. *J. Virol.* **57**, 246–257.
34 McCULLOUGH, K. C. & BUTCHER, R. N. (1982). Monoclonal antibodies against FMDV 146S and 12S. *Arch. Virol.* **74**, 1–9.

35 McCULLOUGH, K. C., CROWTHER, J. R., CARPENTER, W. C., BROCCHI, E., CAPUCCI, L., DE SIMONE, F., XIE, Q. & McCAHON, D. (1987). Epitopes on foot-and-mouth disease virus particles. I. Topology. *Virology* **157**, 516–525.

36 FERGUSON, M., SCHILD, G. C., MINOR, P. D., YATES, B. J. & SPITZ, M. (1981). A hybridoma cell line secreting antibody to poliovirus type 3 D-antigen: detection in virus harvest of two D-antigen populations. *J. Gen. Virol.* **54**, 437–442.

37 EMINI, E. A., JAMESON, B. A., LEWIS, A. J., LARSEN, G. R. & WIMMER, E. (1982). Poliovirus neutralization epitopes: analysis and localization with neutralizing monoclonal antibodies. *J. Virol.* **43**, 997–1005.

38 MINOR, P. D., SCHILD, G. C., FERGUSON, M. MACKAY, A., MAGRATH, D. I., JOHN, A., YATES, J. P. & SPITZ, M. (1982). Genetic and antigenic variation in type 3 polioviruses: characterization of strains by monoclonal antibodies and T1 oligonucleotide mapping. *J. Gen. Virol.* **61**, 167–176.

39 WIEGERS, K.-J. & DERNICK, R. (1983). Monospecific antisera against capsid polypeptides of poliovirus type 1 distinguish antigenic structures of poliovirus proteins. *J. Gen. Virol.* **64**, 777–785.

40 CAO, Y., SCHNURR, D. P. & SCHMIDT, N. J. Monoclonal antibodies for study of antigenic variation in Coxsackievirus type B4: association of antigenic determinants with mycarditic properties of the virus. *J. Gen. Virol.* **65**, 925–932.

41 GREENBERG, H., McAULIFFE, V., VALDESUSO, J., WYATT, R., FLORES, J., KALICA, A., HOSHINO, Y. & SINGH, N. (1983). Serological analysis of the subgroup protein of rotavirus, using monoclonal antibodies. *Inf. Imm.* **39**, 91–99.

42 BURSTIN, S. J., SPRIGGS, D. R. & FIELDS, B. N. (1982). Evidence for functional domains on the reovirus type 3 haemagglutinin. *Virology* **117**, 146–155.

43 APPLETON, J. A. & LETCHWORTH, G. J. (1983). Monoclonal antibody analysis of serotype restricted and unrestricted bluetongue viral antigenic determinants. *Virology* **124**, 286–299.

44 GERHARD, W., CROCE, C. M., LOPES, D. & KOPROWSKI, H. (1978). Repertoire of antiviral antibodies expressed by somatic cell hybrids. *Proc. Natl. Acad. Sci., U.S.A.* **75**, 1510–1514.

45 GERHARD, W. & WEBSTER, R. G. (1978). Antigenic drift in influenza A viruses. I. Selection and characterisation of antigenic variants of A/PR/8/34 [H0N1] influenza virus with monoclonal antibodies. *J. Exp. Med.* **148**, 383–392.

46 YEWDELL, J. W., WEBSTER, R. G. & GERHARD, W. U. (1979). Antigenic variations in three distinct determinants of an influenza type A haemagglutinin molecule. *Nature (London)* **279**, 246.

47 LAVER, W. G., GERHARD, W., WEBSTER, R. G., FRANKEL, M. E. & AIR, G. M. (1979). Antigenic drift in type A influenza virus: peptide mapping and antigenic analysis of A/PR/8/34 [H0N1] variants selected with monoclonal antibodies. *Proc. Natl. Acad. Sci., U.S.A.* **76**, 1425.

48 WEBSTER, R. G. & LAVER, W. G. (1980). Determination of the number of non-overlapping antigenic areas on Hong Kong (H3N2) influenza virus haemagglutinin with monoclonal antibodies and the selection of variants with potential epidemiological significance. *Virology,* **104**, 139.

49 IORIO, R. M. & BRATT, M. A. (1983). Monoclonal antibodies to Newcastle disease virus: delineation of four epitopes on the HN glycoprotein. *J. Virol.* **48**, 440–450.

50 NORRBY, E., CHEN, S.-N., TOGASHI, T., SHESHBERADARAN, H. & JOHNSON, K. P. (1982). Five measles virus antigens demonstrated by use of mouse hybridoma antibodies in productively infected tissue culture cells. *Arch. Virol.* **71**, 1–11.

51 SHESHBERADARAN, H., CHEN, S.-N. & NORRBY, E. (1983). Monoclonal antibodies against five structural components of measles virus. I. Characterisation of antigenic determinants on nine strains of measles virus. *Virology* **128**, 341–353.

52 SHESHBERDARAN, H. & NORRBY, E. (1985). Characterization of epitopes on measles virus haemagglutinin. *Virology* **152**, 58–65.

53 ORVELL, C., SHESHBERDARAN, H. & NORRBY, E. (1985). Preparation and characterization of monoclonal antibodies directed against four structural components of canine distemper virus. *J. Gen. Virol.* **66**, 443–456.

54 McCULLOUGH, K. C., SHESHBERDARAN, H., NORRBY, E., OBI, T. U. & CROWTHER, J. R. (1985). Monoclonal antibodies against morbilliviruses. *Rev. Sci. Tech. Off. Int. Epiz.* **5**, 411–427.

55 GIMENEZ, H. B., CASH, P. & MELVIN, W. T. (1984). Monoclonal antibodies to human respiratory syncytial virus and their use in comparison of different virus isolates. *J. Gen. Virol.* **65**, 963–971.

56 WIKTOR, T. J. & KOPROWSKI, H. (1980). Antigenic variants of rabies virus. *J. Exp. Med.* **152**, 99–112.

57 LAFON, M., WIKTOR, T. J. & MacFARLAN, R. I. (1983). Antigenic sites on the CVS rabies virus glycoprotein: analysis with monoclonal antibodies. *J. Gen. Virol.* **64**, 843–851.

58 VOLK, W. A., SNYDER, R. M., BENJAMIN, D. C. & WAGNER, R. R. (1982). Monoclonal antibodies to the glycoproteins of vesicular stomatitis virus: comparative neutralizing activity. *J. Virol.* **42**, 220–227.

59 PAL, R., GRINNELL, B. W., SNYDER, R. M. & WAGNER, R. R. (1985). Regulation of viral transcription by the matrix protein of vesicular stomatitis virus probed by monoclonal antibodies and temperature-sensitive mutants. *J. Virol.* **56**, 386–394.

60 CHANAS, A. C., GOULD, E. A., CLEGG, J. C. S. & VARMA, M. G. R. (1982). Monoclonal antibodies to Sindbis virus glycoprotein E1 can neutralise, enhance infectivity and independently inhibit haemagglutination or haemolysis. *J. Gen. Virol.* **58**, 37–46.

61 SCHMALJOHN, A. L., KOKUBUN, K. M. & COLE, G. A. (1983). Protective monoclonal antibodies define maturational and pH dependent antigenic changes on Sindbis virus E1 glycoprotein. *Virology* **130**, 144–154.

62 ROEHRIG, J. T., CORSER, J. A. & SCHLESINGER, M. J. (1980). Isolation and characterisation of hybrid cell lines producing monoclonal antibodies directed against the structural proteins of Sindbis virus. *Virology* **101**, 41–49.

63 ROEHRIG, J. T., DAY, J. W. & KINNEY, R. M. (1982). Antigenic analysis of the surface glycoprotein of a Venezuelan equine encephalomyelitis virus (TC-83) using monoclonal antibodies. *Virology* **118**, 269–278.

64 HEINZ, F. X., BERGER, R., TUMA, W. & KUNZ, C. (1983). Location of immunodominant antigenic determinants on fragments of the tick-borne

encephalitis virus glycoproteins: evidence for two different mechanisms by which antibodies mediate neutralization and haemagglutination inhibition. *Virology* **130**, 485–501.

65 GONZALES-SCARANO, F., SHOPE, R. E., CALISHER, C. E. & NATHANSON, N. (1982). Characterisation of monoclonal antibodies against the G1 and N proteins of La Crosse and Tahyna, two California serogroup Bunyaviruses. *Virology* **120**, 42–53.

66 MASSEY, R. J. & SCHOCHETMAN, G. (1981). Topographical analysis of viral epitopes using monoclonal antibodies: mechanism of virus neutralization. *Virology* **115**, 20–32.

67 NOWINSKI, R. C., LOSTROM, M. E., TAM, M. R., STONE, M. R. & BURNETTE, W. N. (1979). The isolation of hybrid cell lines producing monoclonal antibodies against the p15(E) protein of ecotropic murine leukemia viruses. *Virology* **93**, 111–126.

68 LOSTROM, M. E., STONE, M. R., TAM, M., BURNETTE, W. N., PINTER, A. & NOWINSKI, R. C. (1979). Monoclonal antibodies against murine leukemia viruses: identification of six antigenic determinants on the p15(E) and gp70 envelope proteins. *Virology* **98**, 336–350.

69 BRUCK, C., PORTETELLE, D., BURNY, A. & ZAVADA, J. (1982). Topographical analysis by monoclonal antibodies of BLV-gp51 epitopes involved in viral functions. *Virology* **122**, 353–362.

70 GRANT, C. G., ERNISSE, B. J., JARRETT, D. & JONES, F. R. (1983). Feline leukemia virus envelope gp70 of subgroup B and C defined by monoclonal antibodies with cytotoxic and neutralising functions. *J. Immunol.* **131**, 3042–3048.

71 ROSSMAN, M. G., ARNOLD, E., ERICKSON, J. W., FRANKENBERGER, E. A., GRIFFITH, J. P., HECHT, H.-J., JOHNSON, J. E., KAMER, G., LUO, M., MOSSER, A. G., REUCKERT, R. R., SHERRY, B. & VRIEND, G. (1985). Structure of a human common cold virus and functional relationship to other picornaviruses. *Nature (London)* **317**, 145–153.

72 McCULLOUGH, K. C., CROWTHER, J. R., BUTCHER, R. N., CARPENTER, W. C., BROCCHI, E., CAPUCCI, L. & De SIMONE, F. (1986). Immune protection against foot-and-mouth disease virus studied using virus neutralising and non-neutralising concentrations of monoclonal antibodies. *Immunology* **58**, 421–428.

73 GERHARD, W., YEWDELL, J., FRANKEL, H. E., LOPES, D. A. & STAUDT, L. (1980). Monoclonal antibodies against influenza virus. In *Monoclonal antibodies, hybridomas: a new dimension in biological analysis* (ed. R. H. Kennett, T. J. McKearn & K. B. Bechtol), pp.317–334. Plenum Press, New York.

74 LAVER, W. G. (1982). The use of monoclonal antibodies to investigate antigenic drift in influenza virus. In *Monoclonal hybridoma antibodies: techniques and applications* (ed. J. G. R. Hurrell), pp. 103–118. CRC Press, Florida.

75 NATALI, A., OXFORD, J. S. & SCHILD, G. C. (1981). Frequency of naturally occurring antibody to influenza virus antigenic mutants selected *in vitro* with monoclonal antibody. *J. Hyg. (Camb.)* **87**, 185–191.

76 SHESHBERADARAN, H., NORRBY, E., McCULLOUGH, K. C., CARPENTER, W. C. & ORVELL, C. (1986). The antigenic relationship

between measles, canine distemper and rinderpest viruses studied with monoclonal antibodies. *J. Gen. Virol.* **67**, 1381–1392.
77 WIKTOR, T. J. & KOPROWSKI, H. (1978). Monoclonal antibodies against rabies virus produced by somatic cell hybridization: detection of antigenic variants. *Proc. Natl. Acad. Sci., U.S.A.* **75**, 3938–3942.
78 KOPROWSKI, H. & WIKTOR, T. J. (1980). Monoclonal antibodies to rabies virus. In *Monoclonal antibodies, hybridomas: a new dimension in biological analysis* (ed. R. H. Kennett, T. J. McKearn & K. B. Bechtol), pp. 335–352. Plenum Press, New York and London.
79 FERGUSON, M., YI-HUA, Q., MINOR, P. D., MAGRATH, D. I., SPITZ, M. & SCHILD, G. C. (1982). Monoclonal antibodies specific for the Sabin vaccine strain of poliovirus 3. *Lancet* ii, 122–124.
80 CRAINIC, R., COUILLIN, P., CABAU, N., BOUE, A. & HORODNICEANU, F. (1981). Determination of type 1 poliovirus subtype classes with neutralising monoclonal antibodies. *Dev. Biol. Stand.* **50**, 229–234.
81 PRABHAKAR, B. S., HASPEL, M. V., McCLINTOCK, P. R. & NOTKINS, A. L. (1982). High frequency of antigenic variants among naturally occurring human coxsackie B4 virus isolates identified by monoclonal antibodies. *Nature (London)* **300**, 374–376.
82 McCULLOUGH, K. C., CROWTHER, J. R., BROCCHI, E., De SIMONE, F. & OBI, T. (1986). Application of monoclonal antibodies in veterinary medicine. In *Biotech RIA 86: monoclonals and DNA probes in diagnostic and preventative medicine* (ed. R. C. Gallo, G. Della Porta & A. Albertini), chapter 22, pp. 209–218. Raven Press, New York.
83 POLIN, G. A., (1980). Monoclonal antibodies against streptococcal antigens. In *Monoclonal antibodies, hybridomas: a new dimension in biological analyses* (ed. R. H. Kennett, T. J. McKearn & K. B. Bechtol), pp. 353–360. Plenum Press, New York and London.
84 MITCHISON, D. A. & COATES, A. R. M. (1982). Monoclonal antibodies in bacteriology. In *Monoclonal antibodies in clinical medicine* (ed. A. J. McMichael & J. W. Fabre), pp. 301–310. Academic Press, London.
85 MITCHELL, G. F. (1982). Hybridomas in immunoparasitology. In *Monoclonal hybridoma antibodies: techniques and applications* (ed. J. G. R. Hurrell), pp. 139–150. CRC Press, Florida.
86 COHEN, S. (1982). Monoclonal antibodies in parasitology, with particular reference to malaria. In *Monoclonal antibodies in clinical medicine* (ed. A. J. McMichael & J.W. Fabre), pp. 311–334. Academic Press, London.
87 PHILLIPS, S. M. & ZODDA, D. M. (1984). Monoclonal antibodies and immunoparasitology. In *Monoclonal antibodies and functional cell lines* (ed. R. H. Kennett, K. B. Bechtol & T. J. McKearn), pp. 239–274. Plenum Press, New York.
88 DAVIS, W. C., MARUSIC, S., LEWIN, H. A., SPLITTER, G. A., PERRYMAN, L. E., McGUIRE, T. C. & GORHAM, J. R. (1987). The development and analysis of species specific and cross reactive monoclonal antibodies to leukocyte differentiation antigens and antigens of the major histocompatibility complex for use in the study of the immune system in cattle and other species. *Vet. Immunol. Immunopathol.* **15**, 337–376.
89 BALDWIN, C. L., TEALE, A. J., NAESSENS, J., GODEERIS, B. M., MacHUGH, N. D. & MORRISON, W. I. (1986). Characterisation of a subset of bovine T lymphocytes that express BOT4 by monoclonal antibodies and function. *J. Immunol.* **136**, 4385–4392.

90*a* GOGOLIN-EWENS, K. J., MacKAY, C. R., MERCER, W. M. & BRANDON, M. R. (1985). Sheep lymphocyte antigens. I. *Immunology* **56**, 717–724.

90*b* PURI, N. K., MacKAY, C. R., & BRANDON, M. R. (1985). Sheep lymphocyte antigens. II. *Immunology* **56**, 725–733.

91 McKEARN, T. J., SMILEK, D. E. & FITCH, F. W. (1980). Rat–mouse hybridomas and their application to studies of the major histocompatibility complex. In *Monoclonal antibodies, hybridomas: a new dimension in biological analysis* (ed. R. H. Kennett, T. J. McKearn & K. B. Bechtol), pp. 219–234. Plenum Press, New York and London.

92 BETTS, R. L. & McKENZIE, I. F. C. (1982). Monoclonal antibodies to the major histocompatibility antigens. In *Monoclonal hybridoma antibodies: techniques and applications* (ed. J. G. R. Hurrell), pp. 193–222. CRC Press, Florida.

93 SPRINGER, T. A. (1982). Murine macrophage differentiation antigens defined by monoclonal antibodies. In *Monoclonal hybridoma antibodies: techniques and applications* (ed. J. G. R. Hurrell), pp. 169–175. CRC Press, Florida.

94 SUN, D. & LOHMANN-MATTHES, M. L. (1982). Functionally different subpopulations of mouse macrophages recognised by monoclonal antibodies. *Eur. J. Immunol.* **12**, 134–140.

95 O'NEILL, H. C. (1986). Monoclonal antibodies specific for H-2K and H-2D antigens on cytotoxic T cells can inhibit their function. *Proc. Natl. Acad. Sci., U.S.A.* **83**, 1443–1447.

96 LEDBETTER, J. A., GODING, J. W., TOKUHISA, T. & HERZENBERG, L. A. (1980). Murine T-cell differentiation antigens detected by monoclonal antibodies. In *Monoclonal antibodies, hybridomas: a new dimension in biological analysis* (ed. R. H. Kennett, T. J. McKearn & K. B. Bechtol), pp. 235–250. Plenum Press, New York and London.

97 MASON, D. W., BRIDEAU R. J., McMASTER, W. R., WEBB, M., WHITE, R. A. H. & WILLIAMS, A. F. (1980). Monoclonal antibodies that define T-lymphocyte subsets in the rat. In *Monoclonal antibodies, hybridomas: a new dimension in biological analysis* (ed. R. H. Kennett, T. J. McKearn & K. B. Bechtol), pp. 251–274. Plenum Press, New York and London.

98 REINHERZ, E. L., MORIMOTO, C., MEUER, S. & SCHLOSSMAN, S. F. (1983). Dissection of human immunoregulatory T lymphocytes: implications for understanding clinical disease. In *Hybridoma and cellular immortality* (ed. B. H. Tom & J. P. Allison), pp. 45–66. Plenum Press, New York.

99 McCULLOUGH, K. C. & MARTINOD, S. (1988). Recombinant biotechnology in the control of parasitic diseases. In *Agrobiotech 87* (in press).

100 BOSS, B. D., LANGMAN, R., TROWBRIDGE, I. & DULBECCO, R. (eds) (1983). *Monoclonal antibodies and cancer.* Academic Press, New York and London.

101 GOODFELLOW, P. N., LEVINSON, J. R., WILLIAMS, V. E. II & McDEVITT, H. O. (1979). Monoclonal antibodies reacting with murine teratocarcinoma cells. *Proc. Natl. Acad. Sci., U.S.A.* **76**, 377–380.

102 LENNOX, E. S. & SIKORA, K. (1982). Definition of human tumour antigens. In *Monoclonal antibodies in clinical medicine* (ed. A. J. McMichael & J. W. Fabre), pp. 111–128. Academic Press, London.

103 LEVY, R., DILLEY, J. & LAMPSON, L. A. (1978). Human normal and leukaemia cell surface antigens. Mouse monoclonal antibodies as probes. *Curr. Top. Microbiol. Immunol.* **81**, 164–169.

104 KENNETT, R. H., JONAK, Z. L. & BECHTOL, K. B. (1980). Monoclonal antibodies against human tumor-associated antigens. In *Monoclonal antibodies, hybridomas: a new dimension in biological analysis* (ed. R. H. Kennett, T. J. McKearn & K. B. Bechtol), pp. 155–170. Plenum Press, New York and London.

105 BERTHOLD, F. (1984). Monoclonal antibodies to human neuroblastoma cells and other solid tumors. In *Monoclonal antibodies and functional cell lines* (ed. R. H. Kennett, K. B. Bechtol & T. J. McKearn), pp. 215–238. Plenum Press, New York.

106 STRAND, M., SCHEINBERG, D. A., GANSOW, O. A. & FRIEDMAN, A. M. (1983). Monoclonal antibody conjugates for diagnostic imaging and therapy. In *Monoclonal antibodies and cancer* (ed. B. D. Boss *et al.*), pp. 125–134. Academic Press, New York and London.

107 HASKELL, C. M., BUCHEGGER, F., SCHREYER, M., CARREL, S. & MACH, J. P. (1983). *In vitro* screening of new monoclonal anti-carcinoembryonic antigen antibodies for radioimaging human colorectal carcinomas. In *Monoclonal antibodies and cancer* (ed. B. D. Boss *et al.*), pp. 275–284. Academic Press, New York and London.

108 TAYLOR-PAPADIMITRIOU, J., BURCHELL, J. & CHANG, S. E. (1983). Use of antibodies to membrane antigens in the study of differentiation and malignancy in the human breast. In *Monoclonal antibodies and cancer* (ed. B. D. Boss *et al.*), pp. 227–238. Academic Press, New York and London.

109 GOUSSEV, A. I., YASOVA, A. K. & IEZHNEVA, O. M. (1983). The isolation and characterization of monoclonal antibodies against murine alpha-fetoprotein. In *Monoclonal antibodies and cancer* (ed. B. D. Boss *et al.*), pp. 223–227. Academic Press, New York and London.

110 UOTILA, M., ENGVALL, E. & ROUSLAHTI, E. (1980). Monoclonal antibodies to human alphafetoprotein. *Mol. Immunol.* **17**, 791–799.

111 TSUNG, Y.-K., MILUNSKY, A. & ALPERT, E. (1980). Derivation and characterisation of a monoclonal hybridoma antibody specific for human alpha-fetoprotein. *J. Immunol. Methods* **39**, 363–368.

112 GREAVES, M. F., DELIA, D., NEWMAN, R. & VODINELICH, L. (1982). Analysis of leukaemic cells with monoclonal antibodies. In *Monoclonal antibodies in clinical medicine* (ed A. J. McMichael & J. W. Fabre), pp. 129–166. Academic Press, London.

113 FOON, K. A., SCHROFF, R. W., MAYER, D., SHERWIN, S. A., OLDHAM, R. K., BUNN, P. A. & HSU, S.-M. (1983). Monoclonal antibody therapy of chronic lymphocytic leukaemia and cutaneous T-cell lymphoma: preliminary observations. In *Monoclonal antibodies and cancer* (ed. B. D. Boss *et al.*), pp. 39–52. Academic Press, New York and London.

114 TROWBRIDGE, I. S. (1983). Therapeutic potential of monoclonal antibodies that block biological function. In *Monoclonal antibodies and cancer* (ed. B. D. Boss *et al.*), pp. 53–62. Academic Press, New York and London.

115 FEIZI, T. (1985). Demonstration by monoclonal antibodies that carbohydrate structures of glycoproteins and glycolipids are onco-developmental antigens. *Nature (London)* **314**, 53–57.

116 MAGNANI, J. L. & GINSBURG, V. (1983). Cancer-associated carbohydrate antigens detected by monoclonal antibodies. In *Monoclonal antibodies and cancer* (ed. B. D. Boss *et al.*), pp. 251–260. Academic Press, New York and London.

117 BECHTOL, K. B., JONAK, Z. L. & KENNETT, R. H. (1980). Germ-cell-related and nervous system-related differentiation and tumour antigens. In *Monoclonal antibodies, hybridomas: a new dimension in biological analysis* (ed. R. H. Kennett, T. J. McKearn & K. B. Bechtol), pp. 171–184. Plenum Press, New York and London.

118 FABRE, J. W. (1982). Differentiation antigens of the human central nervous system: identification with monoclonal antibodies and potential clinical value. In *Monoclonal antibodies in clinical medicine* (ed. A. J. McMichael & J. W. Fabre), pp. 397–412. Academic Press, London.

119 CUELLO, A. C. (1982). Monoclonal antibodies to neurotransmitters: potential value in the understanding of normal and abnormal neurological function. In *Monoclonal antibodies in clinical medicine* (ed. A. J. McMichael & J. W. Fabre), pp. 413–430. Academic Press, London.

120 GREAVES, M. F. (ed) (1985). *Monoclonal antibodies to receptors*. Chapman and Hall, London and New York.

121 RICHMAN, D. P. (1984). Monoclonal antibodies directed against the nicotinic acetylcholine receptor. In *Monoclonal antibodies and functional cell lines* (ed. R. H. Kennett, K. B. Bechtol & T. J. McKearn), pp. 17–32. Plenum Press, New York.

122 FUCHS, S., SOUROUJON, M. C. & MOCHLY-ROSEN, D. (1985). Antibodies to the acetylcholine receptor. In *Monoclonal antibodies to receptors* (ed. M. F. Greaves), pp. 163–200. Chapman and Hall, London and New York.

123 MONCHARMONT, B. & PARIKH, I. (1985). Monoclonal antibodies to steroid receptors. In *Monoclonal antibodies to receptors* (ed. M. F. Greaves), pp. 67–86. Chapman and Hall, London and New York.

124 TROWBRIDGE, I. S. & NEWMAN, R. A. (1985). Monoclonal antibodies to transferrin receptors. In *Monoclonal antibodies to receptors* (ed. M. F. Greaves), pp. 235–262. Chapman and Hall, London and New York.

125 JACOBS, S., KULL, F. C. Jr & CUATRECASAS, P. (1985). Monoclonal antibodies as probes for insulin and insulin-like growth factor-1 receptors. In *Monoclonal antibodies to receptors* (ed. M. F. Greaves), pp. 263–278. Chapman and Hall, London and New York.

126 SCHLESSINGER, J., LAX, I., YARDEN, Y., KANETY, H. & LIBERMANN, T. (1985). Monoclonal antibodies against the membrane receptor for epidermal growth factor. In *Monoclonal antibodies to receptors* (ed. M. F. Greaves), pp. 279–304. Chapman and Hall, London and New York.

127 HASPEL, M. V., ONODERA. T., PRABHAKAR, B. S., HORITA, M., SUZUKI, H. & NOTKINS, A. L. (1983). Virus-induced autoimmunity: monoclonal antibodies that react with endocrine tissues. *Science* **220**, 304–306.

128 IVANYL, J. (1982). Analysis of monoclonal antibodies to human growth hormone and related proteins. In *Monoclonal hybridoma antibodies: techniques and applications* (ed. J. G. R. Hurrell), pp. 59–80, CRC Press, Florida.

129 RATHJEN, D. A. & UNDERWOOD, P. A. (1985). Optimisation of con-

ditions for *in vitro* antigenic stimulation of dissociated mouse spleen cells for the production of monoclonal antibodies against peptide hormones. *J. Immunol. Methods* **78**, 227–237.

130 HARRIS, H. (1984). Monoclonal antibodies to enzymes. In *Monoclonal antibodies and functional cell lines* (ed. R. H. Kennett, K. B. Bechtol & T. J. McKearn), pp. 33–66. Plenum Press, New York.

131 FRANKEL, M. E. & GERHARD, W. (1979). The rapid determination of binary constants for antiviral antibodies by a radioimmunoassay. An analysis of the interaction between hybridoma proteins and influenza virus. *Mol. Immunol.* **16**, 101–106.

132 LEW, A. M. (1984). The effect of epitope density and antibody affinity on the ELISA as analysed by monoclonal antibodies. *J. Immunol. Methods* **72**, 171–176.

133 JACOBSEN, C. & STEENSGARD, J. (1984). Binding properties of monoclonal anti-IgG antibodies analysis of binding curves in monoclonal antibody systems. *Immunology* **51**, 423–430.

134 BUCHANAN, T. W. (1984). Immunochemical and diagnostic uses of monoclonal antibodies in leprosy and gonorrhea. In *Hybridoma technology in agricultural and veterinary research* (ed. N. J. Stern & H. R. Gamble), pp. 101–110. Rowman and Allanheld, New Jersey.

135 PEARSON, T. W., CLARKE, M. W., PARISH, N. M., RICHARDSON, J. P., MITCHELL, L. A. & SAYA, L. (1984). Antigenic analysis of African trypanosomes with monoclonal antibodies. In *Hybridoma technology in agricultural and veterinary research* (ed. N. J. Stern & H. R. Gamble), pp. 111–120. Rowman and Allanheld, New Jersey.

136 JORDAN, R. (1984). Evaluating the relative specific activities of monoclonal antibodies to plant viruses. In *Hybridoma technology in agricultural and veterinary research* (ed. N. J. Stern & H. R. Gamble), pp. 257–269. Rowman and Allanheld, New Jersey.

137 ANDERSON, J. (1984). Use of monoclonal antibody in a blocking Elisa to detect group specific antibodies to bluetongue virus. *J. Immunol. Methods* **74**, 139–149.

138 CROWTHER, J. R., McCULLOUGH, K. C., BROCCHI, E. & De SIMONE, F. (1984). Monoclonal antibodies against FMDV: Use and potential application. *European Community Committee for the control of FMD, Brescia, Italy*, pp. 40–51. FAO, Rome.

139 McCULLOUGH, K. C., CROWTHER, J. R. & BUTCHER, R. N. (1985). Alteration in antibody reactivity with foot-and-mouth disease virus (FMDV) 146S antigen before and after binding to a solid phase or complexing with specific antibody. *J. Immunol. Methods* **82**, 91–100.

140 McCULLOUGH, K. C., CROWTHER, J. R. & BUTCHER, R. N. (1985). A liquid-phase ELISA for identification of epitopes on antigen in 'natural conformation'. *J. Virol. Methods* **11**, 329–338.

141 SECHER, D. S., & BURKE, D. C. (1980). A monoclonal antibody for large-scale purification of human leukocyte interferon. *Nature (London)* **285**, 446–450.

142 STENMAN, U.-H., SUTINEN, M.-J., SELANDER, R.-K., TONTTI, K. & SCHRODER, J. (1981). Characterisation of a monoclonal antibody to human alpha-fetoprotein and its use in affinity chromatography. *J. Immunol. Methods* **46**, 337–345.

143 THORPE, P. E., EDWARDS, D. C., DAVIES, A. J. S. & ROSS, W. C. J. (1982). Monoclonal antibody-toxin conjugates: aiming the magic bullet. In *Monoclonal antibodies in clinical medicine* (ed. A. J. McMichael & J. W. Fabre), pp. 167–204. Academic Press, London.

144 KLAUSNER, A. (1986). Taking aim at cancer with monoclonal antibodies. *Bio/Technology* **4**, 185–194.

145 VITETTA, E. S. & UHR, J. W. (1985). Immunotoxins: redirecting nature's poisons. *Cell* **41**, 653–654.

146 MÖLLER, G. (ed.) (1982). Antibody carriers of drugs and toxins in tumor therapy. *Immunol. Rev.*, vol. 62. Munksgaard, Copenhagen.

147 RUBENS, R. D. & DULBECCO, R. (1974). Augmentation of cytotoxic drug action by antibodies directed at cell surface. *Nature* **248**, 81–82.

148 BLYTHMAN, H. E., CASELLAS, P., GROS, O., GROS, P., JANSEN, F. K., PAOLUCCI, F., PAU, B. & VIDAL, H. (1981). Immunotoxins: hybrid molecules of monoclonal antibodies and a toxin subunit specifically kill tumour cells. *Nature (London)* **290**, 145–146.

149 THORPE, P., BROWN, A., FOXWELL, B., MYERS, C., ROSS, W., CUMBER, A. & FORRESTER, T. (1983). Blockade of galactose-binding site of ricin by its linkage to antibody. In *Monoclonal antibodies and cancer* (ed. B. D. Boss *et al.*), pp. 117–124. Academic Press, New York and London.

150 WATANABE, Y., UCHIDA, E., HIGUCHI, M., IMAI, Y. & OSAWA, T. (1987). Preparation and antitumour effect of macrophage activating factor (MAF) encapsulated in liposomes bearing a monoclonal anti-human melanoma (A375) antibody. *J. Biol. Resp. Modifiers* **6**, 556–568.

151 GLENNIE, M. J. & STEVENSON, G. T. (1982). Univalent antibodies kill tumour cells *in vitro* and *in vivo*. *Nature (London)* **295**, 712–714.

152 COBBOLD, S. P. & WALDMANN, H. (1984). Therapeutic potential of monovalent monoclonal antibodies. *Nature (London)* **308**, 460–462.

153 SCHMALJOHN, A. L., JOHNSON, E. D., DALRYMPLE, J. M. & COLE, G. A. (1982). Non-neutralizing monoclonal antibodies can prevent lethal alphavirus encephalitis. *Nature (London)* **297**, 70–72.

154 RECTOR, J. T., LAUSCH, R. N. & OAKES, J. E. (1982). Use of monoclonal antibodies for analysis of antibody-dependent immunity to ocular herpes simplex virus type 1 infection. *Inf. Imm.* **38**, 168–174.

155 McCULLOUGH, K. C., SMALE, C. J., CARPENTER, W. C., CROWTHER, J. R., BROCCHI, E. & DE SIMONE, F. (1987). Conformational alterations in virion capsid structure after complexing with monospecific antibody. *Immunology* **60**, 75–82.

156 McCULLOUGH, K. C., PARKINSON, D. & CROWTHER, J. R. (1988). Opsonisation-enhanced phagocytosis of foot-and-mouth disease virus. *Immunology* **65**, 187–191.

157 LETCHWORTH, G. J. & APPLETON, J. A. (1983). Passive protection of mice and sheep against bluetongue virus by a neutralizing monoclonal antibody. *Inf. Imm.* **39**, 208–212.

158 STAERZ, U. D., KANAGAWA, D. & BEVAN, M. J. (1985). Hybrid antibodies can target sites for attack by T cells. *Nature (London)* **314**, 628–631.

159 STAERZ, U. D. & BEVAN, M. J. (1986). Hybrid hybridomas producing a bispecific monoclonal antibody that can focus effector T-cell activity. *Proc. Natl. Acad. Sci., U.S.A.* **83**, 1453–1457.

160 BERNSTEIN, I. D., NOWINSKI, R. C., TAM, M. R., McMASTER, B.,

HOUSTON, L. L. & CLARK, E. A. (1980). Monoclonal antibody therapy of mouse leukaemia. In *Monoclonal antibodies, hybridomas: a new dimension in biological analyses* (ed. R. H. Kennett, T. J. McKearn & K. B. Bechtol), pp. 275–294. Plenum Press, New York and London.

161 JANOSSY, G., GOLDSTEIN, G. & COSIMI, A. B. (1982). Monoclonal anti-human lymphocyte antibodies: their potential value in immunosuppression and bone marrow transplantations. In *Monoclonal antibodies in clinical medicine* (ed. A. J. McMichael & J. W. Fabre), pp. 71–110. Academic Press, London.

162 LEVY, R., STRATTE, P., LINK, M., MALONEY, D. G., OSEROFF, A. & MILLER, R. A. (1984). Monoclonal antibodies to human lymphocytes: clinical application in the therapy of leukaemia. In *Monoclonal antibodies and functional cell lines* (ed. R. H. Kennett, K. B. Bechtol &T. J. McKearn), pp. 193–214. Plenum Press, New York.

163 NOWINSKI, R., BERGLUND, C., LANE, J., LOSTROM, M., BERNSTEIN, I., YOUNG, W. & HAKOMORI, S. (1980). Human monoclonal antibody against Forssman antigen. *Science* **210**, 537–539.

164 SCHLOM, J., WUNDERLICH, D. & TERAMOTO, Y. A. (1980). Generation of monoclonal antibodies reactive with human mammary carcinoma cells. *Proc. Natl. Acad. Sci., U.S.A.* **77**, 6841–6845.

165 SIKORA, K. & WRIGHT, R. (1981). Human monoclonal antibodies to lung cancer antigens. *Brit. J. Cancer* **43**, 696–700.

166 GIGLIOTTI, F. & INSEL, R. A. (1982). Protective human hybridoma to tetanus toxin. *J. Clin. Invest.* **70**, 1306–1309.

167 BUCK, D. W., LARRICK, J. W., RAUBITSCHEK, A., TRUITT, K. E., SENYK, G., WANG, J. & DYER, B. J. (1984). Production of human monoclonal antibodies. In *Monoclonal antibodies and functional cell lines* (ed. R. H. Kennett, K. B. Bechtol &T.J. McKearn), pp. 295–309. Plenum Press, New York.

168 SRIKUMARAN, S., GUIDRY, A. J. & GOLDSBY, R. A, (1982).Bovine × mouse hybridomas that secrete bovine immunoglobulin G_1. *Science* **220**, 522–524.

169 SRIKUMARAN, S., GUIDRY, A. J. & GOLDSBY, B. A. (1983/84). Production and characterisation of monoclonal bovine immunoglobulins G_1, G_2 and M from bovine × murine hybridomas. *Vet. Immunol. Immunopathol.* **5**, 323–342.

170 CROCE, C. M., LINNENBACH, A., HALL, W., STEPLEWSKI, Z. & KOPROWSKI, H. (1980). Production of human hybridomas secreting antibodies to measles virus. *Nature (London)* **288**, 488–489.

171 SIKORA, K., ALDERTON, T., PHILLIPS, J. & WATSON, J. (1982). Human hybridomas from malignant glycomas. *Lancet* i, 11.

172 CHIORAZZI, N., WASSERMAN, R. L. & KUNKEL, H. G. (1982) Use of Epstein-Barr virus transformed B cell lines for the generation of immunoglobulin-producing human B cell hybridomas. *J. Exp. Med.* **156**, 930–935.

173 HANDLEY, H. H. & ROYSTON, I. (1982). A human lymphoblastoid B cell line useful for generating immunoglobulin secreting human hybridomas. In *Hybridomas in cancer diagnosis and treatment* (ed. M. S. Mitchell & H. F. Oettgen), pp. 125–132. Raven Press, New York.

174 JERNE, N. K. (1974). Towards a network theory of the immune system. *Ann. Immunol. (Paris)* C**125**, 373–389.

175 BONA, C. A. (1981). *Idiotypes and lymphocytes*. Academic Press, New York.
176 HOOD, L. E., WEISSMAN, I. L. & WOOD, W. B. (1978). *Immunology*. The Benjamin Cummings Publishing Co. Inc., California.
177 McCULLOUGH, K. C. & LANGLEY, D. (1985). Anti-idiotope vaccines: can they exist? *Vaccine* **3**, 59–64.
178 SACKS, D. L., ESSER, K. M. & SHER, A. (1982). Immunization of mice against African trypanosomiasis using anti-idiotypic antibodies. *J. Exp. Med.* **155**, 1108–1119.
179 REAGAN, K. J., WUNNER, W. H., WIKTOR, T. J. & KOPROWSKI, H. (1983). Anti-idiotypic antibodies induce neutralising antibodies to rabies virus glycoprotein. *J. Virol.* **48**, 660–666.
180 KENNEDY, R. C. & DREESMAN, G. R. (1984). Enhancement of the immune response to hepatitis B surface antigen. *J. Exp. Med.* **159**, 655–665.
181 FORSTROM, J. W., NELSON, K. A., NEPOM, G. T., HELLSTROM, I. & HELLSTROM, K. E. (1983). Immunization to a syngeneic sarcoma by a monoclonal auto-anti-idiotypic antibody. *Nature (London)* **303**, 627–629.
182 KELSOE, G., RETH, M. & RAJEWSKY, K. (1980). Control of idiotope expression by monoclonal anti-idiotope antibodies. *Immunol. Rev.* **52**, 75–80.
183 MULLER, C. A. & RAJEWSKY, K. (1984). Idiotope regulation by isotope switch variants of two monoclonal anti-idiotope antibodies. *J. Exp. Med.* **159**, 758–772.
184 VENTER, J. C., BERZOFSKY, J., LINDSTROM, J., JACOBS, S., FRASER, C. M., KOHN, L. D., SCHNEIDER, W. J., GREENE, G. L., STROSBERG, A. D. & ERLANGER, B. F. (1984). Monoclonal and anti-idiotope antibodies as probes for receptor structure and function: symposium summary. *Fed. Proc.* **43**, 2532–2539.
185 KENNEDY, R. C., ALDER-STORTHZ, K.,. HENKEL, R. D. & DREESMAN, G. R. (1983). Characteristics of a shared idiotope by two IgM anti-herpes simplex virus monoclonal antibodies that recognise different determinants. *J. Immunol.* **130**, 1943–1946.
186 UYTDEHAAG, F. G. C. M. & OSTERHAUS, A. D. M. E. (1985). Induction of neutralising antibody in mice against poliovirus type II with monoclonal anti-idiotypic antibody. *J. Immunol.* **134**, 1225–1229.
187 ERTL, H. C. J. & FINBERG, R. W. (1984). Sendai virus-specific T cell clones. II. Induction of cytolytic T cells by an anti-idiotypic antibody directed against a helper T-cell clone. *Proc. Natl. Acad. Sci., U.S.A.* **81**, 2850–2854.
188 McCULLOUGH, K. C. & BUTCHER, R. N. (1989). Passive immunization can induce both anti-idiotype and idiotype-bearing antibody. *Immunology* (submitted).

Index